COSMETIC DERMATOLOGIC SURGERY

SECOND EDITION

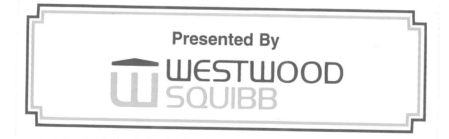

COSMETIC DERMATOLOGIC SURGERY

SECOND EDITION

Samuel J. Stegman, M.D.

Associate Clinical Professor of Dermatology
University of California at San Francisco
San Francisco, California

Theodore A. Tromovitch, M.D.

Clinical Professor of Dermatology
University of California at San Francisco
San Francisco, California

Richard G. Glogau, M.D.

Associate Clinical Professor of Dermatology
University of California at San Francisco
San Francisco, California

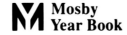
Mosby Year Book

St. Louis   Baltimore   Boston   Chicago   London   Philadelphia   Sydney   Toronto

A Year Book Medical Publishers imprint of Mosby-Year Book, Inc.

Mosby-Year Book, Inc., 11830 Westline Industrial Drive, St. Louis, MO 63146.

2   3   4   5   6   7   8   9   0   PR   94   93   92   91

Library of Congress Cataloging-in-Publication Data

Stegman, Samuel J.
    Cosmetic dermatologic surgery / Samuel J. Stegman, Theodore A.
Tromovitch, Richard G. Glogau. — 2nd ed.
        p.   cm.
    Includes bibliographical references.
    ISBN 0-8151-7920-0
    1. Skin—Surgery. 2. Surgery, Plastic.   I. Tromovitch, Theodore
A. II. Glogau, Richard G.   III. Title.
    [DNLM: 1. Skin—surgery. 2. Surgery, Plastic.   WO 600 S817c]
RD520.S733 1990
617.4'770592—dc20   89-22576
DNLM/DLC   CIP
for Library of Congress

Sponsoring Editor: Nancy E. Chorpenning
Associate Managing Editor, Manuscript Services: Deborah Thorp
Production Project Coordinator: Gayle Paprocki
Proofroom Supervisor: Barbara M. Kelly

Preface

This is an entirely new book. A few of the drawings and photographs are repeated, but most are new and all of the text is new. A great deal has transpired on several planes since the first edition was published in 1984. In areas such as liposuction, blepharoplasty, and hair transplantation, fresh and innovative techniques have been developed. Chapter 6, Surgical Management of Alopecia, contains material on tissue expanders, and Chapter 7, Filling Agents, includes discussions of Fibrel, and Microlipoinjection, which were not even in use in 1984. Browlift and the use of tissue expanders for scalp reduction and tattoo removal are new subjects.

This is still a book for the dermatologist who is interested in surgery and cosmetic procedures. Our specialty has always included these subjects, and, appropriately, we are practicing them more and more frequently. Operations, treatments, and procedures on the skin and subcutaneous fat suitable for outpatient surgery are well within the purview of our specialty. Unfortunately, we have not totally overcome the resistance to this expansion from some of our competitors. They have hindered us by preventing us from obtaining hospital privileges or medical malpractice insurance for certain procedures. There has also been a cry in the media that the public must be "protected" from us. Gradually, however, we are convincing cooler, unbiased heads on the governing boards of hospitals and regulatory bodies to vote our way, and our detractors have yet to show that surgical complications and unsatisfactory results in our specialty occur at rates greater than those in other specialties.

Finally, we have joined the world of computer literacy. This is our first book to be completely composed, edited, and annotated on an Apple Macintosh II. As this book goes to the printer it is as up-to-date as possible, and we hope that it is easy and enjoyable to read.

Samuel J. Stegman, M.D.
Theodore A. Tromovitch, M.D.
Richard G. Glogau, M.D.

v

Contents

One

General Principles of Office Cosmetic Surgery

The Goal

The patient visit for a cosmetic procedure is much different from a visit for a physical ailment or medical examination. In cosmetic surgery, the patient's real goal is often subjective and sometimes obscure—even to the patient. Consequently, excising, changing, or correcting an obvious defect does not necessarily guarantee the patient's happiness. Therefore, it is worth the physician's time and effort to try to discover the patient's true motivation for cosmetic surgery and exactly what the patient hopes it will accomplish. Much of the time, the patient's wishes and goals will be straightforward. For example, if a patient says, "My eyes look tired," blepharoplasty may be needed. On the other hand, if the patient says, "What can you do for me?" the physician must ask careful questions to learn more about the patient's thoughts before rushing in to make specific suggestions.

Even though all medical visits are personal, patients consider cosmetic procedures especially personal, sometimes embarrassing, and even foolish. Approach each cosmetic patient as one who has a delicate personal problem. Avoid the unproductive and unpleasant mistake of confronting patients about problems about which they are uncomfortable. Although it is all right for a physician to walk into an examination room and say, "How did you get that rash?" or "How did you cut your cheek?" it is not appropriate to say, "Boy, do you need your eyes done," even if the patient has scheduled a blepharoplasty consultation. The consultation is the physician's opportunity to be gentle, nonjudgmental, and considerate. Patients may have feelings of guilt or vanity which they should be allowed to express in whatever way they wish. They should be permitted to verbalize their rationalizations for having cosmetic procedures. The physician

then can use such appropriate reassurances as, "Many others have had this." Or, "This is what growing old gracefully means." Or, "Why not look your best?" There are some patients who by the nature of their personalities (and yours) are potential problems. Tardy compiled these traits in an article discussing face-lifts. The list is reproduced here (Table 1–1).[1]

Scheduling Cosmetic Consultations

A cosmetic consultation must not be hurried, or even seem hurried. Even for the simplest problem, allow a little extra time to fully discuss the proposed procedures and answer all of the patient's questions. Most patients have never had a cosmetic surgery consultation and will appreciate the change of pace and extra attention.

Although a few dermatologists limit their practices to cosmetic work, the majority combine cosmetic procedures with general and surgical dermatology and regular patients are an important source of small and large cosmetic procedures. Do not be caught off guard by the patient who says, "By the way, Doctor, while I've got you here, what do you think about this?" If time permits, sit down and talk about the problem, but if the problem is complicated, give these patients an idea about what might be done, discuss whether or not they are good candidates, and then schedule a separate consultation appointment. Some patients will think you are putting them off, and if you detect this feeling, suggest that they wait until after you have seen other patients who are waiting. They will appreciate your extra effort and rapport will quickly improve.

Office assistants, particularly booking assistants, need to be aware of the difference in the amount of time necessary for cosmetic proce-

TABLE 1–1.*
Potential Problem Patients

1. The patient with unrealistic expectations
2. The obsessive-compulsive, perfectionistic patient
3. The "sudden whim" patient
4. The indecisive patient
5. The rude patient
6. The overflattering patient
7. The overly familiar patient
8. The unkempt patient
9. The patient with minimal or imagined deformity
10. The careless or poor historian
11. The VIP patient
12. The uncooperative patient
13. The overly talkative patient
14. The surgeon shopper
15. The depressed patient
16. The "plastic surgiholic"
17. The price haggler
18. The patient involved in litigation
19. The patient you or your staff dislikes

*From Tardy ME, Klimsensmith M: Face-lift surgery: Principles and variations, in Roenigk RK, Roenigk HH (eds): *Dermatologic Surgery.* New York, Marcel Dekker Inc, 1988, p 1249. Used by permission.

dures. If they are scheduled skillfully, cosmetic patients can be handled smoothly and appropriately along with regular medical patients. Some physicians like to block out certain days or times for cosmetic work, and this is another way to allot the proper time and attention to these patients. The physician and the business manager must consider that cosmetic consultations can mean a loss of money, but it can be made up with the surgical fee.

Follow-up visits for cosmetic patients are just as important as initial visits and often just as time-consuming. Failure to recover from a medical illness after a single office visit does not surprise most patients. Cosmetic patients, however, may become frustrated and angry at the physician if they do not recover and see the benefits of cosmetic surgery within the time *they* consider appropriate. Rarely can follow-up visits from cosmetic procedures be charged. It is critical that somewhere or sometime it be communicated to the patient *before* the procedure what the fee in-

cludes in terms of follow-up visits. We agree to a specific time period for follow-up visits as part of the fee. After that, it becomes a new problem or a complication for which we bill the patient's medical insurance company.

Make yourself available to patients in the postoperative period. The first night and next day after any major procedure are critical for the patient, both mentally and physically. We give patients our home phone numbers or, if we are going to a restaurant, tell them where we will be. Although they seldom actually call, patients appreciate having this information. And, if a patient does have a problem, you want to be the first to know, so you can deal with the problem properly. Sometimes a patient with a problem will go to the hospital emergency room. There, well-meaning physicians who are ignorant about most cosmetic procedures may make the wrong diagnosis and alarm the patient. We have had postop peel patients call from a medical intensive care unit and tell us they have third-degree burns on their faces and why did we do that to them? In fact, the emergency room physician had never seen a peel. In other cases, the ER doctor may seek consultation with the surgeon on call who may also be ignorant of cosmetic procedures, or who may be a competitor, or unaware that dermatologists do surgery. The result may be to plant doubts in the patient's mind about the procedure you did or whether you should have been doing that type of surgery in the first place.

Although the temptation is strong not to reschedule troublesome patients frequently, that is exactly what should be done. If these patients need more support, ask them to return more frequently and schedule the extra time you know they will need. It is a good idea never to completely dismiss cosmetic surgery patients. Always leave the door open for follow-up. If there is a real or perceived delay to full recovery, offer to have the patient seen by another physician for consultation. The consultant can be one of your partners or a colleague whose practice is nearby. It is a helpful gesture for everyone: the patient is reassured, your treatment plan is reinforced, and the consulting physician learns firsthand about the range of recovery times.

The Consultation

The Patient Speaks

The first thing we do is give the patient a hand mirror and a cotton-tipped applicator. We ask the patient to use the wooden end of the stick as a pointer to indicate exactly where the problem is. The patient may hesitate or give you a funny look, but a simple statement such as, "It's important that we both see exactly the same things so I can best help you" quickly mollifies the patient. Do not be taken in by, "Why doctor, don't you see my problem?" Too many times we have seen a problem but it was *not* the problem the patient was concerned about. This can be an awkward way to begin the consultation.

We gently encourage patients to describe and point to what they see as bothersome or in need of correction. At the same time, we ask patients to tell us *why* something bothers them. It is surprising what some patients see and do not see on their faces. They can be concerned about their eyelids, yet not see three huge dark freckles and realize how unsightly they are. You may want to do the neck and chin; the patient may want only a little filler for the glabella. Do not underestimate the value of having patients tell you *why* something bothers them. It is the quickest way to get them to talk about pertinent matters, and you will also more quickly uncover any irrational thoughts, such as, "My heart medicine caused this," or "I've always hated this scar because it came from an accident." In fact, the scar may be tiny and almost unnoticeable but the patient's post-acne scarring may be horrendous. This tells more than you could ever uncover by questioning: the patient is seeking relief from a bad memory—something surgery seldom cures—or the patient wants to blame someone or something for an aging face. It helps you tailor your informed consent to know what the patient thinks.

The Examination

Look at the area in question, but check anything else that may help provide information about healing ability, scarring potential, or pigmentary problems. This is the time to gently suggest other cosmetic problems that may benefit from treatment. We usually ask first by saying, "Since you asked about matters concerning your appearance, you might want me to mention other procedures that may help you."

As you mention different things, pay attention to the patient's response. For example, if you point out an ugly mole, say it can be removed, and get a response like, "That mole is a family trait; my aunt has one like that," you know not to pursue it. Most of the time, however, patients are gratified at your thoroughness and glad to hear that certain growths can be treated.

The Informed Consent

At this point, the physician becomes the main speaker. First address the problem the patient came in for, and then discuss other problems that may have been uncovered in the interview or examination. Do not discuss any further issues the patient did not pursue.

Have in mind a complete and thorough explanation about each procedure, which can be complemented with printed handouts, videotape presentations, and other materials. The time that physician and staff spend providing explanations is the most important part of the visit.

An orderly discussion should include four main points. The first point includes the details of the *procedure*—what is done, how it is done, anesthesia, preparation, operative time, and immediate and long-term follow-up. The second point is the *prognosis,* where you try to communicate to the patient what you think will be the result. The third point is a discussion of the *complications.* Not all complications need to be mentioned—just the most common ones *and* those that may be more likely for that particular patient. Also discuss any complications a reasonable person would wish to know about in order to make an intelligent, informed decision about the procedure. And last, mention the *alternative* procedures available.

As important as communicating verbally with the patient is recording on the chart exactly what you said. Although there are many good ways to document the information that the patient received, all can be attacked by lawyers, and all can be ignored by juries. There is no such thing as perfect informed consent. The best kind of informed consent demonstrates diligence, reasonable recording, and a sincere effort to tell the patient what can be expected. How society and the jousting of the adversary system view the physician's work is too unpredictable to worry about, and is the reason for carrying malpractice insurance.

The Fee

In addition to the usual variables that dictate fees including office location, overhead costs, and the physician's experience, cosmetic work carries the following special considerations

Time. All phases of the procedure use up more time than comparable medical and surgical visits. Time must be allotted for consultation, review and discussion immediately prior to the procedure, and early and long-term follow-up.

Malpractice Insurance. All insurance companies charge more when more than 5% of the practice is cosmetic.

Equipment. Special equipment for each procedure is mandatory. We are reminded how many new sets of liposuction cannulae we have purchased in the last 5 years just to keep up with the latest developments.

Training. For dermatologists, cosmetic surgery meetings and training seminars are seldom held in conjunction with regular general dermatology meetings, which means additional expensive trips away and time spent out of the office.

Attitude. Cosmetic procedures are elective and discretionary. When it comes to cost, patients want to hear one round number and not be bothered with itemization and tack-ons. These factors must be built into the fee for the procedure.

A fee payment schedule agreement with the patient is strongly advised. We ask for one-half the fee at the time the appointment for the procedure is made, and the rest on the day of surgery. Other physicians ask for the whole fee at scheduling or at a fixed time before the surgery. Any schedule is good as long as the patient has read and agreed to it. It is a service to patients to force them to commit their money ahead of time. They will have made the decision to have the procedure and not worry about it further. Advance payment also decreases (nearly eliminates) no-shows or late cancellations.

The Day of Surgery

We see the patient personally before any analgesics or anesthetics are administered. At this time we answer all questions, review immediate follow-up care, and make sure the patient has transportation home. At this time we also review the patient's recent medical history and make sure that preoperative photographs have been taken.

On the day of surgery, the physician, the staff, and the mood of the office should be unhurried but efficient. Because most dermatologists perform cosmetic procedures in the office, going to the phone or dealing with charts and staff are tempting while waiting to get started. However, do not attend to other business or do not let the patient see you do it. Give the patient no reason for any disquieting thoughts or memories. These simple steps can remove more patient anxiety than huge amounts of medications.

Reference

1. Tardy ME, Klimsensmith M: Face-lift surgery: Principles and variations; in Roenigk RK, Roenigk HH (eds): *Dermatologic Surgery.* New York, Marcel Dekker Inc, 1988, p 1249.

Two

The Skin of the Aging Face

In a systematic examination of the facial skin of a patient who is seeking cosmetic work, the physician will focus attention on what can be corrected. This will lessen the chance that appropriate treatments will be overlooked. When these treatments are explained to the patient, expectations will be more realistic. The systematic examination we have used for several years and which we discuss below can be accomplished in only a few seconds, once the physician is familiar with it.

We have never encountered a set of definitions for what much of cosmetic surgery is directed to correct—wrinkles. Therefore, the following definitions satisfactorily communicate our understanding of what wrinkles should properly be called. These definitions are based on macroscopic morphology as outlined in Table 2–1.

The broad division is into lines and wrinkles. Lines further divide into creases, folds, and furrows. A crease is a linear, discrete depression with a depth that extends no deeper than the dermis (Fig 2–1, A and B). A furrow is a depression of the skin that includes the dermis and the immediate subcutaneous fat (Fig 2–2, A and B). A fold is an elevation of the skin that includes the dermis and the immediate subcutaneous fat (Fig 2–3, A and B). The difference between a crease and a furrow is the amount of skin involved in the depression. The crease is narrow, with sharp walls, and involves only the dermis, while a furrow is broad, has more gentle, sloping walls, and includes full-thickness skin and subcutaneous fat. Folds and furrows are linear or curvilinear. Wrinkles are multiple, partial thickness, multidirectional elevations, or depressions in the skin (Fig 2–4, A and B). They are soft (easily pressed out) and sometimes cross each other, creating a checked appearance.

These definitions, when used, are added to the anatomic location—for example, vertical glabellar creases, deep medial cheek furrows, or upper lip wrinkles. Such statements denote more exact images. The smile line is complex in location (from the base of the nostril to the oral lateral commissure, or the cheek to the chin) and in morphology (furrow and fold, furrow and crease). With these new terms and mention of the anatomic location, exact terminology is possible. Previously the smile line was referred to as a fatty fold near the nose. Now it can be described as a shallow furrow near the commissure that runs onto the chin as a sharp crease. This describes exactly how the smile line appears, and as a result, communication—written or spoken—between physicians, or between physicians and patients, is much more accurate.

The Primary Factors

Aging, actinic damage, and loss of subcutaneous support tissues are the primary factors that contribute to changes of the facial skin (Table 2–2).

TABLE 2–1.
Morphology of Wrinkles

Lines
    Creases
    Folds
    Furrows
Wrinkles

Inherent Aging

All systems apparently are affected by the "biological clock." Whatever the biological clock is or does affects the inherent construction of the skin. Several investigators have separated biological age changes from sun damage, and have shown that the quality of elastin and collagen fibers deteriorates with age.[1-4] Some people as young as 40 years old and all people by age 70 lay down new elastic fibers that are loosely and haphazardly arranged, and minimal elastin is formed. In the microvasculture of the skin, the veil cells produce excessive basement membranes and gradually decrease in number, which eventually leads to a thinner vessel wall.

The clinical manifestation of the above-mentioned changes and probably many others keyed to the biological clock is skin with much less resilience and snapback. This is skin that is slack and that hangs loosely. At present, we are not aware of any way to stop or alter these changes. Whether or not the induced generation of "new collagen" by the application of topicals such as Retin-A (tretinoin) or vitamin C will be significant is not known.

Actinic Damage

The second primary factor—actinic damage—is now largely preventable and it is hoped that most people will at least begin to reduce this type of damage. A quick and simple way to demonstrate to patients how much sun damage they have is to ask them to look at the buttocks or medial upper arm and compare that skin with the face, the V of the neck, and the dorsal hands and arms.

The effects of the sun are probably more pervasive than had been suspected. Changes are variable but present in all layers of the skin.[2] The

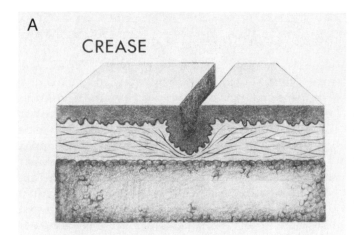

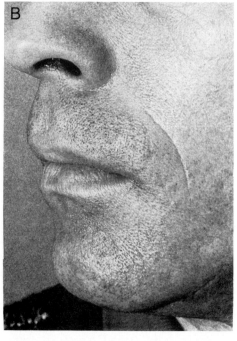

FIG 2–1.
A, diagram of a crease showing the narrow, straight walls; the depth is within the dermis. **B,** 35-year-old man with discrete crease smile line.

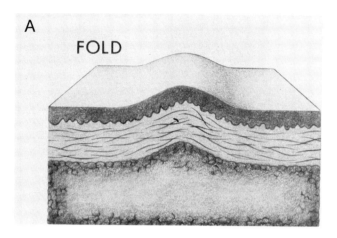

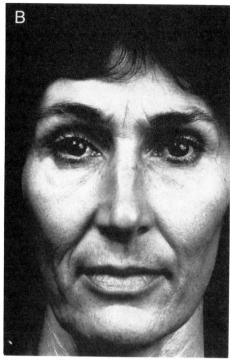

FIG 2–2.
A, diagram of a fold showing the mound elevation of full-thickness skin, including the subcutaneous fat. **B,** 45-year-old woman with smile-line folds.

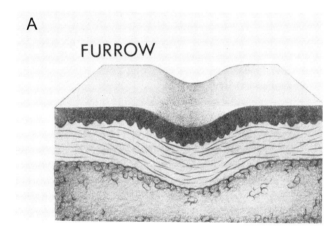

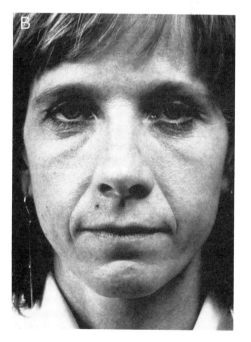

FIG 2–3.
A, diagram of a furrow showing the gentle sloping walls of full-thickness skin including subcutaneous fat. **B,** 40-year-old woman with smile-line furrows.

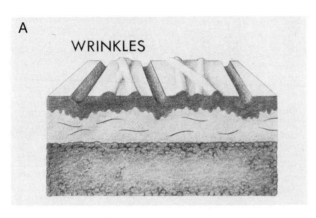
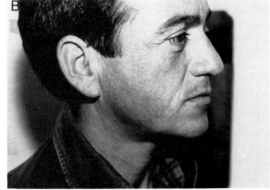

FIG 2–4.
A, a diagram of wrinkles showing the small, multidirectional elevations and depressions. **B,** 35-year-old badly sun-damaged man with wrinkles on the cheeks.

TABLE 2–2.
Factors That Contribute to Changes in the Skin

Primary Factors
  Inherent aging
  Actinic damage
  Loss of subcutaneous support
Secondary Factors
  Gravity
  Facial movement
  Sleep position

epidermis develops focal irregularities in keratin maturation, creating a rough texture and also actinic keratoses. The coloring is affected by the poor dispersion of pigment (melanosomes), and the light reflection to and from the dermis is irregularly altered by the thinner epidermis. Histologically, the papillary dermis appears to be affected least and is the most able to repair itself. However, 5-fluorouracil, Retin-A, and chemical peels all markedly affect the thickness and consistency of the papillary dermis, with resulting clinical improvement in the color and texture of the skin.

Dermal changes range from minimal to moderate to nearly complete replacement with an amorphous mass of degenerated elastic fibers. Clinically, there is circumstantial evidence that severe sun damage contributes to loss of elasticity and accentuates the retention of move-

ment and sleep-related lines (see below). Sun damage also probably produces the dull, muddy skin color so often seen in patients.

In addition to protection from the sun, which fortunately is becoming more common for all ages, treatments are better understood and more readily available. Natural or self-healing, a newly discovered phenomenon,[5] will repair mild sun damage if the area is totally protected. Topical tretinoin and 5-fluorouracil metabolically induce orthokeratosis and less melanosome aggregation, as well as new collagen deposition in the papillary dermis.[6, 7]

Chemical peel and dermabrasion wounds heal with a nearly normal (histologically) epidermis, a thickened and more collagenous papillary dermis, and partial or complete replacement of dermal elastosis with a band of materials which stain deeply positive for elastin, glucosaminoglycans, ground substance, and new collagen (Fig 2–5). Which of these changes are responsible for the various clinical improvements in appearance has not been worked out. With all of the new agents now and soon to be available to correct sun damage, there will be enough keys to deduce which histologic findings correlate with the clinical alterations.

Support Loss

The third primary factor is the loss of subby movement lines, gravity effects, or sun damage will show subtle indications of age because of these fat losses. Changes that can be seen across the room or down the block identify that face as older. Pudgy or fat faces do not manifest this early change, which is one of the reasons why pudgy-faced people seem to age so rapidly once they start to lose weight all over. Fat losses progress with age and eventually encompass the periorbital fat, all of the cheeks and chin (excluding the mental fat pad which produces the "witch's chin") and nose. Eventually, the support tissues are lessened to such as extent that the facial skin is too big and hangs loose and is redundant, while the eyes sink, the nose droops, and the perioral skin puckers.

Autologous fat-grafting or microlipoinjection (Chapter 7) is the treatment of choice for early fat-loss changes. Trying to "pull" out these concavities during a face-lift often results in a mask-like face; excessive augmentation of the malar prominence produces an appearance that is equally artificial. The replacement substance must be soft and voluminous, and right now fat grafting seems the best answer.

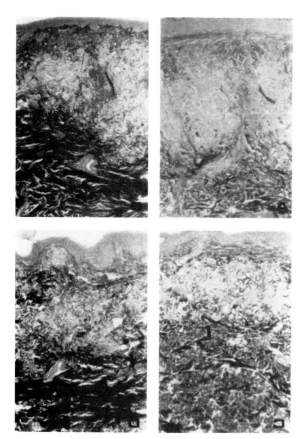

FIG 2–5.
Colloidal iron stains on sun-damaged skin. A normal control *(top left)*; 120 days after treatment with trichloracetic acid 50% *(top right)*, phenol 100% *(bottom left)*, and Baker's formula phenol mixture *(bottom right)* and occluded for 24 hours. Note the normalized epidermis, thicker papillary dermis with new collagen, and the dermal replacement of elastosis with new collagen and ground substance.

cutaneous support tissues which include bone and cartilage, and subcutaneous fat. Bone loss is an event of the sixth decade or later, and is noticed most around the mouth and chin. Loss of cartilage in the nose leads to falling of the tip of the nose and accentuation of the bony structures, producing in some patients the poly-beak, hanging-tip, narrow-nose appearance. Some of these effects are correctable with surgery or implants.

The earliest natural event on the aging face is loss of subcutaneous fat from the cheeks, followed in a few years by fat loss in the temples (Fig 2–6, A to C). Faces otherwise not marked

Secondary Factors

Gravity

When there has been loss of skin elasticity either from natural aging or severe sun damage or both, secondary factors appear. These are the effects of gravity, facial movement, and sleep position.

Gravitational pull on progressively less resilient skin manifests as ptotic eyebrows and eyelids, and formation of jowls and double chins; even the earlobes become longer and floppy (Fig 2–7).

The surgical techniques invented to correct the ravages of gravity have been some of the most successful in all of cosmetic surgery. Brow-lifts, blepharoplasty, rhytidectomy, and in some cases rhinoplasty all remove redundant skin and pull the important cosmetic features upward. When these operations are performed to correct gravitational drift, they are universally successful. But when they are used to improve sun-damage wrinkles, movement lines, or sleep lines, the results range from less than acceptable to unacceptable.

Movement Lines

Another group of secondary factors includes the creases, folds, and furrows that result from facial movement (Fig 2–8). The face is expressive from birth on, but not until loss of resilience from age or other factors is present do movement-related lines appear. Anatomically, a teenager has nearly an adult face. After a teenager smiles or squints, the face returns immediately to its former smoothness. By age 40 or 50, however, smile and frown lines remain longer and longer and eventually become permanent markers.

Movement lines are easy to detect and simple to show to the patient. Ask patients to make faces in front of a mirror, or, to show them the more subtle lines around the mouth and on the lower cheeks, just have them talk while watching the mirror. Once patients realize the cause of the lines, they will more likely be realistic about the results of surgery and the longevity of correction.

The cosmetic physician should discriminate when discussing and treating expression lines.

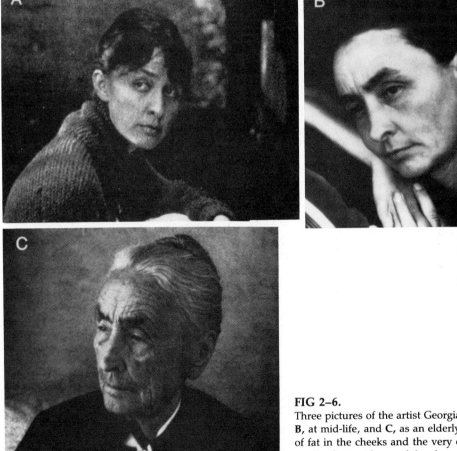

FIG 2–6.
Three pictures of the artist Georgia O'Keeffe; **A,** in her 20s, **B,** at mid-life, and **C,** as an elderly woman. The subtle loss of fat in the cheeks and the very early jowl formation in **B** are the first evidence of the changes of aging. (Courtesy of The Cleveland Museum of Art.)

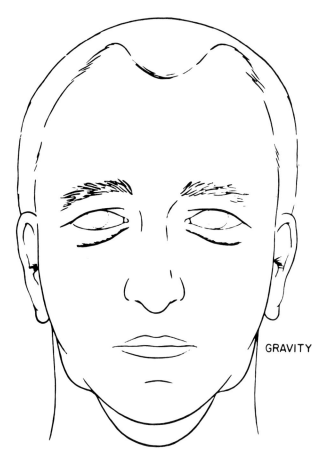

FIG 2–7.
Gravity changes.

furrows is being evaluated. Fat-grafting replaces fat loss and is not indicated for pushing out fine wrinkles in cheeks and foreheads.

The vertical forehead lines, selected parts of the smile line, and perioral lines are all easily corrected with fillers. Effacing a few key lines changes remarkably the mood the resting face portrays. Most faces look best when smiling because the muscles of expression literally lift the sagging skin and esthetically fold it into gentle curves on the cheek and around the eyes. It is the resting face, with some or all of the lines that remain from past decades' expressions, that appears angry, sad, or drawn. The attractive folds and furrows from the active smile drop unevenly and irregularly into the jowls and chin folds and eyelids. The curves also drop out and the lines are generally straight, which broadcasts harshness and anger. Straight lines have more power to catch and trap the viewing eye, and therefore

Many lines are pleasant-looking or attractive, and mirror the individual's personality. On the other hand, some lines imply bad humor or make the face unattractive. It is surprising how a few minimal changes will markedly alter the entire aspect of the face. For example, obliterating the vertical glabellar creases alone removes an angry look. When the smile line extends to or beyond the oral commissure, the lower face is accentuated, sometimes producing what is called a "bulldog" look. Correcting only that portion of the smile line inferior to the oral commissure may be adequate, just as correcting the crow's feet lateral to the orbital rim is often very helpful in the reducing the "cat's whiskers" look.

Filling agents are the most common treatments for movement-related lines. Silicone has been used the longest, but Zyderm collagen is now the most frequently used. Fibrel is newly available and its effectiveness for creases and

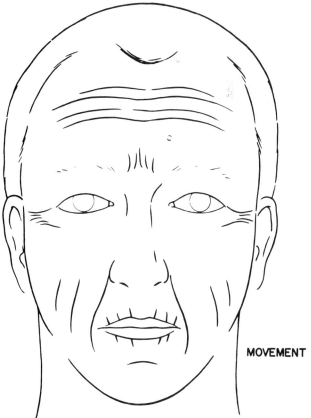

FIG 2–8.
Movement-related lines.

become the dominant features on the face. Cartoonists use straight lines to denote strong emotion and curved lines for gentleness and happiness. When redundancy is not the major defect, fillers erase those lines and brighten the face.

Fillers help the relatively young face of 35 to 50 years old by removing (keeping from view) the initial lines. Fillers help older faces by hiding those lines or portions of lines that detract cosmetically. For example, we call some of the secondary smile lines located lateral to the smile line "pointer lines." These short, straight lines point to the smile line and accentuate it. Obliterating these lines cleans up the lower one-third of the face, making it no more dominant than the other two-thirds of the face and thus returning it to esthetic balance. The same is true when many small lines around the mouth are removed. The point is that not all lines need to be treated to improve the patient's appearance or to lessen a haggard look.

Many patients are relieved to know that something can be done to make them look better without their having to undergo a "complete job." Financially and emotionally, many dread major cosmetic surgery and have well-founded serious reservations about a radical alteration in appearance. Looking younger is properly not the main goal; looking good or as good as possible is the *better* goal. Patients who need major work usually seem to know it, and are resolved before they come in. Others are gratified to find a physician who has the ability to subtly and simply correct the offensive lines of aging and leave the attractive ones. Filling agents do just this task.

Facial exercises are another way to prevent and treat movement-related lines. We discuss this with some reticence because facial exercises are associated with the work of lay "facialists" who usually make people look better temporarily but imply that their renderings do a lot more. Indeed, most facial exercises that we have seen demonstrated or have read about are not only not helpful but also detrimental. Pursing the lips, stretching the neck, pulling the skin over the chin all *add* to the changes of aging rather than correcting them. Slack skin is not the result of loss of muscle tone and is not helped by further stretching.

One of us (S.J.S.) has developed a theory about certain facial exercises, which is based on using one muscle or facial expression (and mastication) to counter other muscles of expression. The muscles of expression are not balanced with opposing muscles as are the skeletal voluntary muscles. Gravity must pull back the smile-folded cheek. As the primary factors lead to loss of skin elasticity, gravity no longer can pull out the smile fold completely. Thus the fold remains. By using the obicularis oris muscle(s), the residual undulations of the smile are tugged smooth. The obicularis is a complex group of muscles with voluntary control to produce various movements. One part of the muscle will pull the upper lip down, thus counteracting the sneer part of the smile; the lateral corners of the mouth can be pulled medially (a fish mouth) to counteract the cheek part of the smile. These movements should be practiced in private, in front of a mirror to make sure that other puckers are not created, and only a few times after long periods of smiling. The exercises should not be overdone so that the skin is stretched. Use discretion before suggesting these exercises to patients. It takes an intelligent and insightful patient to understand your instructions and use them judiciously. S.J.S. thinks they work on people with non-sun-damaged skin who are just starting to develop smile lines.

Full-face, deep chemical peels will remove some movement-related lines which have been more deeply etched in sun-damaged skin. After a deep peel, the lines upon lines in the crow's feet and the lines on folds lateral to the mouth are removed, leaving only the major folds and furrows that are the result of skin's movement with expression. The major lines return fairly quickly, usually within 6 to 12 months. The many accompanying small lines that were to a large extent related to sun damage do not return for a long time. There is some tightening of the skin, noticed especially at the jawline. This may be the result of the mid-dermal changes rather than true, increased elasticity.

Sleep Creases

Creases resulting from the position of the head on the pillow or mattress is the third and final secondary factor.[8] In men, sleep creases are

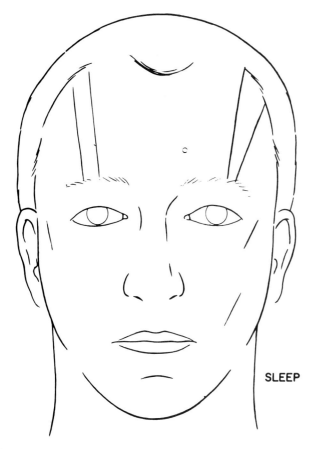

FIG 2–9.
Sleep creases.

long lines on the glabella that extend out on the forehead. It is easy to separate the two lines by having the patient frown. The corrugator muscle develops the central folds and nothing happens laterally. Conversely, having the patient lie on a pillow as when sleeping will fold the lateral forehead and bring the sleep creases into relief (Fig 2–11).

The same technique will differentiate the oblique straight line caused by sleep at the lateral canthus from the crow's feet. When a patient smiles the crow's feet are formed and when the patient lies down the sleep crease is formed.

The treatment and prevention of sleep creases are identical. The patient should stop placing the head in the position that causes the creases. Ask the patient to take a hand mirror to bed, assume the favored sleeping position, and look into the mirror. The cause of the lines

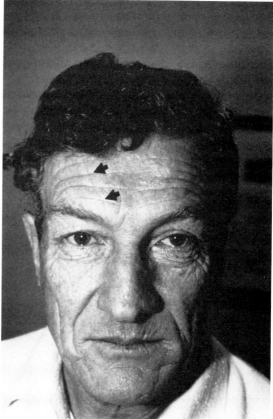

FIG 2–10.
56-year-old man with sleep creases *(arrows).*

commonly located on the lateral forehead and start just above the eyebrow and streak obliquely toward the temporal recede of the hairline (Fig 2–9). The creases are straight, and when deep, make the man look diabolic (Fig 2–10). Women occasionally will develop sleep creases but they are shorter and more shallow and also cross the crow's feet. Rarely, women will develop vertical, straight creases on the medial cheek which are secondary to sleep position. The onset of these lines is coincident with loss of elasticity; babies and teenagers awake with "pillow tracks," but these fall out by breakfast. Adult sleep lines last longer into the day and eventually become permanent marks.

Sleep creases are separate from the central and more vertical forehead lines caused by the corrugator muscles. Once in a while, a person will have corrugator muscle insertions located as far laterally as the mid-eyebrow which cause

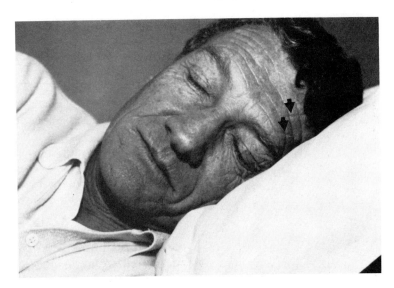

FIG 2–11.
Same man as in Fig 2–10 lying in favored sleep position that induces the sleep creases *(arrows)*.

will be obvious. It is difficult for patients to alter a favorite sleeping position, but it can be done over a period of about three months. Sleeping only on the back is not necessary, despite the suggestions of some 1930s Hollywood starlets. Lying on either side (the best position orthopedically) the patient should look into the mirror and shift the weight of the head on the pillow from the offending position more posteriorly so the weight is borne by the parietal scalp, the ear region, or even the zygoma. The sleep creases will soon disappear and in a few months the new position will be as comfortable as the old. Ask the patient to memorize the wrinkle-preventing position and get into it upon first going to bed. Ask the patient to remember and assume that position again at the earliest twilight awakening in the morning. Gradually, the memory will occur earlier each morning and eventually it will become the new position all night. When not repeatedly refolded, sleep creases will fall out. Within a few weeks of having a seventh nerve stroke, the movement-related lines will fade on the affected side.

Fillers help sleep lines, especially on the softer and thinner skin at the lateral canthus, but improvement does not last long in the thick forehead skin. Also, the smile is a flash and then the fold is released, whereas sleep positions are

held for 20 to 40 minutes and firmly fold the skin; therefore, the filler must resist that long-term pressure.

It is worthwhile for patients to prevent sleep creases because of the harsh lines they make above the eyebrows. No matter how pleasant the rest of the face, the oblique gashes on the forehead can make a face look mean.

Conclusions

Communication is improved and thinking sharpened by the use of descriptive terms. The terms fold, furrow, crease, and wrinkle, as defined in this chapter, will be used throughout this text. The terms are morphologically based, and when combined with anatomic location, accurately define the "lesions" the cosmetic surgeon treats.

A system for examining the aging face induces a thoroughness that might be lost when one or more aspects of the face are dominant. With the six factors in mind, reading a face takes only seconds. Separating sun-damage changes from movement-related changes, or loss of fat from inherent laxity, surely will lead the physician to suggest and perform appropriate procedures.

With so many new procedures and tools available to the cosmetic surgeon, and with increased public sophistication, the physician who gives an enlightened, logical, and practical consultation will be successful that much sooner.

References

1. Braverman IM, Fonkerfo E: Studies on cutaneous aging: The elastic fiber network. *J Invest Dermatol* 1982; 78:434–443.
2. Gilchrest BA: *Skin and Aging Processes*. Boca Raton, Fla, CRC Press, 1984.
3. Kligman LH; Photoaged skin is different. *Dermatol Focus* 1987; 5:3–4.
4. Bouissou H, Pieraggi MT, Julian M, et al: The elastic tissue of the skin: A comparison of spontaneous and actinic (solar) aging. *Int J Dermatol* 1988; 27:327–336.
5. Marks R, et al: Spontaneous remission of solar keratoses: The case for conservative management. *Dermatology* 1986; 115:649–655.
6. Kligman LH, Duo CH, Kligman AM: Topical retinoic acid enhances the repair of ultraviolet damaged dermal connective tissue. *Conn Tissue Res* 1984; 12:139–152.
7. Weiss JS, Ellis CN, Heddington JT, et al: Topical tretinoin improves photoaged skin: A double-blind vehicle controlled study. *JAMA* 1988; 259:527–532.
8. Stegman SJ: Sleep creases. *Am J Cosmetic Surg* 1987; 4:277–280.

Three

Benign Facial Lesions

During a consultation for any cosmetic procedure, in addition to looking at the problem the patient came for, look closely at the patient's face, neck, and hands for unsightly benign (or malignant) lesions. Unsightliness may, in part, result from one or several types of benign lesions that develop with age. As the face accumulates lines and wrinkles, benign lesions, some new and some old, can detract from a patient's appearance. Glasses, loss of skin color, and less vibrant hair all add to the impression of an aging face. The benign lesion is one contributor that usually can be treated easily. A well-done blepharoplasty, a face peel, or dermabrasion alone will not achieve the best potential cosmetic improvement if ugly lumps and bumps remain. Most benign lesions can be treated simultaneously with the main cosmetic procedure.

Because these lesions grow slowly, are recognized as benign, and often are family traits ("Grandmother had the same kind of bumps"), the patient will tolerate a surprising number of them without realizing what a cosmetic liability they are. As part of the consultation, the physician has the chance to point them out (patients sometimes do not even "see" these lesions) and suggest treatment. Be sure the patient gives permission for removal of the lesion(s) and be sure to send for histopathology even if it is a non-billed item.

Telangiectasia

A single telangiectatic vessel, if large and bright red, as well as clusters of small ones, detract from an otherwise clear complexion (Fig 3–1). Too often, these vessels are associated with excessive alcohol consumption, although the heavy drinker exhibits them only rarely. Telangiectasia are not only distracting but may indicate acne rosacea, actinic damage, steroid atrophy, or slow healing from surgery or trauma, suggesting that the area is going to scar; likewise, telangiectasia may simply be the result of the increased metabolic demands and neovascularization associated with wound healing. Although the management of telangiectasia is similar no matter what they are associated with, simultaneous treatment of all factors is critical. Other than treating the above-mentioned conditions, we do not know how to prevent them. The patient needs to understand that treatment of the existing vessels in no way affects the development of subsequent lesions.

For treating telangiectasia, it is difficult to improve on the old Birtcher hyphrecator and an epilating needle. Other damped, high-voltage, low amperage instruments work just as well, and the newer Birtchers do, too. However, we prefer the older models, which we can set to a very low current. Unipolar electrodesiccation is adequate for most vessels, but for recurrent or

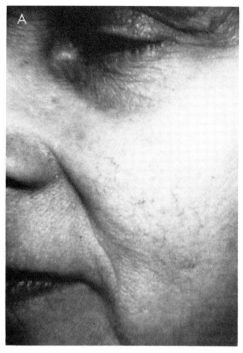
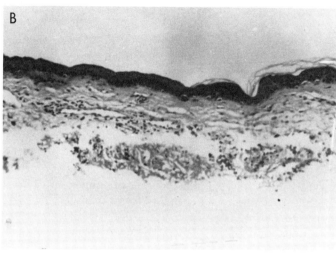

FIG 3–1.
Telangiectasia on the face. **A,** clinical appearance. **B,** microscopic appearance.

refractory ones, bipolar current is more destructive. We start out with the setting as low as possible, and adjust upward until enough spark is produced to jump into the vessel. If many lesions are being treated, the setting may require adjustment because of changes within the machine or in the line current because other machinery is being used in the building.

No special preparation is necessary. Avoid wiping the field with alcohol, so the spark does not ignite the residual surface fluid. Topical anesthetics are not generally effective through keratinized skin, although continued research on new topicals is under way. EMLA (Eutetic Mixture Local Anesthetic, Astra, Sweden), a topical anesthetic now used in Europe, causes vasoconstriction, making it inappropriate for this problem. New ionophoresis devices are being tested which use direct current and lidocaine with or without epinephrine for a painless delivery system. If these devices prove to be valid, they will be most helpful for treating this condition.

The new needles partially coated with non-conducting material work for superficial vessels,[1] but are unnecessary. They are best used for larger (1.0 mm diameter) leg vessels which must be canalized with the needle. For us, the one-inch, bent, disposable epilating needle works perfectly. With the advent of acquired immunodeficiency syndrome (AIDS) and the concept of infective aerosolized virus, we have switched to putting a one-half-inch 30-gauge needle on a Bernsco adapter (Bernsco Medical Supply Company, Seattle) (Fig 3–2). The device fits into the hyphrecator handle and accepts a disposable, metal-hubbed needle on the other end, providing the patient with a new instrument tip and the doctor with a tiny tip which desiccates so little tissue that no visible smoke plume is generated (Fig 3–2). The 30-gauge needle with its more pointed tip is better than the reusable epilating needle used for ultra-fine vessels. It does seem to have a short usability span, however. Probably, the tip melts and oxidizes. After 10 or 20 vessels have been treated, the current must be increased for the device to work. At that point, we just change disposable needles.

It is not necessary to actually probe or cannulate the tiny vessel. The current jumps to and through the skin into the more conductive blood in the vessel. The current will travel some distance within the vessel and seems to go either with or against the flow of blood. It is presumed that the high-energy damped current leads to cell disruption and head coagulation of the proteins. Although most vessels do not reopen, some will, and the patient must understand that.

After explaining the procedure, we encourage the patient to relax. Starting out on the mid- or lateral cheek with one or two short current bursts gains the patient's confidence and cooperation. We deliver ten bursts to ten vessels and then pause. If patients are tense, we ask them to count with us; that way they know when the procedure is going to end. Because the procedure is most painful around the nose and eyes, these areas are treated last. Treatment around the columella or on the nasal ali induces a tearing response and a sneezing reflex.

We treat as many vessels in one visit as the patient can tolerate. Most prefer to have about 20 or 30 treated and then return for more. If the treatment fails twice, we increase the current or consider another modality. If the patient has thick, sebaceous skin around the nasal ali, the technique will sometimes leave a depressed trough that is of the same pattern as the pre-existing vessel. Therefore, ask patients if they

prefer the vessel or the risk of a small trough. Rarely, a tiny scar in the form of a white dot will develop at the entry site of the current. Again, most people prefer to have the vessels removed; the scar is so tiny that it is not a cosmetic problem (except for perfectionists, who are just the ones who seek removal of minimal vessels).

Telangiectasia anywhere on the body resolve with electrodesiccation, but as with any injury, scarring is worse and the cosmetic importance is less the farther telangiectasia are located from the head. Electrical treatment of fine vessels on the neck, the anterior chest, and the backs of the hands has a positive risk-benefit ratio, but the same treatment on the legs commonly produces a line of white-dot scars often called a "string of pearls." Other methods are better for the legs (see Chapter 14).

Other treatments include the pulsed tunable dye laser which only offers less pain than the much less cumbersome and less costly hyphrecator. We have seen patients who developed scarring secondary to lasers, but that may have been the fault of the operator and not the instrument. The bigger drawback of the laser is persistent redness and longer recovery time. After electrodesiccation, a little reactive erythema is gone in minutes; after laser treatment, however, the wounds may be red and swollen for days. When the vessels are massive and cover large areas, dermabrasion will remove them. Predictably, this is a bloody procedure. Very large telangiectasias on the lateral face—usually found on men—are big enough to treat with sclerotherapy. We do not treat vessels close to the eyes or around the bridge of the nose with sclerotherapy because of theoretical retrograde flow into and damage to a retinal vessel. We are not aware, however, that this has ever happened.

Spider Nevi

Electrodesiccation of spider nevi often enough leaves a small white scar that the patient should be forewarned about. Nevertheless, this is the treatment of choice (Fig 3–3). Like telangiectasia, these vascular lesions cannot be anesthetized with any agent that contains epinephrine because any vasoconstriction—from

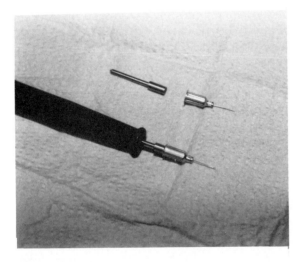

FIG 3–2.
Bernsco adaptor for using disposable needles on the Birtcher hyphrecator.

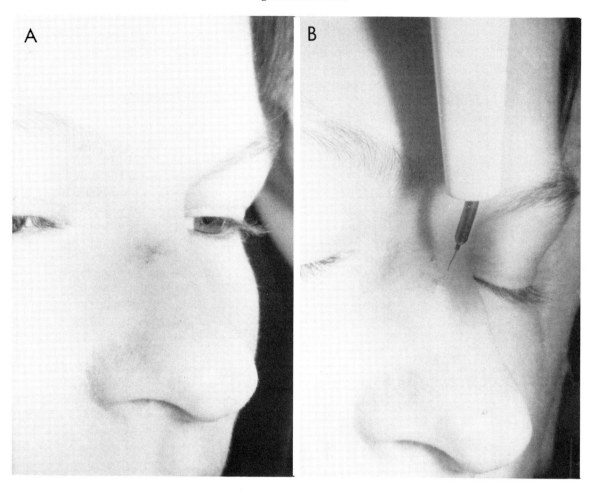

FIG 3–3.
Spider nevus. **A,** clinical appearance. **B,** treatment with electrodesiccation.

fluid, cold, or epinephrine—will obliterate the lesion. For a large spider nevus with the central arteriole clearly visible, lidocaine without epinephrine injected circumferentially or deep into the lesion is acceptable. However, the central feeder vessel must remain visible because the treatment is directed toward it. When the central vessel is destroyed, the smaller arms fade spontaneously.

If the nevus is large, with fully developed arms, treat both the central vessel and the arms. Larger nevi and recurrent or refractory ones are destroyed with a bipolar current or by holding the current in place longer than the usual flash. Anesthesia is required for a longer burst of electricity, and scarring can be expected. When electrodesiccation fails and if the patient wishes it,

a punch excision works. A 2- or 2.5-mm punch excision aimed directly over the central vessel followed by one suture removes the nevus but replaces it with a scar.

Cherry Angiomas

These benign 2- to 5-mm round red lesions are made up of mature ectatic vessels. They appear at midlife on the upper trunk and arms and occur in a large percentage of the population. Most patients are satisfied to be advised that the lesions are benign, will always be benign, and can be removed if the patient wishes.

A quick blast of the electrodesiccator at a low setting, with or without anesthesia, according to the patient's preference, destroys the angioma. A scalpel shave removal followed by a chemical coagulant or a touch of the desiccator also works well. Hot cautery lightly touched to or held just above very tiny angiomas is so quick and easy a procedure that many can be eradicated in one sitting.

Milia

Milia are inclusion cysts, probably of epidermal origin, 0.5 to 2.5 mm in diameter, and nearly always found on the face and neck (Fig 3–4). They appear spontaneously and also are related to accidental or surgical injuries to the skin. Histologically, they are accumulations of concentric layers of keratin produced by squamous epithelium. Some appear to have a pseudocapsule and others do not. They are always found in the dermis.

Milia commonly appear after dermabrasion and occasionally after chemical peel and incision surgery. Post-traumatic milia arise in groups two to six weeks after the injury and remain for weeks or months. A common theory is that post-traumatic milia are entrapped fragments of detached epithelium that continue to keratinize. They will resolve spontaneously or they can be treated if the patient requests. Post-traumatic and naturally occurring milia look alike, and are difficult to distinguish clinically from closed comedones of acne.

The treatment of milia is to unroof and drain them. A small nick made with the tip of a #11 scalpel blade and a little pressure works well but is tedious because the milia move away from the blade and are so small that it is difficult to get enough pressure to pinch them out. Another technique is to stabilize the milia with two or three fingers and to nick the top with a Hagedorn needle or surgical lancet and then use a comedone extractor (Schamberg crimped-type) to express the creamy or inspissated contents. If there is a thin-walled sac, try to express the wall as well.

Whenever the milia are close to the surface and small (less than 1.0 mm to 1.0 mm), hot cautery is the treatment of choice. The fine tip of the hot cautery is heated to a dull red—not bright red or white hot—and touched lightly to or held just above the top of the milia for a fraction of a second; the sac then breaks and the contents may boil out; if not, a comedone extractor will squeeze out the contents, or it can be left alone to dry up in a day or two. The

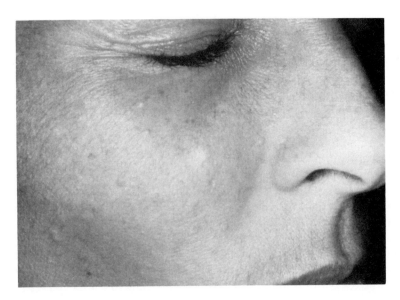

FIG 3–4.
Milia—small, whitish inclusion cysts on the cheek.

hyphrecator with an epilating needle set at low current works in nearly the same way as hot cautery.

All of these methods heal without scarring and seldom require local anesthesia. With the hot cautery, 30 to 60 tiny milia can be treated in a minute or two. Treatment of larger, deeper ones takes longer. The only disadvantage with hot cautery is that the patient realizes a hot instrument is being used, and if a postinflammatory hyperpigmentation arises in the area, it is difficult to convince the patient that it was not caused by the cautery. We make a special point to tell the patient we are not touching the skin, but only the "white bump." Cohen has reduced the incidence of milia formation after dermabrasion by immediately scrubbing the patient's face with a gauze pad and copious amounts of saline.[2]

Intradermal Nevi (Moles)

It is not unwarranted to discuss mole removal in a text on cosmetic surgery. Rarely is a mole thought of as a beauty mark these days, and multiple moles detract from a good appearance. Watch the television for pictures of populations where medical care does not include mole removal—e.g., Russia and England—to see how unsightly aging moles can be. Also, the natural history of many moles is to pedunculate, become sessile, or more deeply pigmented. In less enlightened times, this natural maturation, plus other aging changes on the face, created the visual stereotypes of the witch, or the ogre.

If the patient comes to the office specifically for mole removal, it is a simple matter. However, if an unsightly mole is near or within the field of a proposed cosmetic procedure, offer the option of treating it before or during the cosmetic surgery. Patients are so accustomed to their moles that they are surprised when removal is suggested. It is appropriate to raise the subject during a cosmetic consultation, but do not press too hard. If a hypertrophic scar results, or any untoward result occurs, patients will remember that the physician "pressured" them about mole removal.

Patient and doctor alike consider mole removal extremely simple; the patient thinks removal means that the mole is gone; the doctor thinks that removal does not usually leave much scar. When scarring does occur, there is usually not enough damage for such a case to go to court, but there are many mole removal patients who wish they could go to court. Mole removal often means exchanging the mole for a scar. The chances of that scar's being minimal are related to where the mole is located anatomically, the patient's coloring, and the depth to which the nevus cells extend into the skin. Share with the patient the information that hypertrophic scars are not uncommon on the upper trunk and upper arms, that some moles go deep and removal may leave a depressed scar, that some nevus cells may have migrated deeper and that small brown spots may recur, and that like *any* wound, it may become infected.

Whether mole removal is done during the cosmetic procedure or before it, whether or not a separate fee is charged, whether the physician or the patient suggested removal, it is extremely important to send the tissue for histopathology.

Whenever possible, a shave excision is the best method of mole removal (Fig 3–5). The technique varies with the shape of the base of the mole. If it is sessile or pedunculated, expand the base with local anesthesia and scissor or scalpel it off. If the base is flat, hold three-point finger pressure, or have the assistant hold the skin taut and use repeated gentle, small, sweeping strokes to feel across the base of the mole. If the mole is large enough, lift one edge with a small-toothed forceps to see the junction of the mole with the skin more clearly. With this technique, little of the surrounding skin is lost, and the incision depth can be adjusted as necessary. It is a clinical decision whether or not to chase out any remaining nevus cells at the depth of the wound. Using the scalpel to dig out those few cells may lead to a more noticeable scar, but leaving them increases the chance of recurrent pigmentation. After the mole is out, use the belly of the #15 blade to scrape or dermabrade the edges of the defect. This helps to shave down the margin and reduce the dell and the ensuing depressed scar. Monsel's solution, aluminum chloride, Oxycel cotton, and pressure all are adequate for hemostasis. Only simple dressings are required, and they should be removed in 24 hours. If the dressing is left on too long, the skin will ma-

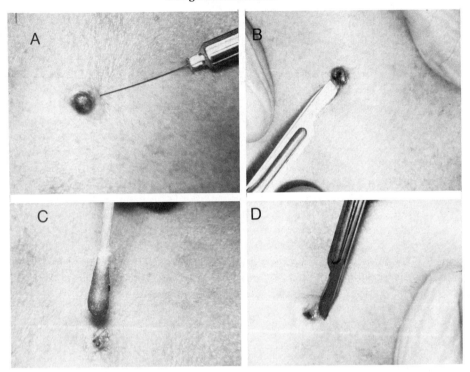

FIG 3–5.
Shave excision technique for an intradermal nevus. **A,** injection of local anesthesia. **B,** shaving of nevus by cutting at junction of normal skin and lesion. **C,** chemical cautery with Monsel's solution. **D,** dermabrading the wound to make it smoother and to tease out any remaining nevus cells.

cerate and the likelihood of infection will increase.

If there is any clinical sign that a nevus may be active or that it has degenerated into a melanoma, it should be removed by excision. Margins for an excision biopsy need to be only 1 to 2 mm because the recommended safety margins will be used on a re-excision once the diagnosis, accurate size and volume, and staging have been completed if the mole is malignant. The lesion must come out in one piece, with special attention paid to cutting well beneath it. Both depth and volume are important prognosticators. Cutting across a pigmented lesion too large to remove in toto is acceptable, but the darker "active" areas should be selected if only a part of the lesion is being removed for histologic examination.

Lentigines (Liver Spots)

A lentigo and a freckle are different histologically, but may look the same clinically. The removal technique is different for each. The freckle is predominantly a pigmented lesion, whereas the lentigo includes epidermal acanthosis and papillomatosis and is slightly elevated above the surface of the skin. Both unwanted marks appear with age and sun exposure. Not surprisingly, the results of removal are better on the face than on the chest or dorsal hands. For unknown reasons, the thicker facial skin heals faster, with fewer complications.

For true lentigines (which are sometimes difficult to distinguish clinically) heat separation with hot cautery limits the wound depth to the dermal-epidermal junction and the wound size to that of just the lesion (Fig 3–6). After local infiltrative anesthesia, set the hot cautery to dull red, and (with magnification) pass the hot tip back and forth just above the lesion, as if coloring it in. The epidermis will blister off, taking the lentigo with it. Follow with a very light curetting, using a ring curette, or rub the site with a gauze-covered finger to remove the remaining charred lesion.

The wound heals by forming a small crust, which is followed by erythema for several weeks. Uncommonly, the area will hyperpigment, usually temporarily. On the neck and the backs of the hands, the healing process is longer, with the development of thicker crusts, longer erythema, and a greater occurrence of hyperpigmentation. The same technique is possible using a hyphrecator and epilating needle, turned on its side and passed over the lentigo, with the side of the needle just touching the surface.

Dermabrasion with a small (4 mm diameter) fraise touched lightly will abrade away the lentigo. Dental garnets, disposable emory or sand-

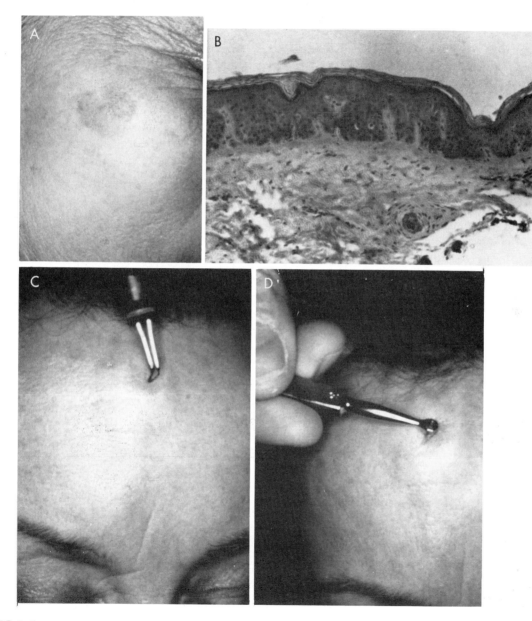

FIG 3–6.
Lentigo. **A,** clinical appearance of the lesion. **B,** microscopic appearance of the lesion. **C,** removal by first passing the hot cautery tip just above the lesion to heat-separate it from the dermis. **D,** the char is wiped away with a curette or gauze wrapped around the surgeon's finger.

paper wheels, or a saucer-shaped, fine diamond fraise attached to the Bell hand engine or other dermabrasion machine all will lightly abrade the skin. Different operators prefer different tools. Technically, it is much more difficult to abrade the exact epidermal-dermal junction and keep it strictly within the confines of the lesion than it is to heat separate. However, for some of the thicker lesions, it is preferable. We have found that healing on the backs of the hands is less complicated and quicker if we cover the treated areas with a semipermeable dressing such as Op-Site for five to seven days.

Others recommend peeling with trichloroacetic acid (TCA) 50% or phenol full strength as the treatment of choice for removal of lentigines. Although we use peeling interchangeably with the other techniques, we use it on the face but not on the hands. The area may not need local anesthesia; degreasing with acetone permits better penetration of the chemical; the application covers the lesion and a tiny border of normal skin; and many lentigines can be treated at one setting. In our experience, chemical peeling agents have proved to be somewhat less successful than hot cautery. With the cautery, the lesion is gone for sure. With the peel, the lesion may not be wounded deeply enough and may heal back rather than heal away. As with full-face peels, persistent erythema and hyperpigmentation follow in a certain annoying percentage of cases. For hyperkeratotic lesions, peels are less helpful.

Liquid nitrogen, applied with a cotton-tipped applicator or sprayed on, blisters the lesion off and is better at bleaching the more flat, almost frecklelike lentigines. Keeping the wound limited to the lesion and controlling the depth of the wound are much harder with liquid nitrogen than with any of the other modalities. However, hyperpigmentation is less likely with this method.

We do not recommend "dry" curetting, or curetting after freezing with one of the spray refrigerants, because the chance of making a wound far deeper than necessary is high and the deeper wounds may scar. The freeze/curette technique, however, is excellent for other exophytic growths, as discussed below. Bleaching agents, either proprietary or prescriptive, seldom work on true lentigines. These agents bleach freckles that occur on the hands and face and also arise with age.

Seborrheic Keratoses

These lesions are quickly recognized by the experienced dermatologist, and when they are typical, are correctly diagnosed by most physicians. The only treatment contraindicated is to excise them and close primarily. The seborrheic keratosis is an *exophytic lesion* and need only be separated at its rather well-defined base (Fig 3–7).

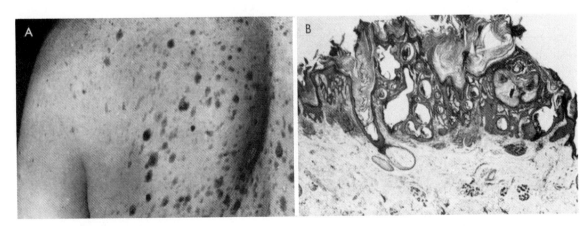

FIG 3–7.
Seborrheic keratoses. **A,** clinical appearance. **B,** microscopic appearance, showing that the lesion is exophytic (above the surface of the skin). This allows treatment to be very superficial.

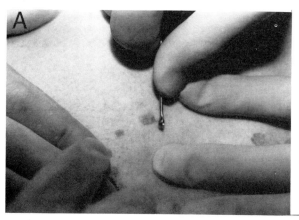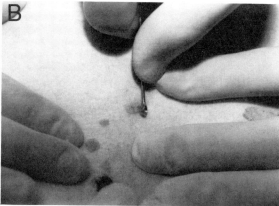

FIG 3–8.
Treatment of a seborrhic keratosis by the "fast curette" technique. **A,** the skin around the lesion is held taut and the curette is brought in quickly with a flip of the wrist. The curette strikes the keratosis at its edge. **B,** the curette is passed right through the lesion with a follow-through stroke like a golf shot; the keratosis chips off.

The quickest, easiest, and best-healing method is what we call "the fast curette method" (Fig 3–8) which we learned from Frederic E. Mohs, M.D.[3] However, this is a very old method. Poor removal of the smaller lesions (0.3 to 1.0 cm) may not require anesthesia unless they are located on sensitive or thin skin. Larger lesions (1.0 cm or larger) need several passes of the curette and can become tender, although we have treated many large lesions without using anesthesia. A spray with one of the refrigerants such as Frigiderm or a touch of liquid nitrogen stiffens the skin and keratosis, which makes it possible to snap off the keratosis more easily.

The method is to stabilize the skin with two- or three-point finger pressure and to hold a ring curette tightly in the dominant hand, holding the curette not like a pencil but like a golf club, with the thumb extended onto the shaft of the instrument. The tight grip and thumb leverage are necessary to keep the knife steady when it strikes the lesion. Starting well behind the keratosis and moving both the arm and wrist, swing the curette at the base of the keratosis with a sweeping movement, hit the lesion, and keep moving in a follow-through motion. Sometimes, the whole keratosis will pop off; at other times, several identical, repeat strokes are needed. The curette does not dig into the underlying skin; it only hits the lesion at an edge and lifts it up. The rest of the action is a blow that knocks it off. Somehow this force chips the lesions off with minimal pain to the patient, and in such a way that scarring is minimized or eliminated. Hemostasis is necessary and can be accomplished with Monsel's, aluminum chloride, Oxycel cotton, or finger pressure. Literally dozens of these keratoses can be removed at a single visit. Try to encourage the patient not to have anesthesia if there are many, because the pain of anesthesia is greater than the total pain of keratosis removal and hemostasis. As expected, some lesions will heal pigmented, some will heal hypopigmented, and rarely with scar or recurrence. This is a great technique.

If the method does not work, the error is most likely in technique—not holding the skin taut, not striking hard and fast enough, or not following through. This sounds like a golf or tennis lesson, because essentially the same arm/wrist hit-and-snap motion is used. Seborrheic keratoses apparently are attached at their bases differently than other lesions, because they will separate by this technique and heal with less or no scarring; with a scalpel shave removal, however, lesions heal slower, with ensuing redness and sometimes scarring.

Experienced cryotherapists can raise a blister just below a keratosis, which will later separate with little morbidity. Although a few thin, flat keratoses will separate after peeling, most will not.

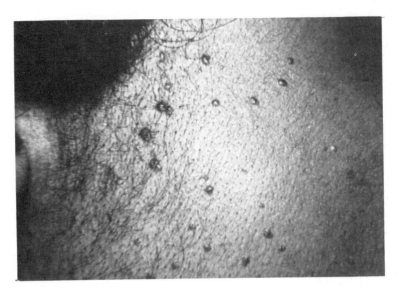

FIG 3–9.
Dermatosis papulosis nigra, clinical appearance.

Dermatosis Papulosis Nigra (DPN)

These lesions develop around the eyes, cheeks, and temples in some darker-skinned families (Fig 3–9). Tens to hundreds of lesions may arise, and patients are amazingly tolerant of them. Be careful when suggesting removal, because many patients consider them normal or "in the family." When the patient suggests removal, give the usual warnings about uncertain results and possibilities of recurrence of hypo- or hyperpigmentation. The fast curette method, using a very small curette, unseats these little brown lesions with dispatch. For pedunculate DPNs, scissor removal with a small scissors such as a Gradle or any small scissors with serrations on one blade causes hardly any bleeding and at most leaves only a small dot blemish or scar. Also, small (0.5 to 1.0 mm) pedunculated lesions shrink down and char quickly when touched by the hot cautery or the hyphrecator tip. Many of these patients have dark skin and may hyperpigment either temporarily or permanently. Patients need to know the risks.

Dermatofibroma (DF)

These are benign lesions and once they reach their full size of around 0.7 cm remain static,

occasionally pigmenting. It is important to know that they are dermal lesions, which means that treatment must remove or injure the dermis (Fig 3–10, A and B). Patients who hear from the physician that a DF lesion is completely benign and that treatment will most likely leave some type of blemish or scar, but who still want the lesion removed, must be carefully quizzed on their understanding of informed consent. If the patient is concerned enough to insist on removal of a benign, unobtrusive lesion, the physician needs to consider how a patient will react to a scar and/or hyperpigmentation that are the same size as the lesion, or to a linear scar two to three times longer than the diameter of the lesion. Much grief can be avoided by leaving these lesions undisturbed.

Once the patient and physician decide on surgical treatment, excision with histopathology is required. The physician is responsible for that lesion forevermore, once the patient has mentioned it and it has been examined. The elasticity of the skin and the location and size of the DF dictate the orientation and length of the ellipse. The depth need only be through the dermis unless there is a clinical finding that indicates the biopsy should be deeper.

Liquid nitrogen freezing—enough to build an ice ball to the full depth of the DF—flattens

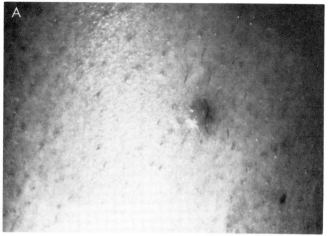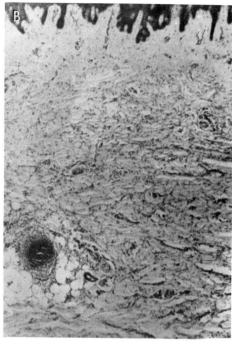

FIG 3–10.
Dermatofibroma. **A,** clinical appearance. **B,** microscopic appearance.

it and sometimes removes it. Freezing is the treatment of choice for elevated and pruritic DFs, and greatly decreases the pigmentation.

Most patients are satisfied with the pronouncement of benignity and the knowledge that removal means exchange of the lesion for a scar. Telling these patients about the "insect bite" reaction theory smooths the way to a "let it alone" decision on their part and answers their questions about why the lesion developed in the first place.

Sebaceous Hyperplasia

Clinically, these benign lesions occur at mid- to late life and appear on the face, upper trunk, and upper extremities. They are not known to relate to systemic disease. Sebaceous hyperplasia produces dermal lesions that may grow up through the epidermis. The color range of creamy pink to yellow depends on the amount of epidermis and papillary dermis that covers the hypertrophic sebaceous tissue (Fig 3–11).

Excision or deep curettement will remove the tissue but produce a significant scar. Chemical peeling, however, removes the lesion and seldom leaves a scar. This is one type of lesion removal that makes the doctor seem like a magician. The theory of the dynamics of peeling is discussed at length in Chapter 4. Briefly stated, however, the wound produced by the escarotic needs to be at or deeper than the pathology being treated. Therefore, to obliterate sebaceous hyperplasia, the peel must be below the mid-dermis. TCA 50%, full-strength phenol applied repeatedly or with occlusion creates mid-dermal wounds.

Consequently, we recommend using a cotton-tipped applicator to apply the agent until it frosts. A drop of the agent sitting on the lesion for 15 to 30 seconds will produce the desired result. Simple adjuncts like gently scraping off the keratin with the wooden end of the applicator stick or vigorous rubbing with acetone preconditions the lesion for deeper penetration of the agent. The residual agent should be diluted or wiped off, and if the hyperplasia is perceived

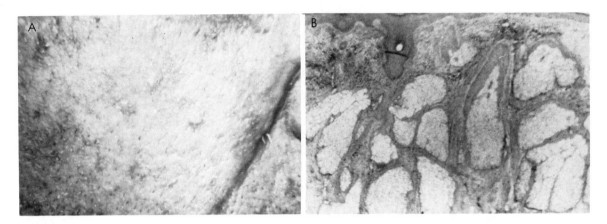

FIG 3–11.
Sebaceous hyperplasia. **A,** clinical appearance. **B,** microscopic appearance.

to be deep, occlusion for 24 hours will deepen the wound. Healing is similar to that of a mid- to deep-level peel, with all of the same possible side effects. As with the peel, the healing is often without any side effects and the physician again turns into a magician. Repeat peeling once or twice is worth a try, but because the process is unaltered by treatment, new hyperplasias may continue to arise.

Judicious use of the hot cautery produces equally good results but also a slight risk that a small scar may develop.

Xanthelasma

This is another benign lesion found on or around the eyelids. Solitary xanthelasmas less than 0.5 cm in diameter are the most easily treated, but often they grow larger, are multiple, and recur. Rarely are they related to systemic conditions; occasionally the patient may have hypercholesterolemia. Excision, scalpel, or laser marsupialization, electrodesiccation, and chem-

ical cautery make up the list of possible treatments. Each has advantages and disadvantages; none prevents new or recurrent lesions from forming.

Excision is indicated for long-standing, static lesions when the eyelid skin is redundant enough to permit it. The eyelids heal beautifully with fine, almost unnoticeable scars. Do not choose excision for newly erupted xanthelasmas, because others may appear and the redundant eyelid tissue will be used up. There is no reason why xanthelasma removal cannot be designed to become like standard blepharoplasty if the criteria for both are met. The incision depth need only be just through the dermis. Xanthelasmae do not extend deeper than that. The technique can be the same as for blepharoplasty, with approximation of the wound with quick-dissolving gut, subcuticular running, or a few vertical mattress sutures and Steri-Strips.

Because healing is so good around the upper eyelids and canthi, the technique of exteriorizing or burning and leaving to heal by second intention creates fine-line, acceptable scars. Insertion of the hyphrecator epilating needle into the center of the xanthelasma, with the current applied for a second or two, shrinks the lesion almost completely. These approaches are best for patients with multiple recurring lesions and little or no extra eyelid skin.

Peeling xanthelasmas require the same technique described above for sebaceous hyperplasia (Fig 3–12). Full-strength phenol or 50% TCA is applied until deep frosting occurs, then is diluted or wiped off, occluded if the lesion is thick, and allowed to heal.

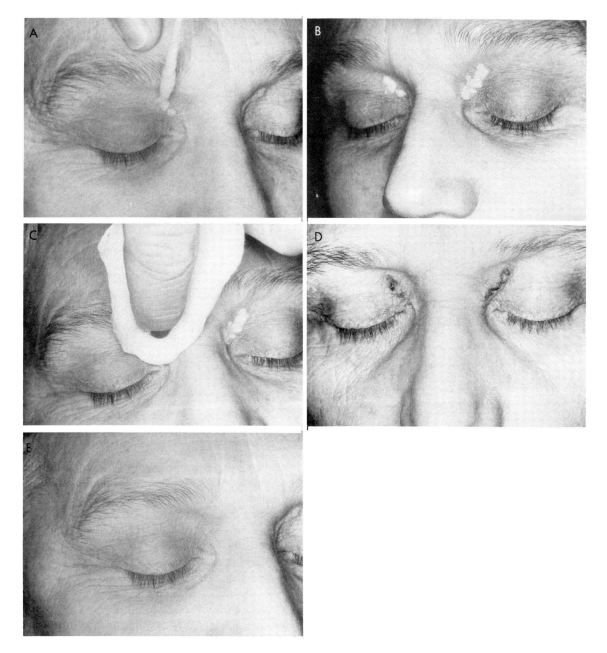

FIG 3–12.
Xanthalesma. **A,** lesion on medical upper eyelid is painted with trichloracetic acid. **B,** entire lesion with an even, white frosting. **C,** cotton gauze pad soaked in tap water applied to cool the area. **D,** two weeks later crusts have formed. **E,** the area after crusts have sloughed off.

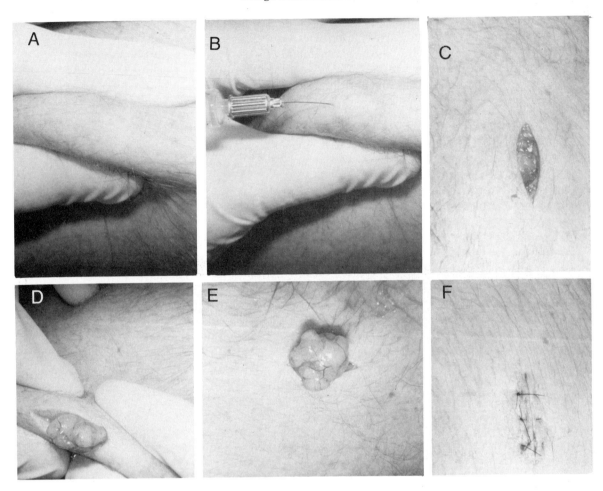

FIG 3–13.
Lipoma, excision technique. **A,** the lipoma is grasped between the thumb and forefinger. **B,** the skin overlying the tumor is anesthetized. **C,** the full thickness of skin is incised to the level of the lipoma. **D** and **E,** pressure of thumb and forefinger is applied on the bulk of the lipoma, causing it to extrude. **F,** the incision is closed with sutures.

Lipomas

Lipomas are appropriate to a discussion of cosmetic procedures when they are prominent or large on the face and neck and when there are great numbers of them on the trunk and extremities. Many physicians have recommended the "best" technique for removing lipomas and have demonstrated fine results, but often do not report the lipoma(s) that is fibrotic (a fibrolipoma) and will not pop out easily, or describe the lipoma that has a significantly sized vessel feeding it through the base which, if left unattended, can produce everything from rapid wound filling to a late-onset hematoma.

It is always worth trying to squeeze out the lipoma through an incision one-quarter of its diameter (Fig 3–13). Grasp the whole lipoma between the thumb and index finger, inject local anesthesia into just the incision site, incise through the skin, and squeeze. Out it pops. Then examine the tumor. Palpate the site for a residual lipoma, check to make sure blood is not welling up, and close. If there is brisk bleeding, use skin hooks to open the small incision and move that opening around to provide a view of the entire base. Identify and stop any bleeders. If the source of bleeding cannot be found, open the incision wider until it can be located.

We always advise patients that we will *try* the squeeze-and-pop method, but if there is bleeding or if the lipoma turns out to be fibrous, we may need to make a longer incision.

Most of the time, the dead space does not need to be obliterated with stitches, packing, or pressure dressings, and surprisingly, does not heal with a depressed scar. As always, the scars have the most acceptable appearance on the thin skin of the face and neck and are more obvious on the extremities and the lower trunk.

Liposuction is indicated for giant lipomas (larger than 3 or 4 cm diameter). The "wet technique" (see Chapter 13) of injecting dilute lidocaine, saline, and hyaluronidase into the lipoma until it is tumescent, followed by cannula liposuction through a stab incision, will remove many such masses and leave a relatively tiny scar and ultimately no depression, providing that the underlying tissues were not pressure-atrophied and the overlying skin was normal. The lipoma fat does *not* usually boil out like fatty pockets elsewhere do. The pseudocapsule and more fibrous stroma between lobules prevent easy flow into the suction cannula. What in fact happens is a mechanical assault on the lipoma with the cannula, ramming it repeatedly through the mass of the tumor which breaks down, and bits of fat break off. Eventually, the lipoma is small and deflated enough to squeeze out through the small opening.

Removal by suction of multiple lipomata that are closely adjacent in one area spares marking that area with many scars. A field or regional anesthesia is given and the cannula is inserted through a stab wound central to several lipomata. The lesions are pumped up with the saline solution, and after a wait of 10 to 15 minutes, the suction and assault begin. Select cannulas that have large ventral openings to accommodate the *blobs* of fat that are different from the cottage cheese-type of fat that is aspirated during regular body-contouring liposuction. A newly designed open-ended cannula (called the cobra tip) works well in this situation. All of the tumors accessible from this one entry site are suctioned; another entry site is selected if needed.

Liposuction is fine if a giant lipoma can be withdrawn through a small incision or if many

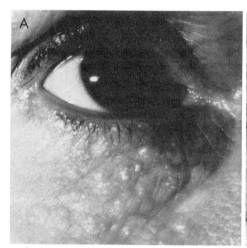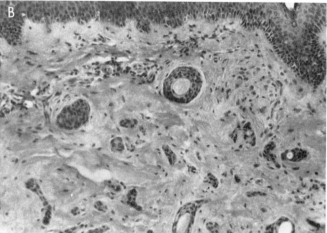

FIG 3–14.
Syringoma. **A**, clinical appearance. **B**, microscopic appearance.

can be removed from one opening. The patient, however, must understand that there is no guarantee that success will occur as hoped.

Syringoma

The histology of this hamartoma with differentiation toward the sweat ducts reveals lesions anywhere in the dermis from the epidermis to the fat (Fig 3–14). It is curious that these sweat-duct-like growths are not affected by peeling or freezing. Possibly the survival of ductal tissue through chemical and cold injury adds credence to the theory that regeneration comes from the ductal linings.

Excision or destruction by laser, electricity, or cautery are the only treatments we know of. All have limitations, because most syringomas are in the area of the lower eyelid. Usually there is limited excess skin on the lower lids, and therefore excision is preferable for a few lesions but not for multiple lesions. If the patient could benefit from a lower-lid blepharoplasty, it can be designed to remove as many lesions as possible. Otherwise, it is helpful to offer the patient removal of selected lesions. It is surprising to realize that certain lesions bother patients more than others. Ask patients which lesion(s) they hate and they will point to one or two and be satisfied if just these can be removed. (However, often the one or two lesions the patient does not like will not be the same ones the physician does not like.)

Destructive methods, such as electrodesiccation, leave scars and are only acceptable if the lesion is small and superficial.

Melasma

Wood's light (320 to 400 nm) examination of melasma helps to clinically differentiate the types of pigment deposition.[4] If the color contrast is enhanced under Wood's light, compared to visible light, the majority of the melanin is located in the basal and suprabasal layers of the epidermis. The melanin can even be as high as the stratum corneum. This type of melasma commonly responds to treatment with bleaching agents and peels. If the color contrast is not enhanced, the melanin is locked in the dermal macrophages, much like a tattoo, and is extremely resistant to therapy. A few people have a mixed variety, and not all cases react to Wood's light. The majority of cases, however, do fall into the epidermal or dermal groups.

The histologic differences in what is clinically called melasma account in large part for the variable response to treatment. Therefore, temper your enthusiasm when discussing treatment with the patient. The Wood's light test is a start. If the color enhancement is not present, tell the patient that the chances of improvement are limited. A small (2 mm) punch biopsy stained for melanin may help determine where the melanin is located and help with the prognosis. That biopsy site can be filled in with a punch transplant from behind the ear.

A long period of treatment with sunscreens and hydroquinone is the first step. The hydroquinone formula may include Retin-A or hydrocortisone or may be dissolved in a solvent such as Neutrogena Vehicle-N. We have had good success with hydroquinone 6% in mild Vehicle-N, or the formula developed by Albert Kligman, which includes hydroquinone, Retin-A, and triamcinolone.

Peeling is probably the first choice for surgical treatment of the epidermal type of melasma. Multiple light peels four to six weeks apart, with 20% to 30% TCA, deep peel with full-strength phenol, with or without occlusion, and a Baker's formula mixture peel, with or without occlusion, all have had limited success. We use the word limited because a significant percentage of patients do not respond, and there is always the rare patient who pigments more. Therefore, when peeling or dermabrasion are used, the patient must be told in no uncertain terms that worse hyperpigmentation is a possibility.

Light dermabrasion also has helped lighten some melasma. It would be the preferred treatment if the patient had other problems which could be improved by abrasion. Because it is suspected that the freezing which accompanies dermabrasion may also affect the melanocytes, the method is double jeopardy for the pigment cells. Because it is technically more difficult to abrade just the area of melasma, it is best to abrade the whole cosmetic unit that contains the dyschromia. Peels, however, can be painted only on the involved areas.

Benign Facial Lesions

The melanocytes' poor resistance to cold is the rationale for a light liquid nitrogen treatment for melasma. Sometimes, it works. The difficulty is in the poor control of wound depth with liquid nitrogen.

The list of complications for each of the above modalities applies to spot treatments as well as full face treatments. Because of predictable complications, limited results, and the knowledge that in some patients the pigment is locked in the dermal melanocytes, detailed informed consent is essential. It bothers us to hear our colleagues on talk shows or to see them quoted in the lay beauty magazines, commenting on the many and wonderful treatments for melasma. What these physicians say may be true 50% of the time. For us, the problem is that it is difficult to know, even with the Wood's light test, which 50% the patient who sits expectantly before us will fall into. We have seen each of the treatments mentioned above make some patients worse.

References

1. Kobayashi, T: Electrosurgery using insulated needles: Treatment of telangiectasias. *J Dermatol Surg Oncol* 1986; 12:936–942.
2. Cohen BH: Prevention of postdermabrasion milia (letter). *J Dermatol Surg Oncol* 1988; 14:1301.
3. Mohs FE: Seborrhic keratoses: Scarless removal by curettage and oxidized cellulose. *JAMA* 1970; 212:1956–1958.
4. Sanchez NP, Madhu A, Pathak MB, et al: Melasma: A clinical, light microscopic, ultrastructural, and immunofluorescence study. *J Am Acad Dermatol* 1981; 4:698–710.

Four

Chemical Peels

History

A dermatologist, George Mackee, reported in the *British Journal of Dermatology*[1] that in 1903 he began using a phenol solution for the treatment of acne scarring. The solution was applied and washed off with ethanol one-half to one minute later. This treatment was repeated every two to three months, from four to six times in all. Dr. Mackee followed some of these patients for up to 30 years and found no serious side effects. He and the patients believed that acne scarring was reduced.

It is generally believed that in the United States our exposure to this treatment came from German dermatologists who immigrated in the 1920s and 1930s. A report in the British literature in 1950 told of using 20% phenol in ether to remove freckles.[2] Physicians began to pay attention to peeling for improving the appearance of the aging face when they began to see the complications that resulted from the efforts of the lay peelers. Full-thickness loss of skin and hypertrophic scars were numerous. Although physicians learned about phenol face peeling by observing how it could go wrong, they did recognize that the method had merit.

The work of Thomas Baker, M.D., of Miami, elevated chemical face peeling to a generally accepted medical procedure.[3-7] Baker's classic studies on the various formulae, his careful toxicity studies, and his long-term follow-up of hundreds of patients established this procedure as scientific, and as one that could be offered with a favorable risk-benefit ratio.

Originally liquified phenol United States Pharmacopeia (USP) was used in its most concentrated strength—88%. This strength is still used for what we call a medium-depth peel. In the 1960s, several groups of physicians developed formulas designed to reduce the irritability of the phenol. We suspect they were looking for a less potent solution. Brown and colleagues[8]

published the following formula in 1960, using oil to reduce the strength or phenol to increase it:

Phenol	60% to 95%
Saponated cresol	0.3%
Olive or sesame oil	0.25%
Distilled water q.s.	100.%

Sperber offered a "buffered" formula in 1963[9]:

Phenol	15.00 ml
Sodium salicylate	.05 ml
Camphor	.025 ml
Anhydrous glycerine	1.25 ml
Ethanol (100%)	.50 ml

Baker originally published his formula in 1961[1] and later modified to:

Phenol U.S.P.	3 ml
Distilled water	2 ml
Croton oil	2 drops
Septisol	5 drops

Baker's formula is simple and has become one of the most popular formulas in use today. Baker made two important discoveries: (1) phenol is most penetrating—thus producing a deeper wound—in a 50% aqueous concentration, and the addition of epidermal irritants such as croton oil enhances the penetration of the active ingredient.

Studies of other popular formulae have been published by experienced peelers. Ayres[10] used equal mixtures of phenol, trichloracetic acid, and alcohol. Aronsohn[11] used phenol with saponated cresol (Lysol) and croton oil. Litton recommended 50% phenol with glycerin, water, and croton oil because it remained stable for three to four months.[14]

It is critical for each physician to learn what to expect from each formulation. How much is actually applied is thus far unquantified in the literature. Therefore, each physician develops a technique that works but without knowning the amounts of escarotic being applied.

Peeling, with chemical and physical modalities, has been a successful treatment for acne for many years. Trichloroacetic acid 20% to 30% (TCA), B-napthol, pancreatic enzymes, plant enzymes such as pineapple and papaya, resorcinol 20%, and salicylic acid all have been used to remove the stratum corneum around impacted follicles.[12] The effect is helpful but temporary. Peeling for acne is not used as much today as in the past, not because it is troublesome or ineffective, but because more effective treatments have been developed.

Light has also been used to lightly desquamate. Cold quartz machines, which used to be found in every dermatologist's office, produce 95% of their rays in the 250 nm range and the rest in the sunburn spectrum. Zein Obaji, M.D., has successfully used light in conjunction with TCA peels to correct the changes of the aging face.[34] The fear of the potential long-term effects has made light-induced peeling unpopular, although it has been shown to be effective for both acne and aged skin.

Dynamics

Little is known about the specific cause-and-effect relationship between the peel and its resulting clinical effect. It has been assumed for years that the wound is the result of protein precipitation. Basically, the peeling agent induces a wound that because of its nature or because of its failure to wound below a certain critical depth heals with the resulting skin architecture different from the pre-existing sun-damaged skin and also different from normal skin. Recent studies suggest that all of the most common agents do *not* wound in the same way, or that they at least affect the skin differently.[36] Most investigators realize that peels induce changes in the epidermis, the papillary dermis, and the upper portions of the reticular dermis, depending on how deep the wound extends.

The literature contains little information on the microscopic alterations induced by peels. It is difficult to obtain multiple biopsy specimens from the faces of patients who are seeking a better appearance. However, it is important to study facial skin because it is unique histologically, it is the area most badly sun-damaged, and thus is the area where peels are almost exclusively performed.

Mackee and Karp in 1952[1] and Ayres in 1960[10] obtained biopsies after phenol treatments. They both found a subepidermal band of "new collagen." Brown[13] acquired biopsies from the face of a single patient who had had a peel 15 years earlier. He commented that the primary change was subepidermal laminated "fibrosis." In 1962[14] Litton reported a marked widening of the "stratum papillare" three months after a peel. In 1970 Spira and colleagues,[15] studying the effects of various agents, noted dermal thickening and the deposition of new collagen without lamination. Baker and coworkers[16] took biopsies from patients who had been peeled 6 months to 13 years before they underwent face lifts. They concluded that the effects of peeling last many years and also reported a band in the dermis that stained deeply with elastic stains.

Stegman peeled or dermabraded 16 areas, each 1 cm diameter, on the neck of a 55-year-old man.[17] One-half of the areas were on sun-damaged skin and the other half were on protected skin. Some of the areas were occluded by tape for 24 hours and the others were left open. The effects of 50% TCA, full strength phenol, and Baker's formula phenol were compared by biopsies taken at 3, 30, 60, and 120 days post-peel. The results suggested that the depth of the wound was related to the strength of the agent used; for example, Baker's formula wounded deeper than full-strength phenol, which wounded deeper than 50% TCA. The effect of tape occlusion increased the depth of the wound for phenol and Baker's formula but made little difference with TCA. Elastosis did not seem to be a barrier to the agents, because sun-damaged and normal skin wounded the same. The depth of the wounds also correlated with the clinical signs of wounding and healing. The deeper wounds developed a thicker scar and were slower to lose edema and erythema.

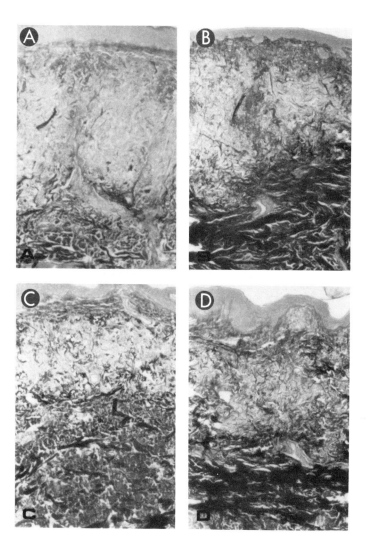

FIG 4–1.
Colloidal iron stains on sun-damaged skin. **A,** a normal control. **B–D,**
120 days after treatment with TCA, 100% phenol, and Baker's formula
mixture, respectively, and occluded for 24 hours.

Brody performed single vs. multiple applications of 35% TCA on the human cheek and compared the effects both clinically and histologically.[37] As expected, the wound was much more severe on the area of multiple application, taking nearly three times as long to heal. Under the microscope, the wound was much deeper into the reticular dermis. This work confirms Stegman's animal and human studies done on other anatomic areas, which show a relationship between dose and wound depth.

Brodland and Roenigk studied the effects of 20%, 35%, 50%, and 80% TCA on the back of a Yucatan hairless minipig.[36] The wounds increased in depth with increased concentration of the agent. The study also looked at the effects of occlusion and confirmed earlier findings that occlusion does not at all appear to affect the wound made by TCA. These studies help us understand why the former experienced clinicians used phenol and tape when they wanted a deeper peel, and used TCA for the lighter peels.

The histologic studies did reveal that the healed postpeel skin is significantly different from the nonpeeled skin in two aspects. The new or regenerated papillary dermis is thicker, with parallel, deeply-staining "new" collagen bundles (Figs 4–1 and 4–2). The thickness of the

Chemical Peels

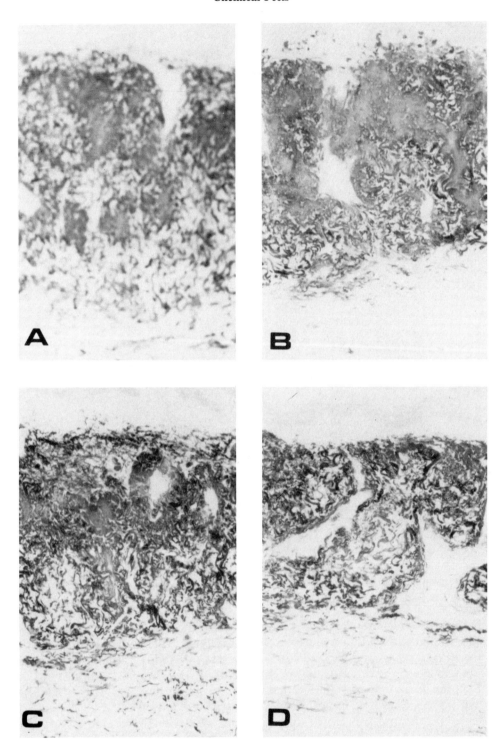

FIG 4–2.
Non-sun-damaged skin, stained with Verhoeff's elastic stain. **A,** a normal control. **B,** 60 days after treatment with 100% phenol left open. **C,** 60 days after treatment with 100% phenol occluded for 24 hours. **D,** 60 days after treatment with Baker's formula mixture occluded for 24 hours.

new papillary dermis is related to the strength of the agent used: the stronger agents produce a thicker new papillary dermis. For the deeper wounds, such as those from occluded Baker's formula, the new papillary dermis is thicker than matched, untreated, non-sun-damaged controls.

The second significant change noted is the development of a band in the dermis that stains heavily with elastic stains and has more dense, thick bundles that are in more closely parallel alignment than in the elastosis the band replaced. In medium-depth peels (full-strength phenol) the new band overlies the remaining elastosis. This band also develops de novo in non-sun-damaged skin.

Kligman, Baker, and Gordon published a study in 1985[18] which sampled the skin normally discarded during face-lifts from 11 patients who had undergone face peels 15 to 20 years earlier. These investigators noticed that a new, wide band of dermis 2 to 3 mm in width had formed beneath the epidermis, which was sharply demarcated from the underlying elastotic mass that represented the old, unpeeled dermis. This newly formed band consisted of thin, compact, parallel collagen bundles aligned horizontally to the surface. Numerous fine elastic fibers coursed through the band in a random fashion and were sometimes parallel, conforming to the collagen bundles. The ground substance within the band was considerably less than it was in nonpeeled skin. The epidermis was altered toward a more normal pattern, showing a basal layer of columnar cells and a return of polarity. The cells were more orderly, without the cytologic irregularities of unpeeled skin.

It is likely that the dermal band is what most investigators have seen and described in various ways, and is probably the same band that Baker and coworkers reported as present some 13 years postpeeling. The clinical significance of the dermal band is unknown.

Recent histologic studies matched to the clinical improvement from the use of Retin-A show that a regenerated and thickened papillary dermis smooths out fine wrinkling. This new and thicker papillary dermis is a hallmark of chemical peels and may be the most significant histologic change that accounts for the clinical improvement. The improvement in the "feel" of sun-damaged skin after a peel and application of Retin-A may be the result of a more ordered and normal epidermis.

In an unpublished report, Stegman biopsied several patients approximately 60 days after they had been treated with a full three-week course of 5% 5-fluorouracil. Although there were no pretreatment control biopsies, the papillary dermis showed "new" pink collagen and was thicker than would be expected. Clinically, post 5-FU patients have fewer wrinkles and smoother skin. Thus, there is more circumstantial evidence that the papillary dermis may play an important role in cosmesis. The antiwrinkling effect of 5-FU does not persist as long as it does with a medium or deep peel. The changes in the dermis and the formation of a thick papillary dermis may contribute to the long-lasting effects of a peel.

Toxicity

Studies in animals and man prove that phenolic compounds are quickly absorbed percutaneously.[19, 20] In animals, the absorbed phenol rapidly produced generalized stimulation of motor nerve endings or spinal motor centers with possible central depression. Animals also developed marked hemoglobinuria, possibly owing to widespread intravascular hemolysis. The severity of these effects is worsened by the dilution of phenol with water.

The highest concentrations of phenol did not necessarily produce the most serious toxicity. A combination of phenol and water 2:1 was the most toxic.[15] A similar dilution-to-effect relationship can be observed clinically. An aqueous mixture that has a final concentration of phenol of 50% produced a deeper wound than full-strength (88%) phenol.

The only serious toxic response to the medical use of phenol has been cardiac arrhythmias. Some arrhythmias have been life-threatening and are presumed to have caused several sudden deaths during peeling procedures. This relationship was first proven by Truppman and Ellenberg,[21] who demonstrated that rapidly applied phenolic mixtures will lead to seriously dangerous arrhythmias. These arrhythmias apparently were not related to the age of the patient, to the amount of anesthesia and thus to the perceived

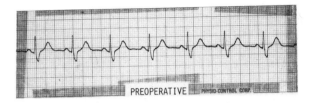

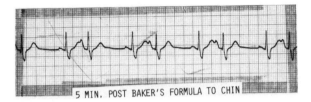

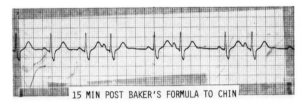

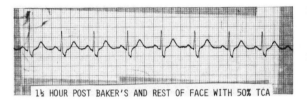

FIG 4–3.
Electrocardiogram tracing from 61-year-old woman preoperatively, 5 and 15 minutes after Baker's formula mixture was applied to the chin, showing an atrial bigeminy, and 1½ hours after Baker's formula mixture was applied to the chin, showing a return to the preoperative state.

pain, or to the clinical reasons for the application of the peel. The arrhythmias were related only to the speed with which the phenol was applied.

In 1984, Gross published the results of monitoring 154 patients during face and neck peels with phenolic mixtures.[22] His protocol was altered after the first 54 patients had been treated because an unacceptable incidence of arrhythmias occurred. The remaining 100 patients were treated in two stages one day apart, or with ten-minute intervals between segmental applications of the phenol. The types of arrhythmias noted by Gross included atrial fibrillation, sinus tachycardia, premature ventricular contractions (PVCs), and ventricular bigeminy. None of these findings was present when the mixture was applied more slowly. It is curious that Gross chose to alter the study by dividing it into a two-day procedure. That was how the dermatologists who originally did the procedure did it.

Since we have been monitoring patients any time we have used phenol for a full face peel, we have noticed PVCs at a more frequent rate than before peeling, and also some sinus tachycardia. These changes quickly stopped when we allowed a longer interval between applications. However, we had one case of a 61-year-old woman who developed an atrial bigeminy after the first application of Baker's formula only to the chin area (Fig 4–3). After treatment stopped, the rhythm returned to normal within one hour.

Stagnone, Orgel, and Stagnone compared the cardiac effects of Baker's formula with 50% TCA on the shaved abdomens of 15 rats.[23] Definite cardiac alterations were demonstrated in the phenol-treated rats; no alterations developed in the TCA-treated cases.

All of these studies have answered an absolutely critical question about the safety of using phenol for peeling. Most likely all of the cases of sudden death can be explained by the development of a serious cardiac arrhythmia. Not many other events cause death within three to five minutes except failure of the heart to pump, as happens when its rhythm is severely distorted. Past theories of drug idiosyncratic reaction, anesthesia death, or "splash reflex" reaction all pale when compared to published evidence that shows the relationship between the speed with which phenol is applied to the development of benign arrhythmias that progress to life-threatening dysrrhythmias.

Now, it is recommended that a full-face peel be divided into segments and spaced so the entire procedure requires a minimum of one hour; for the most part, this has eliminated the risk of sudden death during the procedure. Also, most physicians who use phenol recommend that the patient be monitored. If a change is noted in the patient's heart rhythm, the speed of application can be adjusted before any serious problems develop.

Another factor that affects the speed of penetration and thus the depth of the wound and the danger to the heart is the condition of the "barrier function" of the epidermis. The addition of epidermal irritants such as croton oil contributed to the initial success of modern formulae. Lately it has become routine to vigorously degrease the face prior to peeling. The rationale (unproven) is that a degreased face will lead to a "more even" peel and the adhesive tape will stick better. However, vigorous degreasing with acetone, soap, alcohol, or any combination of these also injures or destroys the epidermal barrier which allows more penetration of the peeling agent. We are aware of cases where the physician changed only the degreasing step of his routine and the patient subsequently developed a much deeper wound that progressed to scarring. Thus, more complete and rapid absorption of the agent can produce a deeper wound and if phenol is used, there is a greater risk of cardiac toxicity.

The barrier function of an actinically damaged epidermis is impaired, as has been shown many times in absorption studies. Consequently, patients with severe sun damage—the most common indication for a phenol peel anyway—will require more or stronger agents to penetrate the epidermis than will patients with minimal sun damage who might be peeled for other indications.

Patients who are pretreated with medicines that will correct the actinically damaged epidermis, such as Retin-A or the alphahydroxy acids, will absorb the agent better. This must be considered in order to dose the patient properly.

The nephrotoxicity or hepatotoxicity that has been ascribed to phenol has occurred in industrial accidents only, and not from the small, controlled doses of phenol used in the medical arena. Individuals who have suffered spills of phenolic solutions where the leg, the back, or other large area was saturated but absorption was slow enough not to cause cardiac problems have developed subsequent kidney or liver toxicity. These cases are not fully explained in the literature.[19, 20, 24]

Industrial decontamination studies of phenol and phenolic compounds have not been discussed widely in the medical literature, although they might be helpful to the physician who inadvertently applies more phenol than originally planned, or if there is an accidental spill on the patient, a member of the staff, or the physician. The best decontamination procedure is to flood the area with glycol or glycerol. The contaminated area should be swabbed and rubbed liberally with cotton swabs soaked in the glycerol or propylene glycol. In the case of an accidental spill, the patient should be taken to an appropriate medical facility where cardiac monitoring and life support can be carried out.[19, 20, 24]

There is some evidence that olive oil may diminish the penetration and thus reduce the injury and potential toxicity of phenol.

Although having agents such as propylene glycol, glycerol, or olive oil around the operatory when using phenolic preparations has not become routine medical practice, the literature for industrial safety and accident prevention supports these materials as the only ones that will decrease systemic toxicity and localized skin injury.

Indications

Actinic Damage

Chemical peels produce the most consistent and predictable results when used for treating the effects of the sun. Deep peels will attenuate some movement-related lines, but only for a short time. Deep peels will also tighten the skin a little so that some of the effects of gravity are partially corrected. This result is also temporary. However, correcting sun damage by rendering the histologic changes (discussed above under dynamics), replacing some or all of the elastosis, creating a new and thickened papillary dermis, and regenerating a new, normal epidermis seem to be permanent changes, unless the patient receives additional sun damage.

With dermabrasion, the color manifestations of actinic damage are often improved, but the results are less predictable. The sallow coloration is probably secondary to loss of the papillary dermis because coloration is corrected by all of those agents that affect it, such as Retin-A, 5-FU, and light peels. An irregular distribution of melanin, freckles, and lentigines is often corrected by peels of all depths, although the deeper peels more often reduce the total melanin with a resulting hypopigmentation.

The chemical removal of seborrheic keratoses and actinic keratoses is coincidental. Deeper peels will remove most of them and lighter peels will not. Those lesions should be treated separately, although treatment may be done in the same session as the peel.

Acne and Other Scars

Peeling is not the best way to treat most scarring, particularly the deep scars of acne. Superficial acne scars are improved by repeat peeling, and if the patient can benefit from peeling for other reasons, the scars will be lessened somewhat. A combination of procedures, such as using carbon dioxide sticks on the scars followed by regional or full-face peeling, is more successful than peeling alone.

Melasma and Lentigines

Many articles and book chapters on peels list melasma as an indication for peeling, and results are often impressive. We too have successfully treated pigmentary disorders with peels. But we have also had many failures and have seen several cases in which the peeling made the pigment darker. We have seen cases that ended up in the hands of lawyers, in which other physicians promised improvement for melasma by peeling, only to induce much deeper pigment in the skin.

Because melasma is a terrible problem for some patients, we think it is acceptable to try peeling to the lighten the skin color. However, the patient must be fully advised that the procedure is a trial and that results are unpredictable. When peeling for melasma, the test spot is highly unreliable, as it often is for any indication.

Sometimes, freckles, lentigines, and melasma will be unaffected by the peel, while all of the other skin that is treated will become hypopigmented. Then, the pigmented lesions are more noticeable than ever. The same problem in color differential can happen with treatment of intradermal nevi. The skin gets lighter and the moles stay the same color. The patient is therefore sure the procedure caused new moles

to appear. This is another reason to take good preoperative photographs.

To prevent darkening, we have tried a peel followed immediately by the use of bleaching agents. This works in some cases, and that apparently is the best guideline when peeling for color: It works *sometimes,* but we cannot predict *when* those sometimes will occur. And, peeling may make the pigment worse.

Freckles

Medium to deep peeling will often remove freckles, and is particularly effective for those redheaded, massively freckled individuals who tan poorly. The problem is not in the success of the peel that removes the freckles, but in the freckled areas that remain. Often patients are so happy to have a clear complexion that they then want the neck, anterior chest, shoulders, and back treated also. Peeling on areas other than the face is possible if done slowly and carefully, but the results are much less predictable and the incidences of pain and complications are much greater.

Technique

The technique for the Baker's formula peel is similar to that used for occluded full-strength phenol or 50% TCA. After the patient has been properly informed of the risks, alternatives, prognosis and procedure, in previous consultation(s) and before any analgesics are administered, the patient is brought to the operating room. Preoperative photographs are taken if they have not been taken already. Immediate postoperative care is reviewed, including making sure that the patient will be driven home and have someone present for the first 24 hours postoperatively. It is *very important* that the patient know how and where to reach the physician for the first postoperative day. We often give deep peel patients a home phone number or the number of where we are going to be. A major problem is if the postpeel patient comes under the care of another physician who does not perform or know about peeling. Invariably, the emergency room or family physician will conclude that the face is infected and permanently ruined. These untruths are conveyed to the patient, who becomes confused about loyalties and loses confidence in the cosmetic surgeon. That is when trouble starts.

Before surgery, we ask the patient to come to the office with the face freshly washed with soap and water and without makeup. If there is a hint of oiliness or residual makeup, we will rewash the patient's face. Contrary to the advice in the literature, we do not want the face so harshly washed that the epidermal barrier is broken, as discussed above.

Preoperative analgesia varies with the physician's preference, the depth of the peel to be applied, and the patient's preference and state of anxiety. Many patients are given only 75 to 100 mg of meperidine hydrochloride (Demerol) intramuscularly (IM) and 10 mg of prochlorperazine (Compazine) IM, which reduces the incidence of nausea, especially if a second dose of Demerol is needed. Diazepam (Valium) 10 mg given sublingually is also mild, without complications, and helpful to the patient, particularly when lighter peels are done.

Additional analgesia and twilight anesthesia are the standard for other physicians, and some patients will request it. If the physician has the equipment and is experienced in the use of office anesthesia and the regular use of heavy doses of analgesia, there is no reason not to meet the patient's request. However, having a second physician on hand to administer analgesics is extremely helpful to the surgeon.

Field block anesthesia for the entire face can be accomplished with a high rate of success. Lidocaine alone, or lidocaine with one of the longer-acting agents such as bupivacane (Marcain) creates a pain-free area for several hours. The pain from a deep face peel seems to last only four to six hours and stops abruptly. This is an almost universal event, and patients can be told with assurance that the postoperative pain will cease the evening of surgery. Because patients tolerate nighttime pain less well, we try to schedule face peels in the morning and advise patients that the pain will be gone before bedtime. We have had patients who had a successful face blocks tell us that they had no pain until the next day, when they experienced the usual discomfort from swelling, oozing, and crusting.

When using Baker's formula or full-strength phenol for a whole face, a cardiac monitor is strongly recommended. Early changes in cardiac rhythm can be recognized and the length between applications, the size of the segment treated, or the amount of the agent used can be adjusted. This will allow the procedure to progress to completion as scheduled and before cardiac problems become symptomatic. Usually early cardiac arrhythmias can be treated by waiting; severe cardiac irritability can be treated with intravenous (IV) lidocaine.

The patient should be in comfortable, loose-fitting clothes or a gown. For phenolic peels, an open IV is recommended.

For many physicians, part of the recipe for peeling is degreasing of the face. Some physicians use isopropyl alcohol, many use acetone, some even have patients wash the face *four* times before surgery—a sure way to produce chapped, irritated skin which is uncomfortable at least, and which possibly increases the risk of infection and greater absorption of toxins. We gently wipe off the face with acetone before moderate or deep peels. We are aware of a physician who vigorously cleansed a patient's face with acetone, followed with a 35% TCA peel, and the patient developed some hypertrophic scarring. This type of situation is rare but it illustrates the point that the degreasing step, if carried to the point of breaking down the epidermal barrier, must be considered to be one more way to affect the depth of the wound, just the same as if more escarotic agent or occlusion were added.

When using Baker's formula or full-strength phenol, the face must be peeled in segments so divided and spaced that the procedure requires a minimum of 45 minutes to one hour. The operative record should show the segments and times of applications (Fig 4–4). It does not matter how the physician proceeds. The procedure can begin at the chin or the forehead, but it is important to slightly overlap the areas so no skipped areas remain. If a skipped area is noticed during the first few follow-up days, peel the area then. If the facial skin is severely wrinkled and redundant, there is in fact a greater surface area to be peeled. Therefore, an entire cosmetic unit such as the cheek or chin should not be peeled at once. Instead, stretch out the wrinkles and

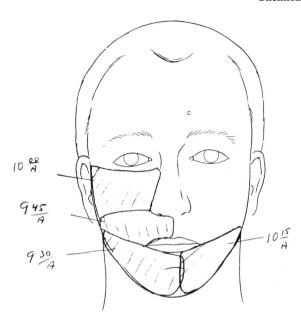

FIG 4–4.
Face peel notation in the patient's record indicating times at which various areas were treated.

divide the segment appropriately into smaller peeling units.

The Baker's formula is a combination of an epidermolytic (croton oil), a soap (Septisol) for emulsification, and the escarotic phenol at a final concentration of 50% to 55%. The mixture is not miscible and separates in the container. Consequently, it needs to be stirred well each time it is used. We make a fresh amount in a dish for each procedure. There is no reason the mixture cannot be made ahead of time, stored, and used from a dark glass bottle.

We use cotton-tipped applicators to apply the escarotic. One, two, or three applications can be held in the fingers to create a cotton "brush" with a one-, two-, or three-applicator width. Across the cheek or forehead, sweep on the mixture with broad strokes. Near the mouth or nose, or on the eyelids, use one or two applicators to work around the furrows and folds. For deep, narrow creases, often found around the mouth, using the wooden end of the stick is a good way to administer a higher dose of the peeling agent to the base of these creases.

It is important to wound the skin evenly all over the face. The salutary result of a peel is secondary to the wound induced. Therefore,

stretch out the wrinkles and furrows and peel all of the skin—in the trough as well as on the crest of each fold. If the redundant skin is not stretched out, the result may be uneven or stripped.

For the application of the escarotic, we dip the applicators into the mixture and stir it very well. Then the applicator tips are pressed dry against the side of the dish (Fig 4–5), aligned abreast, and rubbed over the patient's face with smooth, regular strokes. When the stronger agents such as Baker's formula or full-strength phenol are used, frosting occurs within seconds (Fig 4–6). Although we do not know what the frosting represents in the tissue physiology, it does seem to be related to the depth of the peel. Stronger agents frost a deeper white more quickly, weaker agents frost slowly and faintly. With stronger agents, the frost is a guide to how complete and how evenly the agent has been applied. With the very weak agents, the frost is too slow in appearing and too faint to be a helpful guide for application.

Application of the escarotic varies greatly among physicians and reflects experience. Less experienced physicians should use only one or two applicators and proceed slowly. Experienced peelers can use additional moist appli-

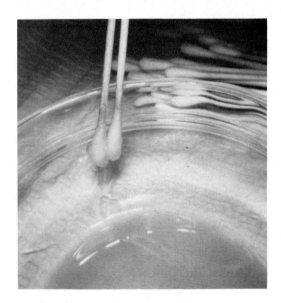

FIG 4–5.
Cotton-tipped applicators are used to stir the peel mixture and then are pressed dry against the side of the dish.

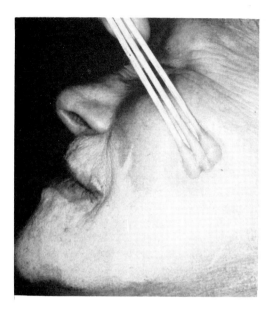

FIG 4–6.
Two or three cotton-tipped applicators are used together to sweep over a broad area of the cheek.

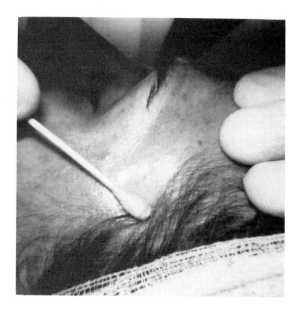

FIG 4–8.
The agent is carried into the hairline.

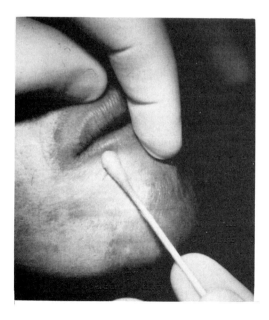

FIG 4–7.
The agent is taken to the vermilion and onto the lip if necessary.

cators and move faster, while remaining cognizant of the dose applied during any one setting. It is difficult to recommend how many applicators should be used for one procedure because the wetness of the applicator tip determines how much agent is applied. We limit our dose to three to five applicators wrung out well for every 15 minutes.

The agent should be taken to and beyond the vermilion border (Fig 4–7). Trying to peel just to the vermilion border does not adequately wound the lip wrinkles and may leave an untreated line around the lip. The lips themselves can be treated. Many of the rhitids of the perioral region extend right onto the lip and will respond to peeling in the same way as the rest of the skin. In women, it is in these radiating creases that lipstick runs, creating red streaks.

The peel must also be carried into the hairline and through the eyebrows (Figs 4–8 and 4–9). Hair is not lost, and even if it were, it would only be a telogen effluvium and would regrow. All edges of the peel should be feathered to lighten the peel or reduce the dose at the margins of the face, or around the eyes or nose (Fig

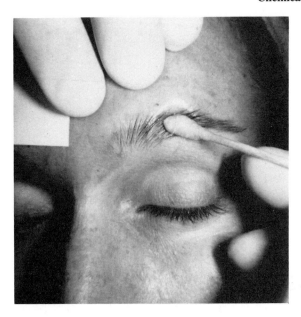

FIG 4–9.
The agent is carried through the eyebrows.

4–10). The peel should be carried irregularly into the unpeeled areas so as not to create a sharp demarcation line. The tragus and ear lobe should also be peeled because both are often wrinkled like the face. Failure to peel these areas only draws attention to them. Also, special attention should be given to the jawline. It is necessary to peel just under the jawline so the cutoff line will be hidden in the submandibular shadow. Observe and mark this line before the procedure starts, with the patient seated. Often, when the patient reclines, that line shifts posteriorly. Also, with the deeper peels there is some tightening of the skin, which tends to pull the jawline skin superiorly. Both actions place the final jawline higher and if not anticipated, will expose the transition line.

Because eyelids are so sensitive, we peel them last. Patients who have tolerated the rest of the procedure well may find peeling of the eyelids almost intolerable. There are different opinions about how strong an agent should be used on the eyelids because the skin is thin, and because when the eyes are open the upper lid folds on itself, creating a natural occlusion. There have been cases of full thickness slough from eyelid peeling although the same agent did not cause problems on the rest of the face. We rou-

tinely use full-strength phenol without occlusion for upper and lower eyelids. However, we know that other experienced physicians will not use anything stronger than 30% TCA. Remember to examine in detail the skin of the infrabrow. Some patients have a lot of noneyelid skin under the brow, which should be peeled with the same agent used on the rest of the face. Others have only thin eyelid skin below the brow and thus a weaker agent is called for.

The technique for peeling the eyelids is for the physician to stand at the head of the table and lean over the patient so that the physician and patient are face to face. Ask the patient to follow your eyes. A single cotton-tipped applicator is applied to the lower lids while the patient looks at the your face. We tell patients they can blink all they want, but when they open their eyes they should look directly at the physician's face. An assistant should stand ready to blot any tears that may escape. It takes only a few seconds to peel the lower lid up to 1 mm of the ciliary margin. The other lower lid and the upper lids are peeled sequentially, with about five minutes between each peel.

We believe the use of eyedrops or ointments to protect the eye from any possible spills is

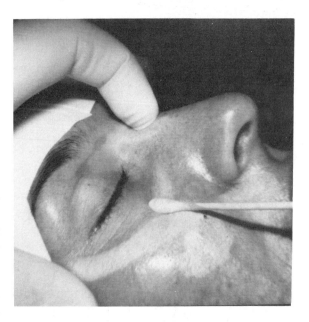

FIG 4–10.
The agent is feathered at all peripheries of the peeled areas.

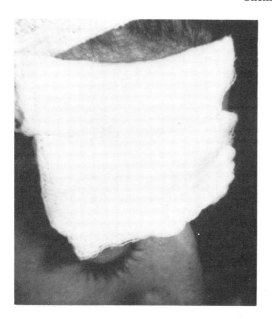

FIG 4–11.
Cool gauze compresses are immediately placed over the treated area to give the patient relief from the burning.

unnecessary. First of all, the applicator is nearly dry and will not drip. Likewise, the peeling agent should be on a nearby stand, *never in the physician's hand.* The most common problem from peeling around the eyes is when tears run onto the surrounding skin. The tears dilute the peeling agent and leave streaks of less peeled or unpeeled skin streaming from the lateral canthi. Another problem is that the patient may squint. The skin at the lateral canthus rolls up into a tube which acts like a capillary tube and may pull the agent into the eye. When peeling around the canthus, we carefully hold the eye open.

If the agent does get into the eye, it stings but is immediately diluted to ineffectiveness. Nevertheless, flood the eye with water and assure the patient that the stinging will soon stop and that the tears protected the eyes from any damage.

Since the earliest writings on peels, "neutralizing" the escarotic with water or alcohol has been discussed. There is no chemical reaction between TCA, phenol, alcohol, and water because they are aqueous solutions to begin with. There can only be dilution, which in the case of full-strength phenol may actually make the agent more potent. Some physicians recommend care-

fully timing how long the agent is left on before it is neutralized with water to stop the reaction. We have seen this advice in the literature but have never seen any explanation of how water can "neutralize" an aqueous solution.

Immediately after each segment is peeled we apply gauze squares soaked in the cold water, but that is to cool the exothermic reaction—the burning—the patient feels (Fig 4–11). The burning lasts for 15 to 20 seconds. The compresses are comforting, and the continued attention reassures the patient. A fan close by directed toward the patient also helps during the burning phase (Fig 4–12).

The peeled skin begins to burn approximately 20 to 40 minutes later. Patients describe it as severe burning or heat, or just plain pain. Although most patients are fairly comfortable during the procedure, analgesics are needed for this postsurgical pain which lasts six to eight hours and stops abruptly.

Whether or not to peel the neck is a complex question. The first consideration is determining where to stop. The jawline is a natural, shadowed line, but the collar line, the low-cut dress line, or the bra line are not anatomically distinct. A transition line anywhere but the jawline is quite visible. Second, the neck skin is very different from that of the face: it heals more slowly, is much more sore, does not show the clinical improvement, and pigments irregularly. Peeling the neck also has a higher incidence of complications of laryngeal edema. Therefore, we are seldom persuaded to peel necks.

Occlusion is the next step. Whether or not to occlude and how are related to how deep a peel is needed to correct the patient's actinic damage. Some physicians (usually those who have an anesthesiologist present) apply more peeling agent, some occlude with ointments, some break down the epidermal barrier prior to peeling and thus wound deeper with the same agents, and some choose to occlude the skin with tape. All methods are effective.

Tape occlusion is probably the oldest method and most often used. As soon as a segment is peeled or after the whole face is peeled, tape is applied until the whole face or whole area needing a deeper wound is covered. Again, it does not matter where the procedure starts—the fo-

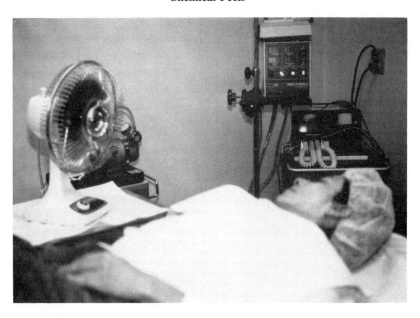

FIG 4–12.
A fan nearby helps cool the burning feeling.

rehead or chin (Fig 4–13). In addition, we are not sure if it makes any difference what kind of tape is used, as long as it is occlusive. It is important to lay the first layers of tape down evenly, with no wrinkles or creases. The tape can be one or one-half inches wide. The mask is built with whatever length strips are necessary. We apply the tape in a scissorslike or sawtooth fashion so that an irregular line is created at the mandibular margin (Fig 4–14). As is well known in cosmetic work, an irregular line is less easily noticed, and thus there is not the sharp contrast between the occluded and unoccluded skin along the mandibular margin. We also use the sawtooth tape pattern at the junction of the cheek and the lower eyelids when the entire face is not occluded. Although some physicians are dogmatic about how the mask is constructed, we have never seen any evidence that the number of layers or the sizes of tapes that are used make any difference.

The entire face—the entire peeled area—does not need to be occluded. Some patients have much more actinic damage on the lower half of the face than on the upper half. Because a heavier peel is required for the lower half, it is taped and the upper area is left open. During the first weeks of healing there is a noticeable differential between the areas that soon evens out.

Some physicians are equally dogmatic about how long the mask should be left in place. The earlier literature recommends 48 hours, but we usually leave it on only overnight. Unpublished animal studies by Stegman showed no difference in the depths of the wounds in the 24-hour vs. the 48-hour occluded peels. Patients are uncomfortable with the mask in place, and most are anxious to take it off. The mask is painful to remove, but no more so than removing tape from a nonpeeled area. The most pain is caused by pulling out the small lanugo hairs. Although the sight of the swelling and oozing makes the patient think that removing the tape will be extremely painful, the peeled skin is actually somewhat numbed and it may only be the pulling on the hairs that causes the pain. We used to give patients Demerol and/or Valium before we removed the tape. We have stopped giving any medications, however, because it takes only 30 seconds to get the mask off and removal does not hurt that much. In fact, the mask is often loosened by the ooze. We ask well-motivated and intelligent patients to take the mask off themselves in the shower the next morning. They

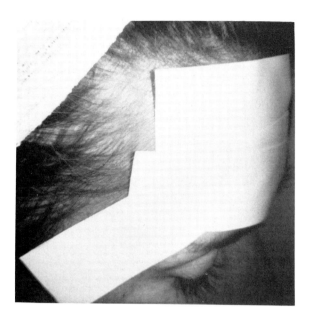

FIG 4–13.
Tape is used to occlude the peel for 24 hours.

up they become. We have seen some patients who were loath to touch their faces and allowed thick crusts to build up. The final result seemed to be the same, but if the wound is kept nearly

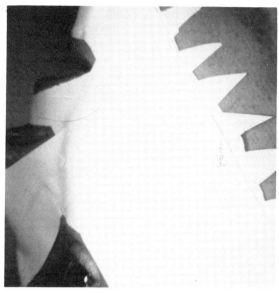

FIG 4–14.
The tape mask is scalloped at the margins to decrease the sharpness of the line between the treated and nontreated areas.

can call us and report that everything is all right and save themselves a trip to the office when they look terrible and feel worse.

After removing the tape, the skin is grayish and edematous, with some areas of desquamation of the damaged epidermis (Fig 4–15). The entire face is massively edematous, with lips protruding and sometimes everting; the eyelids are swollen shut; and there is a generalized serous ooze. To minimize anxiety, this frightening appearance must be explained to the patient and the patient's family prior to the peel. However, regardless of how much preoperative explanation has been provided, most people are not prepared to seem themselves in this condition. At this critical time it is especially important that the patient be able to contact the physician who did the procedure.

Formerly, postoperative care was to induce a thick crust over the peeled areas with thymol iodide or other powders. We prefer to follow the recommendation of McCullogh, who advised his patients to go to the shower the next day and wash the face with soap and water.[25] Washing is followed by application of an antibiotic ointment which a few days later is exchanged for an antibiotic anti-inflammatory cream. The softer the crusts are kept, the less irritating and heaped-

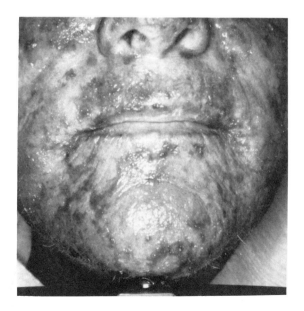

FIG 4–15.
Immediately after the tape has been removed at 24 hours.

crust-free, there is less chance of infection.

Over the next few days scabs form, which fall off in seven to ten days. In rare cases, they will take two weeks to come off. Some pre-existing conditions will lead to slower healing. Previous irradiation, for instance, causes much slower healing[26] and prolonged use of corticosteroids can also delay healing. Pretreatment with trenitoin has been mentioned as speeding healing after dermabrasion and peeling.[35] The end point for comparison and the criteria to judge what is "better" are lacking in these trenitoin studies. The clinical impressions of the investigators are probably valid, but we believe that more investigation needs to be done before we can recommend its use.

As soon as the scabs are off, makeup can be applied over the skin. This can be ordinary over-the-counter makeup which is washed off each day or it can be professionally compounded and applied to help blend out the erythema and the margins between the peeled and unpeeled areas (see Chapter 15).

Complete healing takes nearly six months, but the patient usually looks acceptable enough to go out with light makeup after one month (Figs 4–16, A to C). Advice on the use of sunscreens is appropriate, although most patients who have had a deep peel plan to stay out of the sunlight which was the cause of their need for such a major procedure in the first place.

Light or Freshening Peels

For ease of presentation, we have divided the various peels into light or freshening, medium, and deep. The divisions are arbitrary because with different techniques, combinations of agents, and skin preparations, any wound depth is achievable. In the sections on light- and medium-depth peels, we will not present the technique as completely, but rather point out how these differ from the deep technique.

Light peels include Jessner's or Coombs formulae (which are very similar), TCA 20% to 35%, and most of the peels used by lay peelers and beauticians; these peels are combinations of plant enzymes, salicylic acid, resorcinol, etc. The Coombs or Jessner formula is:

Resorcinol	14.0%
Salicylic acid	14.0%
Lactic acid (85%)	14.0%
Ethanol 95% a.s. a.d.	100.0%

We use these agents to treat mild sun damage, light crosshatch wrinkling, and muddy, irregular pigmentations often found at the end of a long summer of sun exposure. It is likely that regular use of trenitoin decreases the frequency that light peels are needed. There will always be individuals who want results more quickly than can be achieved by creams, and they will request a light peel. Repeated every four to six months, light peels reduce the visibility of acne scars, and also because of low-grade interstitial swelling, make pores look smaller.[27, 28]

The wound depth is not below the papillary dermis. The very light agents such as Coombs only injure the epidermis, but the 35% TCA can wound as deeply as through the papillary dermis. Occlusion with tape is almost never used because using a stronger agent is much easier and more comfortable for the patient if a deeper wound is desired. Many physicians apply ointments immediately after peels to provide some occlusion and deepen the wound.

The light peel technique is similar to the deep peels discussed above, but it is quicker and less painful, and the healing time is shorter. Most patients do not require analgesia unless TCA 35% is used, and then very mild agents are satisfactory. The face is prepared with washing and degreasing. With the agents for light peels, there is no cardiac toxicity, and therefore they can be applied over the whole face in one sitting. The only limiting factor is patient discomfort. The agents sting in direct proportion to their strength. Coombs's formula hardly hurts at all, but 35% TCA stings briskly. Usually the lighter agents are applied two or three times with five-minute intervals between each, until a light frost is observed. Higher concentrations of TCA are applied once and occasionally twice to obtain complete coverage. TCA 35% will frost within a minute or two. If the stratum corneum is too thick to obtain a light frost, a stronger agent can be used immediately. Also, for thick keratotic lesions such as actinic and seborrheic keratoses,

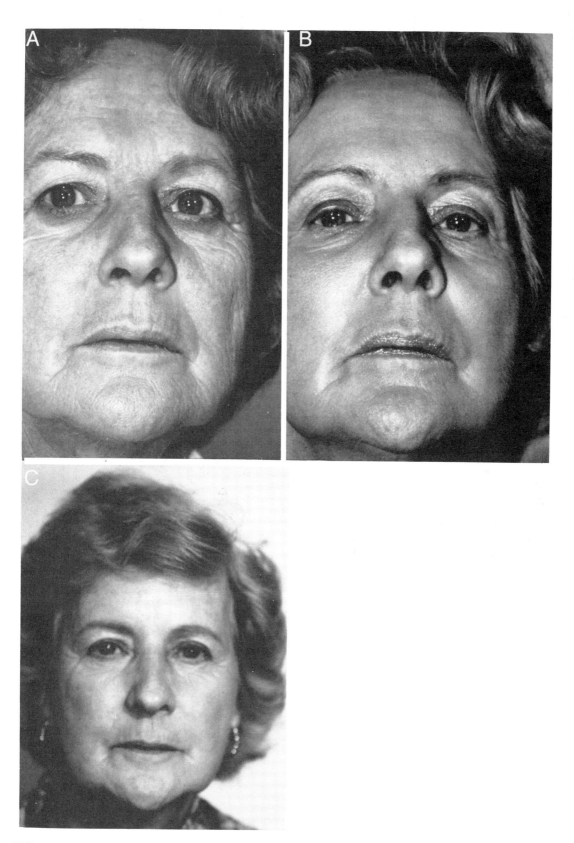

FIG 4–16.
A 55-year-old woman undergoing a Baker's formula mixture face peel which was occluded 24 hours. **A**, prior to peel. **B**, 4 weeks postpeel. **C**, 5 years postpeel.

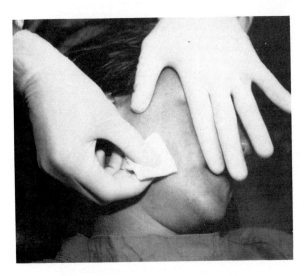

FIG 4–17.
The use of a folded gauze to apply nonphenolic escarotics.

the horn can be scraped off with the wooden end of the applicator or a curette and the area peeled in the same way as the rest of the face.

The application technique using one, two, or three cotton-tipped applicators is fine for light peels, although many physicians use folded gauze squares or cotton balls since they can be applied without worry of too-rapid absorption (Fig 4–17). During the first 30 to 60 seconds the skin burns, so cool compresses or having the fan close by is helpful.

Follow-up care is similar to that for a deep peel only neither as involved nor as long. The pain is less and lasts a shorter time. The crusts are thinner and come off quicker. The complications (discussed below) are fewer, and if present, less troublesome. Transient hyperpigmentation seems more common with the 35% TCA peels, but is almost always present for only three months and fades spontaneously. It can be treated with bleaching agents which may or may not speed its resolution. Hypopigmentation is rare with light peels, as are most complications—they are rare but not unheard of.

Unlike a deep peel, light peels, especially the Coombs's type, can be repeated many times without apparent permanent damage. The wound is superficial and seems to heal completely. We have heard at meetings and read in the literature that repeated peels "thin the skin."

We do not know what "thin the skin" means and have never seen these comments backed up with any scientific proof.

Medium-Depth Peels

Full-strength phenol without occlusion and TCA 40% to 50% are the agents we use for a wound that extends to the mid-reticular dermis. There are physicians who do not want to take the risks associated with the use of phenol; we believe, however, that with cardiac monitoring those risks are well controlled. If the patient's cardiac status prevents the use of phenol, the best substitute is a 50% TCA peel with or without occlusion. For reasons we do not fully understand, concentrations of TCA higher than 50% have an unacceptably high risk of scarring. Also, the results of 50% TCA are seldom as good as with the phenolic mixtures. We have seen good results with TCA but they do not occur as consistently as with phenol for *deep* actinic wrinkles. For a medium-depth peel, we prefer full-strength phenol unoccluded. This is also the peel of choice following a face-lift.

The indications for medium-depth peels are the same as for deep peels, with the choice of agent based on the degree of sun damage. Patients with moderate sun damage or those who are not ready to undertake the long healing of a Baker's peel are treated with medium-depth peels (Figs 4–18, A and B). This level of peel is also used when an attempt is made to lighten hyperpigmentation with a series of peels.

The technique is exactly the same as for the deep peels: there are needs for analgesia, monitoring if phenol is used, staged application, assistance for the patient for the burning, and close follow-up. Medium-depth peels result in 30 days of erythema, and have the same potential complications as deep peels, only they occur less often.

Combinations

Depending on the surgeon's experience, many peels will be performed with a combination of techniques. The most common is to vary the amount of the escarotic agent applied—a heavier application where a deep wound is needed, and a lighter one elsewhere. The wound depth can also be controlled by using different agents, such as 50% TCA on the perioral region and 35% TCA on the cheeks, and by occluding some areas and not others (Figs 4–19 A–D). Other modalities can be combined with peeling. Brody and Hailey popularized the use of carbon dioxide sticks that were dipped in acetone and then rubbed onto areas that needed deeper wounds, such as deep acne scars, followed by a whole-face 35% or 50% TCA peel.[29] Dermabrasion is often used for discrete, radiating perioral creases, and for a peel over the rest of the face.

Complications

The incidence of complications from peeling is fairly high, although most are correctable with time or medication. Nevertheless, it is important to prepare patients for the possibility of complications.

The most common complication is color change. With the deeper phenol peels, hypopigmentation—often not manifest until three to six months postpeel—can be expected, and should be considered a side effect rather than a complication. We have also seen hyperpigmentation—over the entire area but more commonly splotchy—develop at six weeks and be quite resistant to bleaching (Fig 4–20). Clearly, sun exposure increases the risk of hyperpigmentation and careful patient instruction on sun damage prevention is essential.

The line of demarcation between peeled and unpeeled areas becomes more of a problem for the patient whose natural color is darker. Hypopigmentation on the fair-skinned patient is difficult to appreciate, but on olive or brown skin it stands out sharply and is difficult to hide with makeup. That is why we emphasized above the scalloped margins on the taping, the careful preoperative examination of where the jawline would lie, and the feathering of the peel at all margins.

Erythema, sometimes accompanied with itching and burning, can be expected during the first few weeks. That kind of c-fiber itching or burning is helped by aspirin. In the occasional patient, however, the erythema persists for months. It is particularly disturbing because the normal blush response becomes accentuated. Not only are blushes red, but they also become bright red whenever the patient gets warm, embarrassed, or angry. Although this complication always goes away spontaneously, sometimes it can last for six months. Propanolol in low dose will help some of these patients.

Infections can arise, as would be expected

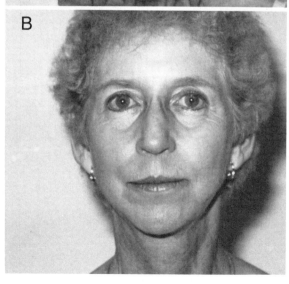

FIG 4–18.
A 53-year-old woman with moderate sun damage undergoing a 100% unoccluded peel. **A,** preoperatively. **B,** 8 weeks postoperatively with light makeup.

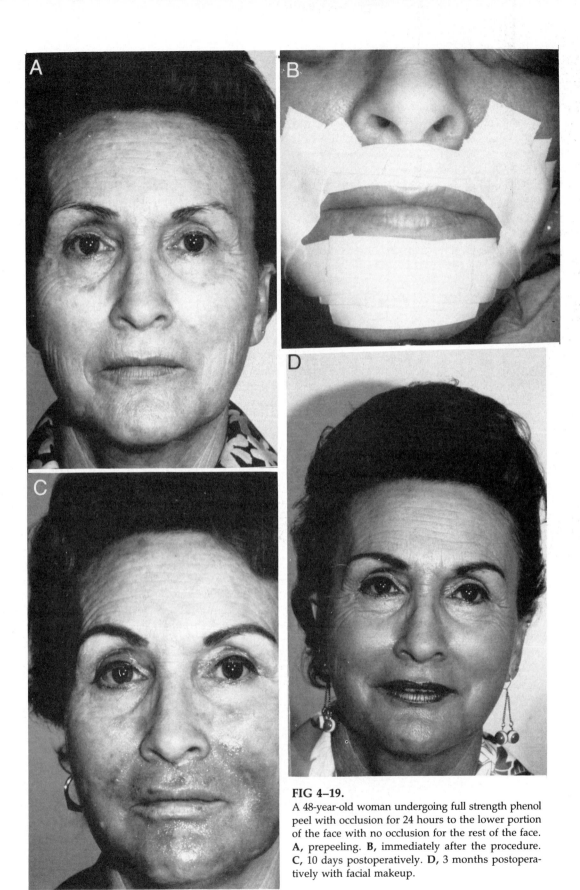

FIG 4–19.
A 48-year-old woman undergoing full strength phenol peel with occlusion for 24 hours to the lower portion of the face with no occlusion for the rest of the face. **A,** prepeeling. **B,** immediately after the procedure. **C,** 10 days postoperatively. **D,** 3 months postoperatively with facial makeup.

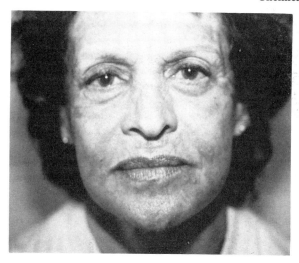

FIG 4–20.
Six weeks after Baker's formula peel, this 48-year-old woman developed marked, blotchy hyperpigmentation that was very resistant to bleaching.

topically and systemically, and it is also important to soak off any remaining scabs which provide a perfect culture medium. Often the patient who gets infected was not following instructions to wash with soap and water followed by antibiotic ointments twice a day. There has been one reported case of toxic shock syndrome after a Baker's formula peel.[30]

Herpes simplex 1 infections were much more of a problem in past years[31] (Fig 4–22). Now these infections can be treated prophylactically if the patient has a history of herpes labialis, or actively, if the patient develops herpetic lesions, with oral acyclovir. Even before acyclovir was in widespread use, the lesions responded well to supportive care and healed without scarring.

Laryngeal edema has been reported following Baker's formula peel in 3 of 245 cases.[32] The symptoms were stridor, hoarseness, and tachypnea, which developed within 24 hours after the peel. The patients who developed this complication were heavy smokers; otherwise, the cause remains unknown. These patients responded to inhalation therapy with heated aerosol mist.

Scarring, fortunately, is infrequent. It is tragic when someone comes in seeking an improved appearance and leaves with a scar. The most

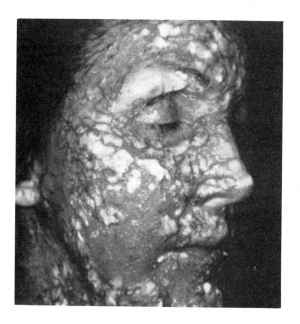

FIG 4–21.
A 44-year-old woman, 6 days after Baker's formula peel, who did not apply antibiotic ointment. The soft crusts all over the face are a combination of eschar, moisturizer, and *Pseudomonas aeruginosa* infection.

with the extensive wounds of peeling. Bacterial infections can come on early or late and are caused by the usual *Staphylococcus aureus* or *Pseudomonas* (Fig 4–21). They respond to antibiotics

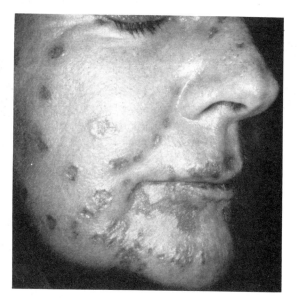

FIG 4–22.
A 53-year-old woman with herpes simplex 1 lesions 9 days after Baker's formula peel.

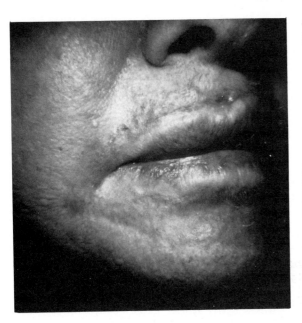

FIG 4–23.
Three years after a peel of unknown nature performed in Mexico. The scars are resistant to intralesional steroids.

common areas of scarring are the upper lip and the angle of the jaw (Fig 4–23). Although there are many theories about why these areas scar, it is probably because the skin is thinner and the physician is trying to wound deeper to remove creases.

We treat scars with time, support, and intralesional triamcinolone acetonide 5 to 20 mg/ml every three weeks. If, when we see patients three weeks postoperatively, we detect areas of slow healing, or areas still scabbed, we will start them on strong topical steroids twice daily. Often this will prevent true scarring. If not, we switch to intralesional steroids at the first sign of true scar development. Early prevention and treatment greatly shorten the time it takes for the scar to mature and nearly dissolve. Most of the time, these scars will almost completely resorb. For these early scars, triamcinolone acetonide 40 mg/ml is too strong and may cause atrophy, or will deposit out as small, milialike droplets.

Other complications that are uncommon include texture change, which is a grainy, porous effect. Some patients who have had more than one deep peel may develop atrophic changes. Telangiectasia sometimes occur after medium or

deep peels, and one physician reported hirsutism in the peeled areas.[33]

Conclusion

After reading this chapter, it would be understandable for physicians who do not do peels

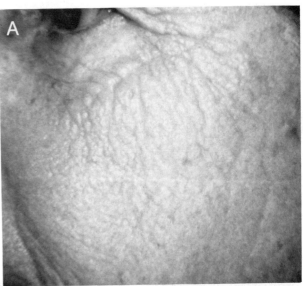

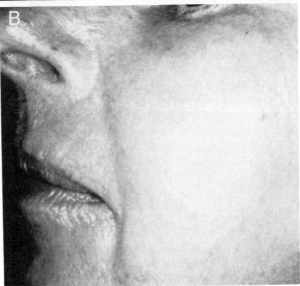

FIG 4–24.
A 45-year-old woman with severe, premature sun-damaged skin who underwent a Baker's formula peel occluded for 24 hours. **A,** preoperatively. **B,** 3 months postoperatively.

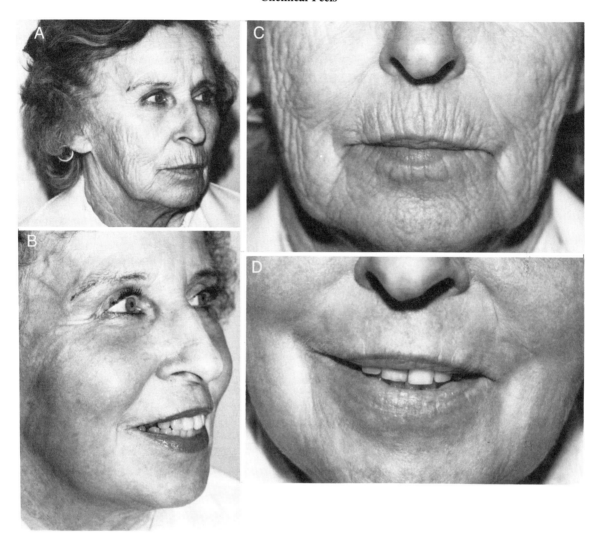

FIG 4–25.
A 67-year-old woman undergoing a Baker's formula peel. **A,** prepeel. **B,** 60 days postpeel. **C,** prepeel close-up, perioral. **D,** 60 days postpeel, close-up, perioral.

to decide they are not worth the effort. However, the primary motivation for performing peels is that they work. They correct prematurely aged skin. They transform patients with dull, crepey skin into individuals who look radiant (Fig 4–24). This is one of the most rewarding of all cosmetic procedures, but also one that requires a great deal of patient support (Fig 4–25).

References

1. Mackee GM, Karp FL: The treatment of post-acne scars with phenol. *Br J Dermatol* 1952; 64:456–459.
2. Winter L: Method of permanent removal of freckles. *Br J Dermatol Syphilil* 1950; 62:83–85.
3. Baker TJ, Gordon HL: The ablation of rhytides by chemical means: A preliminary report. *J Fla Med Assoc* 1961; 48:451.
4. Baker TJ: Chemical face peeling and rhytidectomy. *Plast Reconstr Surg* 1962; 29:199.
5. Baker TJ, Gordon HL: Chemosurgery of the face: Some warnings and misconceptions. *J Fla Med Assoc* 1962; 49:218.
6. Baker TJ, Gordon HL: Chemical face peeling: An adjunct to surgical face lifting. *South Med J* 1963; 56:412.
7. Baker TJ, Gordon HL, Seckinger DL: A second look at chemical face peeling. *Plast Reconstr Surg* 1966; 37:487.
8. Brown AM, Kaplan LM, Brown ME: Phenol induced histologic skin changes: Hazards, techniques, and uses. *Br J Plast Surg* 1960; 13:158.
9. Sperber PA: Chemexfoliation in treatment of acne scarring. *Texas State J Med* 1963; 59:496.
10. Ayers S III: Dermal changes following application of chemical cauterants to aging skin. *Arch Dermatol* 1960; 82:578.
11. Aronsohn RB: Facial chemosurgery. *Eye, Ear, Nose, Throat* 1971; 50:128.
12. Townshend R: Skin peeling: A master's tool in skin care. *Aesthetic's World* 1984; 12:16–22.
13. Brown AM, Kaplan LM, Brown ME: Cutaneous alterations induced by phenol. A histologic bioassay. *J Int Coll Surg* 1960; 34:602.
14. Litton C: Chemical face lifting. *Plast Reconstr Surg* 1962; 29:371.
15. Spira M, Dahl C, Freeman R, et al: Chemosurgery: A histologic study. *Plast Reconstr Surg* 1970; 45:247.
16. Baker TJ, Gordon HL, Mosienko P, et al: Long-term histological study of skin after chemical face peeling. *Plast Reconstr Surg* 1974; 53:522.
17. Stegman SJ: A comparative histologic study of the effects of three peeling agents and dermabrasion on normal and sun-damaged skin. *Aesthet Plast Surg* 1982; 6:123.
18. Kligman AM, Baker TJ, Gordon HL: Long-term histologic follow-up of phenol face peels. *Plast Reconstr Surg* 1985; 75:652–659.
19. Harkness RA, Beveridge GW, Davidson DW: Percutaneous absorption of l-naphthol-(^{14}C) in man. *Br J Dermatol* 1971; 85:49.
20. Conning DM, Hayes MJ: The dermal toxicity of phenol: An investigation of the most effective first-aid measures. *Br J Ind Med* 1970; 27:155–159.
21. Truppman ES, Ellenberg JD: Major electrocardiographic changes during chemical face peeling. *Plast Reconstr Surg* 1979; 63:44.
22. Gross BG: Cardiac arrhythmias during phenol face peeling. *Plast Reconstr Surg* 1984; 73:590–594.
23. Stagnone GJ, Orgel MG, Stagnone JJ: Cardiovascular effects of topical 50% trichloroacetic acid and Baker's phenol solution. *J Dermatol Surg Oncol* 1987; 13:999–1002.
24. Brown VKH, Box VL, Simpson BJ: Decontamination procedures for skin exposed to phenolic substances. *Arch Environ Health* 1975; 30:1–6.
25. McCollough EG, Langsdon PR: Chemical peeling with phenol, in Roenigk RK, Roenigk HH (eds): *Dermatologic Surgery, Principles and Practice*. New York, Marcel Dekker, 1988.
26. Wolf SA: Chemical face peeling following therapeutic irradiation. *Plast Reconstr Surg* 1982; 69:859–862.
27. Resnik SS, Lewis LA, Cohen BH: Trichloroacetic acid peeling. *Cutis* 1976; 17:127–129.
28. Resnik SS, Lewis LA: The cosmetic uses of trichloroacetic acid peeling in dermatology. *South Med J* 1973; 66:225.
29. Brody HJ, Hailey CW: Medium-depth chemical peeling of the skin: A variation of superficial chemosurgery. *J Dermatol Surg Oncol* 1986; 12:1268–1275.
30. Dmytryshyn JR, Gribble MJ, Kassen BO: Chemical face peel complicated by toxic shock syndrome. *Arch Otolaryngol* 1983; 109:170–171.
31. Rapaport MJ, Kamer F: Exacerbation of facial herpes simplex after phenolic face peels. *J Dermatol Surg Oncol* 1984; 10:57–58.
32. Klein DR, Little JH: Laryngeal edema as a complication of chemical peel. *Plast Reconstr Surg* 1983; 71:419–420.
33. Kotler R: Personal communication (letter). April 19, 1988.
34. Obaji Z: Personal communication. July 1987.
35. Mandy SH: Tretinoin in preoperative and postoperative management of dermabrasion. *J Am Acad Dermatol* 1986; 15:878–879.
36. Brodland D, Roenigk RK: Depth of chemoexfoliation induced by various concentrations and application techniques of TCA in a porcine model. *J Dermatol Surg Oncol* (in press).
37. Brody HJ: *J Dermatol Surg Oncol* (in press).

Five

Dermabrasion

History

Dermabrasion is a dermatologist's technique. It was initially performed by dermatologists, who were the first to publish studies of the technique. And the first instruments specifically designed for dermabrasion were made for dermatologists. As early as 1905, Kromayer published the results of his experiments with burrs attached to dental equipment to reduce scarring.[1] He wrote a book published in 1929 about a "leveling procedure" for smallpox scars.[2] (Curiously, we now believe dermabrasion is not helpful for most smallpox scars.) He and a nephew, Ernest Kromayer, Jr., contributed the concept of freezing to make the skin rigid, and the concept that injury above a certain depth does not heal with a scar. These studies were published in 1933.[3, 4]

Cryotherapy with carbon dioxide slush was reported by Karp, Nieman, and Lerner in 1927,[5] and in 1935 the first articles on wire brush planing for tattoos were published by Janson.[6] Scarification plus the application of trichloroacetic acid or phenol for treatment of acne pits was published in 1940 by Cannon.[7] In 1947, Iverson rolled 0 and 00 sandpaper around roller gauze and abraded tattoos, and McEvitt applied the technique to acne pits in 1948.[8, 9] The procedure was limited by hemorrhage during the procedure and the development of silica granulomas later.

It was against this background that Abner Kurtin, a New York dermatologist, developed a procedure for treating acne scars which is not greatly changed today. Kurtin met an instrument maker, Noel Robbins, who was able to make wire brushes that could be sterilized and had sharp tips of adequate strength to withstand the centrifugal forces on the end of a high-speed motor.[10] (Noel Robbins is today still an instrument maker, and owner and president of Robbins Instrument Company, Catham, New Jersey. Throughout his long career he has designed pi-oneering instruments for many physicians, including the Orentreich punch and liposuction cannulae.) Kurtin also added a blower to blast air over the patient's face while the ethyl chloride was sprayed on; this provided the rigid, bloodless field necessary for wire-brush dermabrasion. In 1953, he published a report on his first 273 cases.[11]

Older dermatologists remember hearing about the Friday afternoons around Dr. Kurtin's operating table when he would perform several dermabrasions with this new technique. New York physicians, out-of-town physicians, dermatologists, and nondermatologists alike all came to see this wonder. One of the students was the young Norman Orentreich who later advanced the technique and kept the Friday sanding sessions going after Dr. Kurtin's early death.

The refinement of dermabrasion is the sum of many contributions by many well-known names in dermatology. In the 1950s, Luikart, Ayers, and Wilson had printed by the University of Southern California School of Medicine a short monograph, *Synopsis of Surgical Skin Planing (Dermal Abrasion)*, which is repeated here in part:

1. Wexler pointed out the value of this method in rhinophyma.
2. Lowenthal showed the value of the punch method for pock marks.
3. Orentreich combined the auto-punch-graft and planing technique.
4. LeVan demonstrated the value of the Telfa dressing, and introduced an apparatus to combine a stream of compressed air with the ethyl chloride spray to achieve freezing more quickly and conveniently.
5. Grais used a B.M.R. air tube to avoid ethyl chloride inhalation by the patient.
6. Hubler demonstrated that gentian vi-

olet was valuable to delineate the areas to be planed and the floor of the pits.

7. Lubowe recommended Metaphen for the same purpose and suggested the use of preoperative Demerol.

8. Blau and Rein published a major article in December of 1954 giving an excellent resume of the history of the subject and the findings of men throughout the country who were using the procedure.

9. Wilson, Luikart and Ayers introduced dichlorotetrafluroethane to replace ethyl chloride; thereby eliminating the blower and some attendant hazards.

10. Edelstein and Marmelzat both made careful studies of the complications which may occur.

11. Ayers and Luikart suggested the cotton glove for traction.

12. Eller and Eller recommended the high speed Schreuss motor and introduced the diamond and ruby fraises as well as the stainless steel milled cutter.

13. Beirne and Beirne designed an apparatus for the collection of abraded skin particles, which also acted as a spatter guard.

14. Wilson, Luikart, and Ayers designed the jet-spray handpiece permitting freezing and planing with one hand, and added a spatter guard to obstruct the disagreeable spray and yet permit good vision.

15. Epstein and Kligman delineated the pathogenesis of milia.

16. Levy suggested Nisentil as a good alternate preoperative analgesia, and showed the value of the process in the treatment of adenoma sebaceum and other disorders.

17. Marmelzat wrote stressing the psychological aspects and hazards.

18. Sternberg wrote on freon mixtures.

19. Kligman and Strauss have shown that vellus hair follicles can be formed from human adult epidermis.

20. Wilson, Luikart, and Ayers recorded certain hazards in the use of excessively cold freon mixtures.

21. Epstein published cases showing the value of planing precancerous (sailor's, farmer's) skins.

22. Strauss and Kligman have shown in their experiments on human subjects that the cheek can be frozen for as long as 8 minutes without any lasting untoward effects, and that even very deep planing on the cheek does not remove more than 2.5 mm of tissue, thereby leaving adequate adnexa for regeneration without scar.

23. Burks has published an excellent book entitled *Wire Brush Surgery*.

Today and for the past ten years, the standard for dermabrasion has been refined, practiced, and taught by a core group of dermatologists who join together at an annual course sponsored by the American Society for Dermatologic Surgery. Presenters include John Yarborough, who learned the technique from Dr. Burkes, Henry Roenigk, H. William Hanke, the authors, and others, including Norman Orentreich. This three-day course is given all around the U.S., and teaches basically the same technique Kurtin assembled in 1952—freezing, planing with a brush or fraise, and healing.

Equipment

The operating room should have plenty of space to accommodate the physician, the assistant(s), and the equipment. The room should also have good ventilation and be able to be cooled so that refrigerants will be most efficient. The table should be height-adjustable and comfortable. Lighting that can be directed on the patient's face or tangential to the face is helpful. Face shields, face masks, and head caps are required for the physician and all of the staff who assist at the table (Figs 5–1 and 5–2). Today more than ever, careful attention should be given to where blood and tissue debris are spread. Recent studies using particle physics have demonstrated that the 0.6- to 0.7-micron-sized particles necessary for deposition in the lung are generated by the rotational forces of a diamond fraise at the speeds used for dermabrasion.[12]

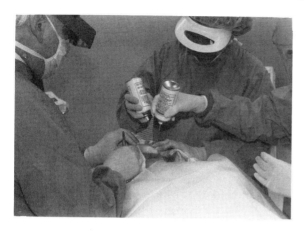

FIG 5–1.
Proper and necessary gowns, masks, face shields, and magnification for the physician.

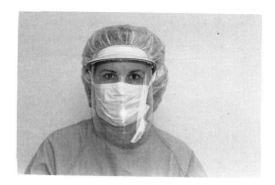

FIG 5–2.
Surgical assistant with necessary protection: mask, face shield, clothing, and hair coverage.

Larger particles do not get to the alveoli, and smaller ones are kept in the air flow and exhaled. Splatter guards located at the site of the abrader, where the physician and the assistants stand, and in the direction that the tools are pointed are part of the technique and eliminate or greatly diminish the exposure to blood and tissues. Surgical gloves are mandatory, although they sometimes make it difficult to hold the skin taut. If this is a problem, cotton gloves can be worn over latex gloves.

There are several different dermabrasion systems made up of a motor (stationary or hand-held), a cable, and a tip. Thousands of successful dermabrasions have been performed with each type of machine. Each physician who uses a dermabrader soon finds a favorite type of equipment and often becomes a dogmatic advocate of that particular system. Others stick with the machinery they learned on. In actuality, dermabrasion is only a controlled skin wound which can be achieved in many ways; whether it is achieved in microseconds or just seconds probably makes little difference to the final outcome.

The cable-driven types of dermabraders were most popular before hand-held engines were developed. The cables were motor-driven and protected with a flexible coil (Fig 5–3). The motor was mounted on a stand or placed on a Mayo stand nearby. The endpiece accommodated the fraise or brush of choice and was knurled for easy gripping. So that no kinks would develop

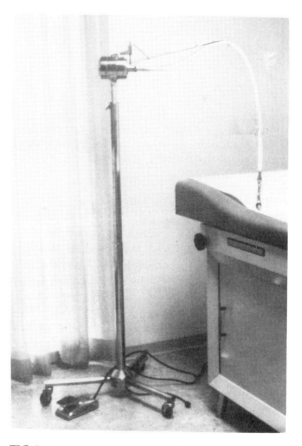

FIG 5–3.
Cable-driven dermabrader designed and manufactured by Robbins Instrument Co. In a different model, the motor sits on a small table holder.

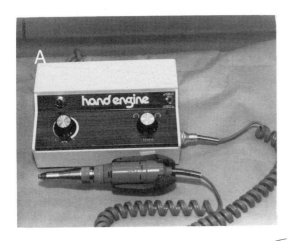

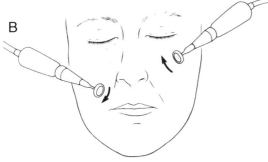

FIG 5–4.
A, the hand engine by Bell International Machine Company, Other types and models are available. **B,** bidirectional rotation demonstrated with Bell hand engine.

advantages are the cable, the necessity of having nitrogen tanks strapped to the wall nearby, and the larger handpiece. The advantages are speed and rotational power. If the physician wishes it, abrasion can progress faster with the air-driven units.

The most recent equipment (although now 15 years old) is the hand engine (Fig 5–4). These instruments have miniaturized motors encased in the handpiece. They are light and have unlimited maneuverability because only an electric cord is attached, as opposed to the coil-wrapped cable of the tools described above. Because the hand engines are so small, they are high-revolution machines that produce a high-pitched whine and some vibration. They turn at 15,000 to 35,000 rpm, depending on the make and model, but easily lose torque when the tip meets much resistance. Several companies manufacture them, and each model has slightly different characteristics. The Bell International hand engine and the engine manufactured by Osada are similar, and Mill-Bilt Equipment Company and Robbins Instrument Company also distribute hand engines. The Dremel Power Tool #370 is a noisy, bulky hand-held engine that we use only as a back-up machine. Clearly, the instrument with the greatest speed and torque is the high-speed Schreuss (Derma III) produced by A. Schumann Precision Manufacturer, Dusseldorf, West Germany.

Importantly, many models have a bidirectional switch that makes it possible to reverse the direction in which the tip rotates. Thus, to have a fraise or brush rotating in the opposite direction, the operator need only flip the switch rather than change position or go to the opposite side of the table. The bidirectional quality is handy when working around orifices because the rotation needs to be toward the lip or eyelid; rotation in the opposite direction may catch and tear the structure. These models can also be used for hair transplantation, and therefore have become quite popular.

Endpieces or Cutting Tools

Currently two types of tips are in regular use: the diamond fraise and the wire brush (Fig 5–5). A tip called a serrated wheel is no longer manufactured. Its design combined features of

in the coil/cable, it was necessary to place the apparatus so the cable moved in a wide, gentle arc as the doctor moved the tip to and fro. Additional friction reduced the speed of the tip, reduced the torque available, and burned out the cable more quickly. The rotating speed was controlled by a foot pedal and the revolutions per minute (rpm) ranged from 800 to 15,000. The handpiece had very little vibration and glided easily over the skin. It also developed good torque, which was only slightly reduced by the friction with the skin. The motor and cable made a high-pitched whine which sounded something like the old dental drills.

Another type of cable tool is driven by air or compressed nitrogen. The Stryker brand is the most popular. These instruments develop great rotational speeds of 40,000 to 60,000 rpm and retain their torque through any drag the skin can provide. They are sturdily built. The dis-the brush and the fraise. Rows of sharp metal points were mounted on a stainless-steel wheel which cut deeply with moderate to heavy pressure, but with light pressure behaved like a fraise.

The diamond fraise is a stainless-steel wheel with diamond chips bonded onto the surface. The chips usually come in two or three grades, depending on how the company labels them; the smaller one is labeled regular or fine; and the larger is labeled course or rough and is the stronger cutting surface. Most experienced abraders use the rougher fraises because the desired depth is reached so much more quickly. Different shapes and sizes of fraises are available (Fig 5–6). Diameters range from 7 to 22 mm, with 17 mm being the most common. The width or sanding surface ranges from 2 mm to 10 or 12 mm. The narrower wheels cut more easily and quickly and while good for abrading deeper around pits and depressed scars, can quickly cut a trough. We often start out with a 4 mm width used on its widest surface, and by rolling it up on its edge, can cut deeper as needed. The wider fraises are good for planing—for large areas that require smoothing, or for use on actinic-damaged skin. These fraises tend to gouge less but have greater drag, and will slow down when pressed hard unless the machine has a strong torque power. The fraises also come in various shapes. The wheel is the most common, but the cylinder with a dome-shaped tip is handy for large surfaces and narrow crevices. Pear- and bullet-shaped tips are designed to abrade around structures like the nose, in and over irregular surfaces like the philtrum, or to spot pits on the cheeks and nose. When using a pear or bullet tip, the instrument should be held like a pencil and the fraise applied in a circular fashion; with the wheels or cylinders, the handpiece should be held like a tennis racket and the cutting surface applied with linear strokes, as described in detail below.

The wire brush is made of multiple wires arranged on a stainless-steel wheel (Fig 5–7). The ends are beveled and trimmed to create a flat or tapered cutting surface. Many experienced abraders prefer the brush, which certainly is the faster cutting tool and has a more efficient tip when abrading thick skin with scars or sun damage. With skill and a light touch it also works well for lighter abrasions. The brush will gouge and run more easily than the fraise, especially if the skin is not well-frozen. Be aware when the skin defrosts, because the brush simply will not cut or will run across the skin. Drag or antitorque forces are greater with the brush, requiring a firmer rein on the instrument. The beginner should be well-trained and proctored when starting to use the brush, or should use the fraise until relatively skilled with the brush technique.

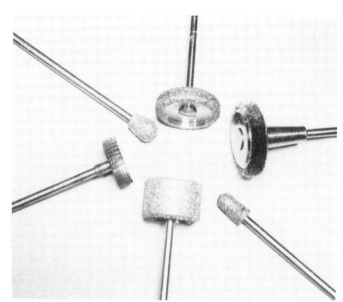

FIG 5–5.
Types of tips used; diamond fraises *(top and bottom)*; serrated wheel *(left)*; wire brush *(right)*; pear- and bullet-shaped fraises *(oblique)*.

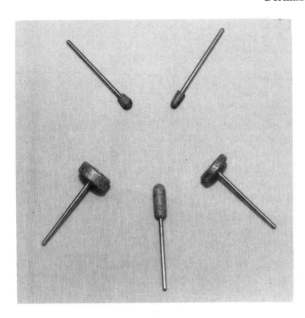

FIG 5–6.
Diamond fraises: bullet *(top right)*; pear *(top left)*; cylinder *(bottom)*; 4 and 7 mm wide, 17-mm-diameter wheel fraises *(right and left oblique)*.

Refrigerants

Light dermabrasions (shallow-depth wounding) are achieved with little or no freezing. Sometimes it is preferable not to use any freeze, as described below. However, nearly all moderate to deep abrasions will require freezing the skin unless local anesthesia or the super-high-speed abraders are used. The freeze serves two functions—for anesthesia, and to provide skin rigidity. The latter is essential when the wire brush is used.

Fridigerm and Fluoro Ethyl are used almost exclusively. Two refrigerants, Cryosthesia (−30°) and Cryosthesia (−60°), are no longer on the market because of the untoward effects of the deep freeze.[13] The chemical composition, physical properties, and effects on the tissues have been worked out in studies of humans and animals (Table 5–1).[14–16] The freon 12 cooled the skin so efficiently that reports of hyper- and hypopigmentation, necrosis, sloughing, and persistent erythema have accompanied its use.[13]

In addition to the type of refrigerant used, several factors affect the efficiency and thus the depth of the freeze wound. The temperature of the facial skin is obviously a factor. Prechilling the skin with cold gel bags is practiced frequently. The patient or the assistant hold the cold bags against the facial skin for 15 to 20 minutes. This prechilling reduces the pain and discomfort of the spray refrigerants which cause significant burning and stinging. Prechilling also speeds freezing time and increases the depth of the freeze obtained from the routine spray refrigerants.

The ambient temperature and room circulation directly affect the ease of freezing. In a hot stuffy room, freezing the skin will take longer and never be as complete as in a room that is cool and well-ventilated. There is a critical distance at which the spray from commercially prepared spray refrigerants is most effective (Fig 5–8). Holding the can farther away freezes less or not at all; holding it closer does not permit full aeration of the freon and thus it is still liquid when it hits the skin, producing a messy field. The liquid form is not an effective refrigerant. Therefore, the distance the spray can is held from the skin surface during freezing clearly impacts on the freeze.

The thickness of the epidermis and the state of the epidermal barrier also affect freezing efficiency. Dzubow[16] demonstrated that refreezing skin that has already been abraded results in an additional wound from the freeze not produced by the abrasion alone. This same study concluded that the short (less than 30 seconds), one-time spray freezes used by most physicians for dermabrasion probably do not add to the

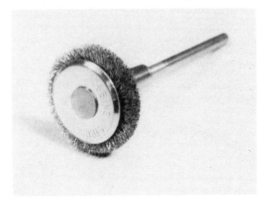

FIG 5–7.
Kurtin style wire brush showing the individual wire construction.

TABLE 5–1.

Skin Refrigerants*

Product	Chemical Components	Boiling Point	Maximum Cooling Temperature
Frigiderm	Freon 114[†]	+3.8°C	−40.6 ± 0.4°C
Fluoro ethyl	Freon 114 (75%)	+3.8°C	−42.8 ± 0.4°C
	Ethyl chloride (25%)	+12.0°C	
Cryosthesia −30	Freon 11[‡]	+23.8°C	−52.0 + 0.5°C
	Freon 12[§]	−29.8°C	
Cryosthesia −60	Freon 12	−29.8°C	−66.0 + 0.7°C

*From Hanke CW, O'Brian JJ: A histologic evaluation of the effects of skin refrigerant in an animal model. J Dermatol Surg Oncol 1987; 13:664–669. Used with permission.
[†]Freon 114 = dichlorotretrafluoroethane.
[‡]Freon 11 = trichlorofluoromethane.
[§]Freon 12 = dichlorodifluoromethane.

depth of a wound or produce a wound that is any deeper than the wound obtained from the abrasion alone. However, spray freezes of longer than 60 seconds or repeat freezes do lead to measurable histologic changes, indicating wounding in addition to abrasion.

It is important to clarify that although repeat freeze-thaws or overlapping refreezes increase the wound depth, a continuous freeze apparently does not. Strauss and Kligman showed that the skin can be frozen for up to eight minutes without damage.[17]

It is clear that a thick, horny keratin layer inhibits freeze penetration, which even the novice abrader can appreciate. Finally, freezing in one area overlaps the adjacent skin, gradually cooling the entire area. Because these many diverse and complex factors affect the depth of freeze, the operator must constantly watch the whiteness of the frozen area and frequently palpate the skin for firmness by tapping on it to monitor the depth of freeze. Making appropriate adjustments to anticipate one or several of the factors discussed above is a critical part of the physician's job during dermabrasion.

Indications

Postacne scarring is the indication for the majority of dermabrasions (Fig 5–9), and was the problem for which the procedure was developed. With widespread use of 13-cis-retinoic acid, however, there may not be as much acne scarring in the future. The other side of the coin is that as fewer people have acne scars, those who do will be more inclined to have them treated. Dermabrasion is very helpful for superficial and shallow, well-demarcated scars. It is less helpful for saucer-like and rolling scars, but because it obliterates or softens the edges of scars, it has a cosmetic value often greater than the actual improvement of the scar itself. Shallow ice-pick scars in thick skin can be completely abraded away. Deep ice-pick scars cannot be abraded away and may look larger if the scar is

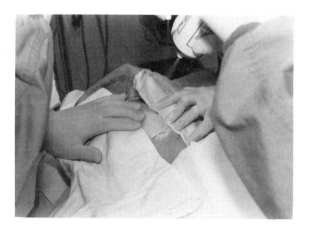

FIG 5–8.
Spray refrigerant. The distance from the skin is critical and only one of several factors that influence the speed and effectiveness of the freeze.

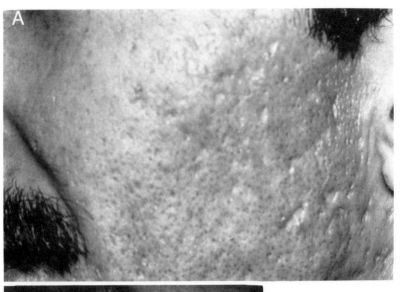

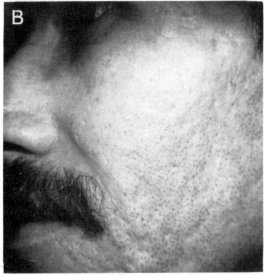

FIG 5–9.
A, 35-year-old man, before dermabrasion; he has several types of scars with shallow, ice-pick type predominating. **B,** three months postabrasion showing improving of most but not all of the scars. Color has returned to normal.

not cylindrical but, instead, an inverted cone.

Because acne scars are seldom homogeneous, close inspection and cataloging of the scar is necessary during the initial consultation. The results of this assessment must be shared with the patient, who should be told and shown which scars will most likely respond to abrasion and which will not (Fig 5–10). As discussed in Chapter 1, the consultation is best made with the patient holding a mirror. Dermabrasion may be the only recommended treatment, or may be one of several parts of a treatment plan for postacne scars.

Posttraumatic and postsurgical scars can be greatly improved by one or several dermabrasions. The technique is valuable for removing ridges at the edge of grafts, second-intention healing, or flaps. It will also blend the texture and coloring, which are often the most obvious evidence of tumor removal or trauma. Elevations from hair transplants, punch-transplant replacements, and varicella scars will plane down, as will sebaceous and fibrous tissue excesses, e.g., rhinophyma, sebaceous hyperplasia, and angiofibromas.

A controversy continues about when is the

ideal time to abrade: soon after the wound (within the first 4 to 6 weeks), or after the scar is mature (6 months)? Yarborough recommends early treatment, but admits to the lack of controlled or comparative studies.[18] It is unlikely that such studies will ever be available because it is an unlikely protocol to treat only one-half of a patients disfigurement, and the characteristics of a scar, especially a traumatic or postdisease scar, change from millimeter to millimeter. It is a well-known clinical fact that simple excisions with primary closures heal better, with less discernible scarring, when done the same day of dermabrasion and within the dermabrasion field. But the critical time in late healing in which to abrade in order to improve scar cosmesis is not known.

Actinic damage is removed by the postdermabrasion healing process. When the wound extends to the lower limits of the elastosis, the elastosis is replaced during healing with a dermal band of new collagen, ground substance, and new elastic fibers. The histologic changes associated with dermabrasion are similar to those seen after deep chemical peeling.[19] In addition to the replacement of elastosis, the epidermis

regenerates with fewer or no irregularities secondary to sun damage, and the papillary dermis is thicker and comprises parallel collagen bundles.

Abrasion for sun damage is indicated when there are other indications for sanding such as scarring, pigmentary problems, and excessive, premature keratoses or basal-cell carcinomas. Abrasion is also indicated when the skin is thick and sebaceous because peeling—even deep, occluded peeling—is not as effective on this type of surface. Abrasion, particularly with a wire brush, will correct the sun damage and sometimes reduce the sebaceous quality. In addition, abrading thick skin is easier because there is less chance of going too deep. Conversely, thin, non-sebaceous skin is better for peeling because on that type of skin it is easier to obtain an even result. The general rule (with exceptions, of course) is to dermabrade men and peel women for actinic damage. (Be careful with either technique on men because the resulting hypopigmentation is more of a cosmetic liability and more difficult to camouflage.)

Melasma or hyperpigmentation sometimes lighten or disappear after dermabrasion. The

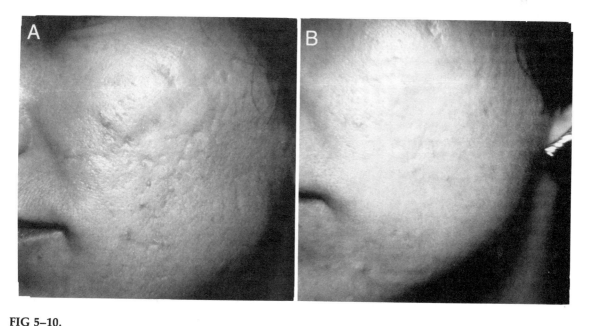

FIG 5–10.
A, 28-year-old woman before dermabrasion; she has a long depressed scar on the high medial cheek and several other irregular depressed scars. **B,** 6 months postabrasion shows some of the smaller scars gone but the long depressed scar still present although significantly improved.

problem is the inability to predict absolutely *when* that sometime will be. Frequently, dermabrasion leads to hyperpigmentation. We have seen cases where the operative indication was hyperpigmentation and the result was lightening of the nonpigmented skin, which made the hyperpigmented skin look darker. It is acceptable to offer dermabrasion as a treatment for hyperpigmentation, but that offer must be made to a patient who is completely informed and willing to risk no change or worsening of the pigmentary problem.

At several American Society for Dermatologic Survey-sponsored courses on peels and dermabrasions, Hanke has presented a list of indications for dermabrasion. This list is reproduced below as published in Roenigk and Roenigk, *Dermatologic Surgery* (Table 5–2).[20]

Anatomic Markers for Dermabrasion Depth

It is possible to visualize the approximate depth of the dermabrasion as it is performed by observing anatomic changes as successive layers of skin are removed (Fig 5–11, A). These observations are best made when using a diamond fraise because it bites less than a wire brush and less freezing is required. Not all patients will show all of the findings, but when they are recognized, they are a great help in determining the depth of the abrasion while it is happening. That way, adjustments can be made and trouble prevented.

In human facial skin, level 1 is reached when there is a change to a lighter color, indicating that the epidermis with its melanocytes has been removed (Fig 5–11, B). Also, the tiny vessels of the subepidermal plexis become visible. Level 2 is seen when the vessels disappear and small yellow dots just begin to be perceived. This indicates that most or all of the papillary dermis has been removed. The yellow dots are the most superficial edges of the sebaceous glands, just visible through a few bands of collagen. Level 3 is reached when larger, more numerous yellow dots are seen, indicating that the middle of the sebaceous glands has been reached; this is essentially the mid-dermis. When the yellow dots become larger, fewer in number, or disappear,

TABLE 5–2.
Various Entities Treated With Dermabrasion*

Postacne scars	Adenoma sebaceum
Traumatic scars	Neurotic excoriations
Smallpox or chickenpox scars	Multiple trichoepitheliomas
Rhinophyma	Darier's disease
Professionally applied tattoos	Fox-Fordyce
Amateur-type tattoos	Lichenified dermatoses
Blast tattoos	Porokeratosis of Mibelli
Multiple seborrheic keratoses	Favre-Racouchot syndrome
Multiple pigmented nevi	Lichen amyloidosis
Actinically damaged skin	Verrucous nevus
Age- and sun-related wrinkle lines	Molluscum contagiosum
Active acne	Keratoacanthoma
Freckles	Xanthalasma
Pseudofolliculitis barbae	Hemangioma
Telangiectasia	Leg ulcer
Acne rosacea	Scleromyxedema
Cholasma	Striae distensae
Vitiligo	Hair transplantation elevations
Congenital pigmented nevi	Linear epidermal nevus
Syringocystadenoma papilliferum	Syringoma
Nevus flammeus	Angiofibromas of tuberous sclerosis
Keloids	Chronic radiation dermatitis
Dermatitis papilaris capilliti	Xeroderma pigmentosum
Lupus erythematosus	Lentigines
Basal cell carcinoma— superficial type	

*From Roenigk HH Jr: Dermabrasion, in Roenigk RK, Roenigk HH (eds): *Dermatologic Surgery, Principles and Practice.* New York, Marcel Dekker, 1988. Used with permission.

level 4, or the lower dermis, has been exposed. Also at this level, the compacted dermis is revealed by the appearance of rope-like collagen bundles. Level 5 is reached when yellow globules of fat appear, indicating that the subcutaneous plane has been exposed. Ideally, this plane will never be seen unless the fraise uncovers an unsuspected cyst and "falls through."

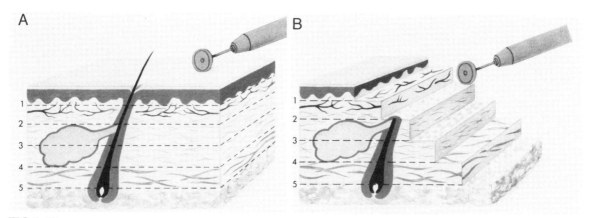

FIG 5–11.

A, the five levels of anatomy discernible during dermabrasion. **B,** stepwise uncovering of the anatomy as viewed by the physician from above the patient.

Try not to become too frustrated if these levels are not easily recognized. They will not be seen in every patient, and the frost, blood, and tissue debris can interfere with a quick inspection. However, in time and with persistence, these anatomic findings will become identifiable and will be important guides for the depth of abrasion. Often, the skin thickness is not what is expected: older women may have extremely thin skin, skin thickness may vary from location to location, or there may be a deep scar that needs deeper abrasion. In that case, anatomic markers can tell how deep the scar is.

To try out new equipment, to learn how to recognize the anatomic levels, and to begin mastering the technique, the grapefruit is the best model. (It is workable for the diamond fraise but not for the wire brush.) As the grapefruit is abraded, the yellow color is removed, revealing the white skin below. This is equivalent to removing the human epidermis with its pigment. Slightly deeper abrasion to the point where the holes or pores of the grapefruit begin to show and look similar to the sebaceous glands, is analogous to the level of the papillary dermis. The next layer on the grapefruit is the white, stringy pith, comparable to the compacted dermis. Finally, the pulp mimics the subcutaneous fat.

Like any model the grapefruit has limitations and during this exercise the room and equipment will become splattered with grapefruit zest and smell like a citrus farm—but this is a good demonstration of how much blood and debris will be splattered in a real operation. It is also a good way to experience the feel of the machines and fraises, and is a good method of training the hand and eye to expose various "anatomic" layers. We believe strongly that simply sanding off the gentian violet (see below) or evenly abrading the entire face is not good technique. Each scar must be examined and sanded until it is gone or until maximum depth has been reached.

Preoperative Evaluation

It has taken years for us to truly understand the limitations of this procedure. *Everyone*—doctors and patients alike—thinks, hopes, and expects that dermabrasion will make more of a difference than it usually does. Granted, there are thousands of patients who have benefitted from this procedure over the years, but there are also thousands who honestly and objectively say it was not worth the trouble, cost, and side effects. Probably as many as one-half would not have it again. Although we have patients who have been ecstatic over the improvement, we also have patients who are disgusted daily when they have to put on heavy makeup to cover the demarcation line between the abraded and unabraded skin.

Consultation(s) before surgery must accomplish the physician's careful scar-to-scar analysis. At this time, the total treatment plan is proposed—seldom should only a dermabrasion be proposed. Not only do many patients need more than one treatment modality (dermabrasion(s), Zyderm collagen, punch transplants, etc.) but the doctor *always* needs an out when patients are not completely satisfied. The next step is more difficult: trying to educate the patient about the procedure, the prognosis, the alternatives, and the risks. We would rather perform two dermabrasions than do one dermabrasion consultation. It is possible that we are overly concerned about informed consent or have become jaded by our troubles and do not remember accurately our many successes. Nevertheless, the pressure to fully inform is present, and unfortunately printed materials are such traps for plaintiff attorneys to use against the physicians that the actual consultation becomes the only way to inform.

Preoperative Medications

This is the time to double check what medicines the patient is taking. Aspirin, nonsteroid anti-inflammatory drugs, and other anti-inflammatory medicines will increase bleeding. Birth control pills and estrogen cause the skin to retain water, making it possible to abrade the skin much more easily and quickly, and probably increase the incidence of hyperpigmentation. Additionally, there might be medicines that should be prescribed before the abrasion—Zovirax (acyclovir) to prevent HS I if the patient has a history of herpes, antibiotic prophylaxis for any valve disease, and Retin-A (tretinoin) to speed healing.

Preoperative Studies

As with any procedure, conservatism and completeness cannot be criticized. Obtaining a CBC, SMA, Hepatitis Ab and Ag, and human immunodeficiency virus (HIV) Ab are routinely ordered by some physicians and only specifically indicated by others. Usually, patients will give necessary medical information in the history. If you doubt the patient's veracity or intelligence, or if you are concerned about protecting your own health, specific tests should be ordered. Hepatitis Ag and Ab and HIV Ab studies are important to know about for a procedure that introduces virus particles into the air. Equally as important, HIV-positive patients may not heal as well as HIV-negative patients, and dermabrasion is contraindicated for HIV-positive patients because of their inability to handle infection. These days, we always wear face shields, caps, and masks when performing dermabrasions.

Test Spots

This is a controversial subject. It is easy to dermabrade a small area near the hairline or in the preauricular area. However, just how much information can be accurately extrapolated from that spot is questionable. If testing for pigmentation, six months' follow-up is necessary. If testing for scarring potential, that potential changes with every location on the face. If testing to educate the patient about the procedure and the results, it is well worth the effort. If testing to establish how careful you are, it looks great on the chart.

Photographs

Good quality preoperative photographs should be taken during the consultation or just prior to the procedure. Often the patient will not want to remove makeup at the consultation visit, but a clean face is important for accurate pictures. Get several angles, and bracket the focus and flash settings so the scars and depressions will show best. Ideally, a room or corner of the office should be equipped with a smooth, light-colored backdrop and side lighting permanently mounted on the walls. Photographs taken only with front flash blanch out so many of the defects that accuracy and documentation of improvement are lost.

We take Polaroids for the chart in addition to the Kodachromes for the files. It is helpful to have the Polaroids during follow-up visits so the patient can see the improvements. Patients can become so discouraged during the long months of recovery that it is a boost for them to see how many scars are gone or improved. Other doctors we know file the Kodachromes in the chart and carry a small hand viewer so the patient can look at slides in the office. Use whatever works.

Dermabrasion

Technique

Analgesia and Anesthesia

The true pain of dermabrasion is the initial cold spray of the refrigerant and some stinging during sanding. There is no deep pain except for the cold on the forehead. The amount of analgesia given is almost entirely to help the physician. Some doctors want the patient to feel and say nothing, and are more comfortable when they do not have to deal with the patient. Thus, these patients get more preoperative and intraoperative medications. If the physician does not mind talking to the patient, however, and wants the patient to be able to cooperate and also leave soon after the procedure, the patient is given less medication.

Usual preoperative medications include Valium the night before, immediately preoperatively, or sublingually at the start of the procedure. Barbiturates the night before and 30 minutes before is an old plan but still valid. We have come to prefer meperidine (Demerol) 50 to 100 mg intramuscularly (IM) and prochlorperazine (Compazine) 10 mg IM 20 minutes before the procedure begins. If a second dose of Demerol is needed, the Compazine eliminates the nausea that commonly occurs.

IV sedation with Demerol, Ketamine, or Sublimase are compatible with this operation. Although we have used IV sedation and known many doctors who use it routinely, many physicians hire a nurse anesthetist or anesthesiologist to administer sedation or anesthesia. These physicians agree that they are much happier and better able to give full attention to the operation. Also, the more sedation, the greater need for monitoring and recovery. Although anesthesia helps meet the needs of the operating physician and the patient, it is not absolutely necessary because dermabrasion can be done with the freeze only, if necessary or desired; thousands of procedures have been done this way.

Local anesthesia with lidocaine or Marcaine is safe and effective. Patients who have had dermabrasion with and without a local prefer the anesthesia. Block the forehead with a ring block just above the eyebrows which hits the supraorbital, supratrochlear, and temporofacial nerves (Fig 5–12). The infraorbital and mental nerves

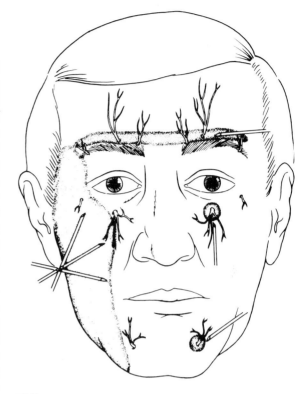

FIG 5–12.
The sites for local anesthesia face block.

are each blocked separately (Fig 5–13). The temporozygomatic nerves are blocked by entering the skin with a long spinal needle just preauricularly and sweeping over the entire lateral cheek. If necessary, the nose is blocked by injecting the bridge at the bony cartilagenous junction, in each alar groove, and at the base of the columella.

Patients do sometimes complain about "those needles" but they learn that a full-face block eliminates the discomfort at the time of surgery and for several hours afterwards. Patients also complain if one area does not become completely anesthetized. Currently we use only the topical freeze, or local face block, or these in conjunction with mild analgesia in the form of Demerol and Compazine IM and local anesthesia.

Once the face is abraded, gauze squares dipped into lidocaine 1% with epinephrine are laid over the abraded area. Because the epidermis is gone, the lidocaine is absorbed and rapidly becomes effective. It stops stinging immediately.

Skin Preparation and Marking

Clean skin is all that is necessary for dermabrasion. We are satisfied if all the makeup has been removed and the face freshly washed with soap and water. There is no evidence that further cleansing in the office with antibacterial cleansers is beneficial.

Painting the entire area to be abraded with 1% aqueous gentian violet has been a standard step for a long time. It serves two purposes: the deep color fills the depths of the scars and pits, drawing attention to every last one of them so they can be treated. It is not difficult to overlook a scar during the procedure because of the presence of towels, blood, tissue debris and frost. Theoretically, when the gentian violet has been dermabraded away from the bottom of the scar, all of the scar has also been completely abraded. However, this is not always true. The gentian violet can be abraded off without the scar having been adequately treated. Although we have used gentian violet painting in the past and have no objections to using it now, our current technique of looking carefully at each scar and the anatomic levels of abrasion makes the paint unnecessary.

Whether or not gentian violet is used, some marking of the limits of the abrasion should be made (Fig 5–14). With the patient seated, hold-

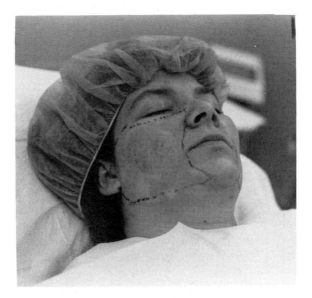

FIG 5–14.
The limits of the abrasion are marked with the patient sitting prior to draping. Note that the line is placed just under the jaw line.

ing a mirror, and watching, and prior to analgesia, mark the limits of the abrasion. Especially mark the line just under the chin so that the abrasion will be carried to that line, placing the demarcation between the abraded and unabraded skin well within the shadow of the jaw. When the patient reclines, that line shifts; therefore, it is important for the patient to sit during the marking. Nothing is more upsetting than to see patients in follow-up and hear them say certain areas "were missed." Thus, they should watch and comment on the marking.

The patient is made comfortable on the table and draped as necessary. The patient should be on the back with the head flat and free to turn from side to side. The light can be overhead or moved to shine tangentially to highlight and bring the depressed and elevated scars into relief. Local blocks are administered if they are to be used. Prechilling with ice packs or cold polyglycol gel bags for 10 to 15 minutes is very helpful for further anesthesia, more efficient freezing, and reduction of the pain of the initial blast of refrigerant.

Dividing and Abrading

Many variations of the technique apparently

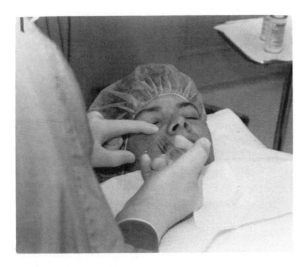

FIG 5–13.
The infraorbital nerves being infiltrated with lidocaine. The index finger of the opposite hand sits over the infraorbital notch and the injection is placed just inferior to it.

produce equally good results. The best way to develop a technique is to observe as many different physicians as possible. Learning is much easier these days because many fine video teaching tapes are available. As with any procedure, the student's technique is a synthesis of many teachers' techniques. What we describe here is what we do now. Our technique may change, and we fully recognize that there are many other successful methods. The best instruction for the actual hands-on dermabrasion is at the table, but videotapes are quite close in learning value.

We currently follow partially the technique of Norman Orentreich and block off segments of the face with towels or gauze squares (Fig 5–15). A square area about 3 cm is partitioned. It is frozen to the desired firmness: a hard freeze for wire brush and deep scars, a lighter freeze for diamond fraises or shallow scars and moderate sun damage. Immediately after the freeze, the towels or gauze squares are lifted and moved back one-half to 1 cm and laid back down and held firmly; this also stabilizes the underlying skin. Abrade within that square, going over it repeatedly until it is finished or until the freeze wears off. The gauze squares or towels are then placed over the next area, with some overlap to the previous and adjacent areas. The sequence of cover, freeze, reposition, hold, and abrade is repeated until the whole face is completed.

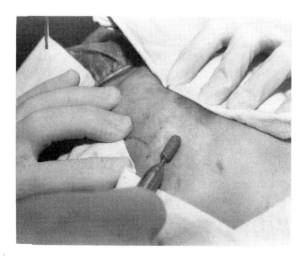

FIG 5–15.
The limits of a segment are established by towels. The assistant holds the skin taut.

Users of towels insist on their importance. Most have caught a gauze square in the wheel or fraise and been permanently traumatized by the event. There is a loud pop, followed by a wrapping-flapping noise that continues until the operator releases the foot pedal. It is not hard to unravel the sponge from a fraise, but it is fairly difficult to get it off a brush. Then the patient has to be retrieved from the ceiling and convinced that everything is all right and the operation can proceed. This is unsettling, and the problem is eliminated by using towels or cloth baby diapers. Disadvantages, however, are that the towels are not disposable and need to be refolded to bring a fresh side to each new area; the gauze sponges are simply tossed away as new ones are brought into the field. The sponges are also more absorbent. But if a surgical laundry and sterilizing equipment are already part of your office, towels may be preferable.

For the beginner, the tip is moved across the skin in a straight line perpendicular to the direction of rotation. The tip is pulled toward the operator rather than pushed away. Pulling instead of pushing and the movement perpendicular to the rotation both help prevent gouging and running. This is especially true of the wire brush, which has more rotational pull and grabbing ability. When using the brush, be sure the patient's skin is well-frozen.

In each area it is probably best to start at one edge and move systematically over the entire patch. Also have your hand and arm in motion before applying the tip to the skin. Do not set the fraise or brush on the skin and then begin to move.

The above two rules are for beginners. With experience, the tip can be moved to and fro and in a circle. You can start wherever you want in the frozen area because you will be much more confident and quick. As is advised in so many endeavors, keep your eye fixed on the skin surface being cut by the wheel.

The endpiece is held like a tennis racket but steadied by extending the thumb and resting it on the shaft of the handle. This gives added leverage in case the instrument begins to run across the skin.

It makes no difference where the abrasion begins: forehead, chin, or nose. Starting at the lowest site and working superiorly minimizes the amount of blood that runs over the field, although the bleeding stops quickly anyway, and is held under gauze or towels. There is no doubt that bony prominences, especially the forehead are much more sensitive to the cold spray, which may be a reason to do those areas last.

It is technically more difficult to abrade the cutaneous upper lip area because it is a narrow, sensitive area between the lip and the nose. We know of no difficulty if patients inhale the refrigerant, but it makes them uncomfortable and disrupts the procedure. Therefore, we pinch the nostrils while spraying in this area, and also use smaller or bullet-shaped fraises.

The nose can be abraded if it is scarred or sun-damaged. It is harder to do, but if the skin is thick enough, it will abrade satisfactorily. It can also be left untreated. Within a few months it is almost impossible to discern that the nose was not treated. During early healing patients are concerned about having a normal, white nose on a face covered with crust, ooze, and the erythema. But it blends out quickly. A combined procedure of peeling the nose with 35% TCA makes it erythematous, and it heals at the same rate as the abraded areas.

The abrasion should be carried onto the vermilion. Trying to stop at the white or red line only accentuates that line, and if any lines extend from the perioral area onto the lips, they become little accent lines around the mouth. No matter what the indication for the abrasion, do abrade onto the lips. When nearing the lips, adjust the tip so the wheel rotates toward the orifice (Fig 5–4B). It does not matter in what direction the doctor moves the entire endpiece—in a straight line, to and fro, in one direction only, or in a circle. It only matters that the tip rotates toward the opening. The same is true near any opening, and on the eyelids. The rationale is that the rotating wheel literally pushes the lip or eyelid margin closed, whereas if it rotates away from the margin it may grab the tissue and tear it. We have seen that happen.

During work around the mouth, it is helpful to have patients stick the tongue behind the area being abraded or insert folded gauze and cover it completely with the lips. This makes the area flat or convex, which is easier to get to than a concavity, and stretches it slightly, which helps stabilize it. The doctor's or the assistant's fingers can be put into the patient's mouth to do the same thing. Placing a little finger in the nostril also helps when abrading the nasal ala.

Although it is technically difficult, the eyelids can be abraded. Only the lower lids ever need it, usually the lateral one-half. Favre-Racouchot, crow's feet, and sun damage are indications for lid abrasion. Slow the rotation of the wheel, set the rotational direction toward the orifice, freeze carefully, and push down lightly. This is tricky, but possible.

We usually do not cover the eyes during dermabrasion because it adds to the patients' feelings of claustrophobia and surrendering of control. However, we are careful to hold towels or gauze over the eyes when we get close to them. Gentle finger pressure over a gauze covering the eye is reassuring to the patient and gives good protection without the need for an appliance. Some doctors like to have patients wear swim goggles or put ointment into their eyes and cover them with eyepads.

Spot Abrasions

Spot or regional abrasions are not usually recommended for acne scars unless the patient has had a previous abrasion. Skin color and texture are so often altered by the procedure that the sum of the cosmetic improvement is seldom positive, even if the scar(s) treated are improved. Once the patient has had an abrasion and experienced the changes in color and texture, the second abrasion causes little change. We do recommend second or even third abrasions to better treat some deep scars if the skin is still thick enough and if there have been no pigmentary problems.

A regional abrasion presents the same problems as a spot, but the different textures and colors are mitigated by the boundaries of a cosmetic unit. If the perioral area is abraded, as is often the case for radiating lip lines, the smile lines, the jaw and chin lines, and the nose separate the treated skin from the rest of the face adequately so that the viewing eye does not readily notice the difference. If a peel is combined with an abrasion, the color and texture changes are slightly different with the two modalities, but the differential is less noticeable.

In addition, on regional or spot abrasions little or no freezing is necessary. Once the skin is anesthetized, the assistants can hold the skin very taut. The fraise, rotating at low or moderate speed, is gently touched to the surface until the desired depth or wound is created.

Dressings

Upon completion of the procedure, the soiled towels and gauze are removed. Usually the oozing has already stopped and the face can be cleansed gently with water, Zephiran chloride, or hydrogen peroxide. It is here that Cohen recommends scrubbing with copious amounts of saline to prevent milia formation.[21] If it has not been done already, cover the abraded area with gauze squares dipped in lidocaine 1% with or without epinephrine for 10 minutes. This will stop the stinging at once.

Our standard routine is to cover the face lightly with an antibiotic ointment, Telfa, and gauze, and hold it all in place with roller or Kling gauze and an outer covering of flexible surgical net. This dressing comes off the next day and the patient is instructed to wash the face and hair—preferably in the shower. We suggest that patients wash their hair and, as the soap and water rolls over the face, they will be convinced that it is all right to wash that wound. They should apply the antibiotic ointment after washing twice daily for two to three days and then switch to an antibiotic and corticosteroid cream.

The Telfa dressing has served us and our patients well for years, although many new sophisticated dressings are now available (Fig 5–16). We and others have tried them for dermabrasion wounds. These new dressings are generally considered occlusive or semiocclusive with the semiocclusive varieties related to the exchange of gases possible through some of them. One of the new dressings, Omni-derm, even allows topically applied medications to penetrate without unsetting the dressing. The penetration of oxygen, originally touted as important, seems to be of little importance.

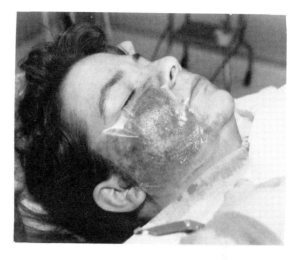

FIG 5–16.
One of the new semipermeable dressings, Omiderm, in place.

Varghese and colleagues showed that fluid obtained from chronic wounds being treated with either an oxygen-permeable or oxygen-impermeable dressing was uniformly hypoxic.

Post-dermabrasion, the reason for the covering is to stop pain, contain serum ooze, protect the skin from bacteria, and speed healing. There are five basic types of occlusive dressings.

1. Films. These are made of thin, transparent, and adherent polyurethane that transports some water vapor and gases. They are not absorbent and do not stick to the wound itself. Accumulation of exudate under the dressing is the worst problem. Dressings need to be changed daily for the first few days. A few of these are Op-Site, Tegaderm, Bioclusive, and Univlex.

2. Foams. These are made of nonadherent polyurethane material that is taped in place over the wound. They will absorb only a little fluid. Examples are Synthaderm and Epilock.

3. Hydrocolloids. These have a water-impermeable polyurethane outer covering separated from the wound by a hydrocolloid material that is different with each particular dressing. They should be applied only on a fresh wound and eventually accumulate enough wound fluid to cause a gradual separation of the dressing.

They also may become malodorous and produce a yellow-brown drainage. Examples are Duoderm and Comfeel.

4. Hydrogels. These are made of a polyethylene oxide gel covered on both sides with a semipermeable polyurethane film. The film is removed from one side and is placed over the wound. These are semitransparent, nonadhesive, and absorbent. They may stick to the wound if allowed to dry out. Vigilon is the prototype of this group.

5. Double-Layered Permeable Membranes. These dressings allow all of the fluid beneath to permeate to the surface and allow penetration of topical medications to the wound below. Omniderm is the prototype of this category.

In a bilateral comparison study of patients after full-face dermabrasion, Pinski evaluated several of these new dressings.[23] By preventing dehydration, they encouraged rapid re-epithelialization. Healing time was sometimes reduced by 50%, and this effect was noticed in the first 24 to 48 hours.

These dressings are not without their problems: slippage, sticking, leaking, possibility of infection, and cost. Also, rapid re-epithelialization does not necessarily translate into better cosmesis. We will continue to monitor their use after dermabrasion and of course try them on our patients.

Postoperative Care

Regardless of the ensuing postoperative care, the patient is most comfortable leaving the office with a dressing that provides full, substantial coverage—a dressing that snugly covers all of the wounded skin and which will absorb serum oozing (Fig 5–17). Such a dressing is constructed on top of whatever is chosen for the base coat, whether Telfa or one of the synthetic skin materials, and includes gauze squares, roller gauze, and an outer fixation layer of Kling gauze or elastic web gauze. In spite of this, the patient can expect that serous or serosanguineous fluid will soak through the dressing, especially at the lower or neck margin of the wrap.

We recommend that the dressing be changed the next day. If something simple like Telfa is used, the patient is encouraged to shower and wash the hair, which causes soapy water to flow over the facial injuries and convinces the patient that washing does not hurt much and is quite refreshing. Then the patient can go ahead and wash the face gently with soap and water. The washing removes the early crusts, cleans up all the surrounding skin, and greatly reduces the bacterial contamination on the surface. After the skin is patted dry, the abraded areas are covered with an antibacterial ointment and left open or dressed lightly for one more day. On day two and henceforth, the skin is washed with soap and water and covered with ointment twice a day until day four or five, when the ointment is switched to antibiotic cream with or without cortisone.

When gel or colloid dressings are used, the patient should be seen in the office on day one or two because of the problems of fluid accumulation under the dressing, as happens with Op-Site, or with potential drying out and sticking, as with Vigolone. Reapplication of these dressings requires skill and experience and four hands. The length of time the semipermeable dressing is left in place depends on how the wound is progressing; if oozing continues, switch to open healing and application of ointment. If

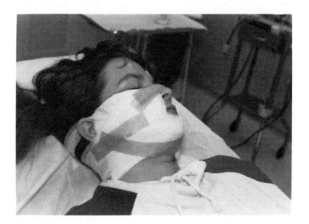

FIG 5–17.
Several layers of gauze are securely fixed just above the semipermeable dressing. The completed wrap is necessary the first night regardless what kind of dressing is used under it.

the wounds are dry and granulating, the dressings can stay on for one to two weeks. It is important to follow the patient closely when using these coverings; the soap, water, and ointment routine, on the other hand, can be followed by the patient alone, without office visits.

In the past few years it has become an unwritten practice among experienced abraders to follow the patient closely for two to six weeks postoperatively. It is in that window that slow or nonhealing patches can be discovered and treated as areas of potential scarring. If an area is purposely abraded deeper to obliterate some deep scars and the operator remembers them, longer healing times can be expected. Conversely, in a field of skin supposedly abraded evenly a few patches may be much slower to heal, noted clinically by failure to re-epithelialize, persistent redness or pinkness, and a palpable interstitial edema. The cause of that slow healing is because the skin was abraded deeper, or is infected, or for whatever reason the blood supply is not as good, or there is excess movement. The cause will probably remain obscure, but the treatment needs to start *immediately* and *may* prevent scarring.

The treatment for areas of slow healing is systemic antibiotics and walking a tightrope with steroids. Antibiotics are used for the possibility of a subclinical infection and can be chosen from a broad spectrum of types. The type of steroid and dosage are determined by trial. If there are massive areas of slow healing or nonhealing, systemic dosages given intramuscularly or orally for a few days are indicated. If there are only patches, they can be covered with steroid-impregnated tape—e.g., Cordran cut out to fit the troublesome area only. If after a week the patch is healing better, topical creams and ointments are adequate. If at any time the patch looks worse, intralesional treatment is indicated, starting at 5 mg/ml triamcinolone acetonide, working up to 20 mg/ml as needed. These patients should be seen weekly and advised that there are areas of slow healing that may scar and that frequent, long-term follow-up is necessary.

Fortunately, the greatest percentage of slow healing areas will eventually heal completely with no permanent markings. Unpredictably—at least clinically—some areas develop into scars. It is

much wiser to treat the potential scar-forming areas early. Treatment does not adversely affect the skin in any way, you have been alert and diligent in recognizing and treating a potential problem, you have maintained the patient's trust, and you and the patient are spared the possibility that some other physician or friend or aunt or beautician will say to the patient, "You've been scarred by that doctor."

Frequent and long-term treatment is the key to all postabrasion scarring. If the patient returns weeks or months later with scarring, start out immediately with intralesional steroids. Give injections every three weeks with gradually increasing doses of triamcinolone acetonide between 5 and 20 mg/ml until there is an adequate response; continue this plan for months and follow the patient for years. Try to resist the patient's request to "cut out" the scars. Time and steroids are the best and only treatment.

Sun avoidance is the most important advice to be stressed during postoperative visits. Protection from the sun for a minimum of 3 to 6 months is mandatory. In some very sensitive individuals, a single episode of extensive exposure can stimulate pigmentation. Remember to warn your patients that after insult the melanocytes sometimes do not become active for several months. It may take 6 to 8 weeks, long after the scabs and erythema have resolved, for the pigment to begin to appear. A rule of thumb is that the earlier hyperpigmentation appears, the more likely that it will spontaneously resolve in 3 to 6 months; the later it appears, the more likely it is to be permanent. Happily for all, sunscreens are being developed which are better protectors and more pleasant to use.

Persistent erythema is only rarely a problem with dermabrasion (it is much more common postphenol or TCA peeling) (Fig 5–18). We have not seen it persist longer than 6 months. If the patient reports that the redness comes on in waves or with certain events like exercise, a hot environment, or showers, consider the possibility of an exaggerated blush response which can be blocked by the beta-blocks such as propanolol. Otherwise, just wait it out.

Makeup is quite successful not only for postabrasion erythema, but for covering the unsightliness of wounded, healing skin. Any time you

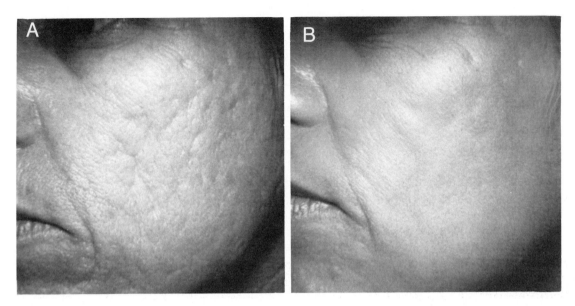

FIG 5–18.
A, 43-year-old woman before dermabrasion, with multiple, varied facial scars. **B,** 4 months postabrasion and still showing erythema although with much smoother skin. The erythema always fades but is slow to disappear in some patients.

can convince a patient to seek professional counseling for makeup, everyone benefits. The patient can return to normal activity much more quickly and the improvement from the dermabrasion is enhanced many times. Makeup can go on as soon as the scabs come off. There are many right ways to provide patient instruction about makeup: train yourself or one of your staff in the use of makeup, develop a professional relationship with an aesthetitian, have good literature available for the patient.

Complications

Scarring is the most serious of the complications (Fig 5–19). It is the result of a wound deeper than the body can heal without turning on the scarring-type of repair, and probably indicates a wound into the deep or compacted dermis or lower; or, scarring can also be the result of something that extends the depth of the wound, such as infection, repeated irritation, movement across the delicate granulations, or an altered substrate such as postirradiation, malnutrition, or systemic disease. When scarring is manifest, the history should be reviewed for possible factors. A few can be corrected or altered.

The appearance of scars can occur "suddenly" 6 weeks to 3 months posttreatment, or slow-healing areas can progress into scars. Postabrasion scars often will develop around the mouth or along the jawline. Time alone will soften many scars, but we recommend treatment as soon as they are noticed. Small, flat scars will respond to tape-impregnated steroids or high-potency creams, but most raised or fibrotic scars need intralesional therapy. As discussed above, the drug to use is triamcinolone acetonide 4 to 20 mg/ml every three weeks until resolution. Frequently, triamcenalone hexacetonide persists in the skin, leading to visible accumulations of the drug and prolonged drug activity that produces atrophy of the surrounding tissues.

We introduce this next complication with reservation. In 1986, Rubenstein, Stegman, Roenigk, and Hanke published a preliminary report on delayed development of scarring postdermabrasion in six patients who had been treated with isotretinoin (Accutane).[24] We had agonized about whether or not to publish that paper and apparently so did the editor of the journal. Wisely, senior dermatologists and experienced dermabraders did not want to see our observations in print in a refereed journal because of the in-

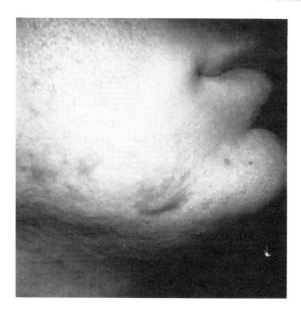

FIG 5–19.
A 25-year-old man 3 months postabrasion. This fibrotic scar was gradually improved with intralesional cortisone injections.

stant medical-legal implications that would be created. On the other hand, if our combined experiences were valid, we wanted to prevent further trouble. One of us (Roenigk) had even previously recommended dermabrasion while the patient was still on isotretinoin and he felt strongly about the need to reverse his advice.

The six cases developed hypertrophic scars 1 to 4 months after abrasion (Fig 5–20). The scars developed on areas of thick skin such as the cheeks, and there were no other obvious reasons for the scars. Also, the scars developed de novo; they were not in areas of slow healing. Actually, healing in all 6 cases was progressing uneventfully when the scars "suddenly" appeared. Each case resolved slowly with standard treatment and time, leaving only small, permanent marks. Our advice then as now was not to dermabrade patients until at least 6 to 12 months following the withdrawal of isotretinoin. It is arbitrary advice.

We do not know and may never know whether or not there is a relationship between isotretinoin and delayed scarring after dermabrasion. We suspect most abraders are waiting 6 months before treatment.

Pigmentary aberrations are the most common complications—so common that hypopigmentation might be categorized as an expected side effect rather than a complication. Hypopigmentation may occur in as many as 50% of all abrasions. The discoloration presents in a variety of ways: even, hypopigmentation of the entire abraded area which is clearly visible at the junction of the treated and untreated borders, splotchy or pinto-pony pattern, or muddy patches that fall on the same areas as melasma. The demarcation line(s) and the splotchy patterns are the most difficult to cover with makeup (Fig 5–21). Otherwise objective, intelligent, grateful patients who have been left with these color changes relate that the need for makeup even before they feel comfortable running errands is a huge burden not offset by the gains of dermabrasion.

Because the problem is loss of color and color differential, the method of correction is to try to bleach the untreated skin or reduce the color differential. Bleaching agents are of minimal value. Re-abrading or peeling the margins sometimes softens the difference between the treated

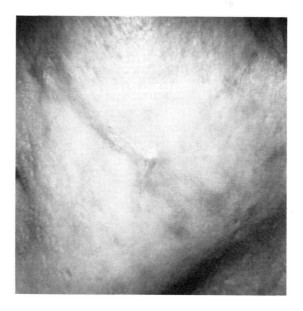

FIG 5–20.
A linear thick, fibrotic scar that appeared three months postabrasion on a 36-year-old woman who had completed a full course of isotretinoin (Accutane) 3 months before abrasion.

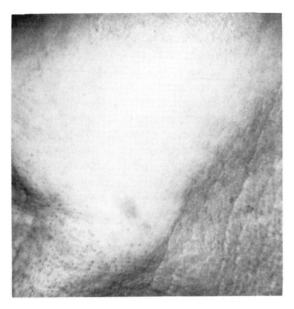

FIG 5–21.
The cheek/neck junction of a 30-year-old man showing the demarcation line of the hypopigmented, abraded skin next to the normal-color, nonabraded neck skin.

and untreated skin, but often does not work. These techniques carry their own risks. We have seen cases in which the neck was peeled in an attempt to depigment it, only to have it hyperpigment—in a splotchy pattern, making things much worse. Fortunately, we have also seen peeling help soften the differential. If the patient is desperate for some help, try wood stains. Pick an appropriate stain color (usually almond) at the paint store, then paint tiny amounts of stain on the hypopigmented areas with a cotton-tipped applicator. The skin stays stained for a week or so until the keratin layer sheds naturally.

Hyperpigmentation is the second pigment problem. Although not uncommon at 3 months postop, it is far less frequent than hypopigmentation. Often the pigment will fade, indicating possible postinflammatory melanin deposits in the corneocytes, and will be lost as those cells mature, move up, and slough off. The sooner treatment is started the better it seems to work—for reasons we do not know. Hydroquinone is the only active chemical for depigmenting that is safe and trustworthy as a medicament. How it is delivered and with which other agents is the physician's choice. Certainly creams with

2%, 4%, or 6% concentrations are old standards. The solvents with 4% to 6% solutions, such as Neutrogena Vehicle-N, are efficacious. And the addition of tretinoin may affect absorption, which increases efficiency. Sun avoidance and regular use of ultraviolet-blocking sun screens is obvious.

Repeated peeling with very light agents such as Jessner's formula can speed the loss of hyperpigmentation. This is an opinion only, but it is based on the experience of several physicians.

Grooving or long troughs in the skin almost always indicate error in physician techniques, and can occur if a surgeon is inexperienced. It is simply the result of abrasion of irregular depth by someone using the linear stroke method. It also is more likely to happen when a firm freeze is used. The only treatment is to re-abrade lightly, trying to even out the depth of wound. With time, the skin will remodel somewhat, but if the troughs are deep, the patient is not likely to want to wait for improvement.

Milia can be expected to appear in almost every patient. They spontaneously disappear in a few months, but simple unroofing with a #11 blade or a touch with hot cautery will eliminate them. A few patients develop massive numbers of milia and only need reassurance. As mentioned above, scrubbing the skin with saline and gauze just after the abrasion may help prevent or reduce the number of milia.

Herpes simplex can colonize the entire wound, or form numerous isolated lesions. Today, acyclovir is effective treatment, and effective prophylaxis if the patient has a history of herpes. Even when sores developed in the days before acyclovir, conservative, nonspecific therapy seemed to work and most patients healed without scarring.

Bacterial infections are rare and most often merely the result of excessive contamination in the eschar. Soap and water work quickly and well, even when the peagreen signs of *Pseudomonas* are present. Naturally, any signs of systemic infection, although quite rare, must quickly be covered with cultures and appropriate therapy.

Acne flares happen with some regularity in those patients who still have active acne or the potential for it. These occurrences are usually short-lived, but seem to be the most persistent in adult women who have the adult form of female acne. The standard acne therapies are indicated. Or, another course of Accutane may be necessary to curtail this condition.

References

1. Kromayer E: Die heilung der akne durch in neves norbenlases operations verfahren. Das Stanzen. *Illustr Monatsschr Aerztl Polytech* 1905; 27:101.

2. Kromayer E: Cosmetic treatment of skin complaints (English translation of the 2nd German [1929] edition). New York, Oxford University Press, 1930, p 9.

3. Kromayer E: Das Frasen in der Kosmetik. *Kosmetologishe Rundschau* 1933; 4:61.

4. Luikart R, Ayres S III, Wilson JW: Recent advances in medicine and surgery: Surgical skin planing. *NY State J Med* 1959; 59:3413–3437.

5. Karp FL, Nieman HA, Lerner C: Cryotherapy for acne and its scars. *Arch Dermatol Syphilol* 1939; 39:995.

6. Janson P: Eine einfache methods der entfernung von Tatauierungen. *Dermatol Monatsschr* 1935; 101:894.

7. Cannon AB: Treatment of x-ray burns and other superficial disfigurements. *NY State J Med* 1940; 40:391.

8. Iverson PC: Surgical removal of traumatic tattoos. *Plast Reconstruct Surg* 1947; 2:427.

9. McEvitt WG: Acne pits. *J Michigan Med Soc* 1948; 47:1243.

10. Robbins N: Dr. Abner Kurtin, father of ambulatory dermabrasion. *J Dermatol Surg Oncol* 1988; 14:425–431.

11. Kurtin A: Corrective surgical planing of skin. *Arch Dermatol Syphilol* 1953; 68:389.

12. Wentzell JM, Robinson JK, Schwartz DE: Physical properties of aerosols produced by dermabrasion. Presented at annual meeting of American Society for Dermatologic Surgery, Ft. Lauderdale, Fla., 1989.

13. Hanke CW, Roenigk HH, Pinski JB: Complications of dermabrasion resulting from excessively cold skin refrigeration. *J Dermatol Surg Oncol* 1985; 11:896–900.

14. Hanke CW, O'Brian JJ: A histologic evaluation of the effects of skin refrigerants in an animal model. *J Dermatol Surg Oncol* 1987; 13:664–669.

15. Dzubow LM: Histologic and temperature alterations induced by skin refrigerants. *J Am Acad Dermatol* 1985; 12:796–810.

16. Dzubow LM: Survey of refrigeration and surgical technics used for facial dermabrasion. *J Am Acad Dermatol* 1985; 13:287–292.

17. Strauss JS, Kligman AM: Acne. *Arch Dermatol Syphilol* 1956; 74:397.

18. Yarborough JM Jr: Dermabrasion by wire brush. *J Dermatol Surg Oncol* 1987; 13:610–615.

19. Stegman SJ: A comparative histologic study of the effects of three peeling agents and dermabrasion on normal and sun-damaged skin. *Aesth Plast Surg* 1982; 6:123–135.

20. Roenigk HH Jr: Dermabrasion, in Roenigk RK, Roenigk HH (eds): *Dermatologic Surgery, Principles and Practice*. New York: Marcel Dekker, Inc. 1988.

21. Cohen BH: Prevention of postdermabrasion milia (letter). *J Dermatol Surg Oncol* 1988; 14:1301.

22. Flanaga V: Occlusive wound dressings: Why, when, which. Presented at Hawaii Dermatology Seminar, Feb 1989.

23. Pinski JB: Dressings for dermabrasion: Occlusive dressings and wound healing. *Cutis* 1986; 37:471–476.

24. Rubenstein R, Roenigk HH Jr, Stegman SJ, et al: Atypical keloids after dermabrasion of patients taking isotretinoin. *J Am Acad Dermatol* 1986; 15:280–285.

Six

Surgical Management of Alopecia

Punch Transplants

History

The curious and perhaps apocryphal story persists that the ancient Japanese transplanted hair centuries ago. It was necessary for a virginal bride to have adequate pubic hair. Those with less sought help, and the "doctors" of the day transplanted scalp hairs successfully.

Reports of transplantation of hair and feathers in animals and humans was published in Austria in 1822 by Dieffenbach.[1] His work was probably influenced by his teacher Dom Unger. Repair of traumatic alopecia with full-thickness, hair-bearing grafts has been reported in the literature since 1893.[2]

Some of the first hair transplantation papers in the United States were published by Butcher, who worked with albino rats.[3] In the 1930s and 1940s, many papers reported how tissue—hair-bearing tissue—was transplanted to study subjects with conditions as varied as pigment formation, wound healing, amyloidosis, scleroderma, drug eruptions, and hyperhidrosis.[4]

In a study published in 1959, Norman Orentreich described multiple transplantations performed on various types of alopecia: alopecia prematura, alopecia areata, alopecia cicatrisata, and other conditions such as morphea, vitiligo, and lupus erythematosus.[4] The biopsies were taken with cylindrical, power-driven punches ranging from 1 to 12 mm in diameter that were especially designed and manufactured by Noel Robbins of the Robbins Instrument Company, Catham, N.J.

In that paper Orentreich introduced the concept of donor and recipient follicular dominance, and proved that alopecia prematura (now called male pattern alopecia, or MPA) was a donor follicular-dominant condition. Eventually, these studies demonstrated that scalp hair would grow when moved from growing areas to bald areas. Hair grew when transplanted by punches smaller than 5 mm in diameter, and seemed to grow for at least the four-year period of follow-up for that study.

Concurrent with Orentreich's work were the hair shaft insertion method of Sasagawa[5] and the full-thickness autografts of hair-bearing skin for the correction of alopecia of the scalp, eyebrows, and moustache area by Okuda.[6, 7] In the days of the Manchurian conquests and military expansion of Imperial Japan, followed by World War II, the publications of these Japanese researchers were lost to the Western world.

In his work during the 1960s, Orentreich realized that there was a genetic difference in scalp hairs; simply stated, fringe hairs are not lost, but frontal and crown hairs are lost in various patterns and at various ages. Now medical science has confirmed that male pattern alopecia (MPA) is genetically determined[8] by receptors for androgens in each individual hair follicle[9] and is only secondarily affected by vascular supply,[10] hygiene,[11] or diet.[12]

The history of the instrumentation, the various techniques, and the ancillary methods for the surgical treatment of MPA are described below.

Instruments and Equipment
Punches

One of the first regular uses of a punch in clinical dermatology was described and published by Edward Keyes in 1879.[13] However, the New York dermatologist and historian Herman Goodman, M.D., stated that B. A. Watson, M.D., used a similar instrument for tattoo removal a decade before Keyes.[14] The first description of a motor-driven rotary punch was published in 1951 by Urbach and Shelley.[15] And as mentioned above, Orentreich's original study used motor-driven punches. As he refined the technique between 1959 and 1967, however, he designed a hand-held punch described as a stainless-steel

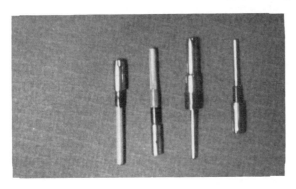

FIG 6–1.
Hair transplant punches. (Left) Orentreich type with long linear grooves parallel to handle; (second left) Resnik-Lewis punch with diamond cross-cut knurled handle; (third left) Australian power punch; (right) American power punch.

cylinder cup with a sharpened rim, attached at its base to a mandril-type handle 3.0 mm in diameter and knurled for good gripping between the thumb and index fingers.[16]

Through the years, several modifications of the punch used for hair transplantation have been made, seeking to produce a plug that is cylindrical rather than conical (Fig 6–1). This was accomplished by making the punch wall thinner than the thick-walled punch that Keyes borrowed from leather workers. Also, the cutting edge was sharpened on the inside, with the bevel on the outside. These punches served well for many years and could be sharpened by machine, making it practical to keep them sharp by sending them out or training a staff person to sharpen them in the office.

Stough designed a thicker handle for the Orentreich punch; Lewis and Resnik added more knurls on the handle to make it easier to hold; Orentreich and Pierce both designed detachable handles so the proximal end of the handle rested against the operator's palm, thus reducing fatigue when many plugs were taken.[17] Arouete of Paris also designed a longer handle which could be attached to the Orentreich punch for the same purposes.[18]

The surgeon's goal in punch transplants is to harvest a transplant with minimal damage to the follicles and to include as many follicles as possible in a plug of a given diameter. Hagerman and Wilson published the results of their tinkering, undertaken in Dr. Wilson's garage, which

produced a thin-walled, cylindrical punch that vastly improved the biopsy sample obtained.[19] In 1972 one of us (T.A.T.) designed and had manufactured a thin-walled, cylindrical punch with the tip sharpened on the outside (internal bevel) in hopes of harvesting a more cylindrical plug of tissue. Two experienced Australian physicians, Richard Shiell and Frank Torok, designed punches of high-density carbon steel, with two holes rather than one for the exit of air and debris, and an end with both the internal and external edges sharpened. Rolf Nordström of Finland and O'Tar Norwood also separately designed punches similar to the ones from Australia. Robbins Instrument Company manufactured these models. Originally the double-sharpened end was honed to a 20-degree angle, but recent communication with Dr. Shiell informs us that he now recommends a 15-degree angle on the external side and a 5-degree angle on the inside lip. He also stresses the importance of proper sharpening: a rotating tapered metal rod for the inside, and a buffing wheel with jeweler's rouge for the outside.

We notice a difference in the shape of the plug produced by the three types of punches. The internal bevel (usually thin-walled and sharpened on the outside edge—the Tromovitch design) gives a cylindrical plug with a slight bulge of fat below. The external bevel (the original Orentreich type—sharpened on the inside, usually a thick-walled punch) produces a slightly conical plug. The double-edged sharpened punch (which is called Australian) produces a cylinder from the surface to the subcutaneous junction and a larger amount of fat below (Fig 6–2).

Because the diameter of the punch is measured from one sharpened edge to the other, the location of the bevel makes a difference in the true width of the plug harvested with an internal vs. external bevel: the external bevel produces a slightly smaller plug. This difference is of little importance except in the fine adjustments of fitting the donor plugs into the recipient openings. Sometimes, although not routinely, we will harvest with an internal bevel and insert the plug into an opening made with a punch of the same diameter which has an external bevel. The plug is only slightly larger than the opening. This small difference is noticeable on scalps where

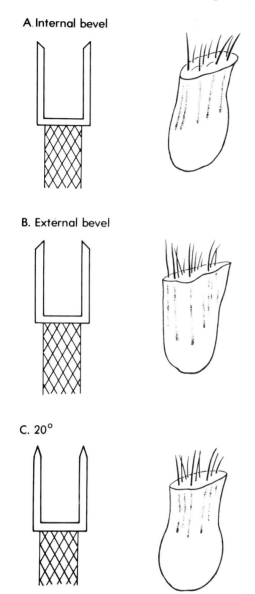

A. Internal bevel

B. External bevel

C. 20°

FIG 6–2.
A, internal bevel punch construction with the type of plug it produces. **B**, external bevel punch and the tapered plug produced. **C**, 20-degree-angle punch with the plug it produces, which has a fat bulge but is otherwise cylindrical.

the Bell hand engine for harvesting; other hand-held machines will work, but for low noise and ease of holding it is hard to beat the Bell (Fig 6–3).

We use the motor-driven punch for harvesting nearly all of our donor grafts. We do not use it to cut the recipient openings, for two important reasons. First, if there is some hair in the recipient area, there is a chance the rotating punch may get caught in that hair and pull some of it out. It does not hurt, because the patient's scalp is numbed, but it is poor form, and a nuisance to pull the hairs off the punch. The recipient-area hairs can be wetted with water or oil to keep them flat and out of the way. Second, the power punch cuts a more cylindrical opening and the hand punch cuts a more conical opening. Thus, the power-punched cylindrical transplant fits a bit tighter into the conical-shaped hand punch opening. It is a small difference, but is often just enough to hold the plug in without having to go to the next opening .5 mm wider.

It is most important to realize that the value of these variations has not been proven. There are technically beautiful photographs taken with a macro lens[20] showing what are perceived to be "good" and "bad" plugs. The angle of the cut, the sharpness of the punch, and the speed of rotation are factors that affect the appearance of the grafts. But to our knowledge the critical study

there is little shrinkage of the plug after harvesting, and little gaping of the recipient holes.

The reintroduction of motor-driven punches was an advance for this type of surgery. The plugs harvested by machine are visibly more cylindrical, have fewer follicles transsected, and have a much lower incidence of lipping. We use

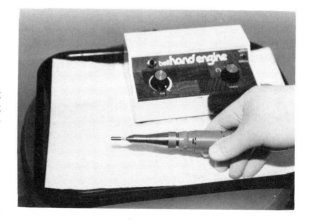

FIG 6–3.
The Bell international hand engine with a mounted transplant punch.

has not been done that answers the question: *do they grow better hair?* It would be a difficult if not impossible study to perform because transplants grow differently depending on the location on the scalp and the number of plugs in a given area. Also for unknown reasons, different sessions produce different successes. Obviously, transsected roots or mangled plugs will not produce as many hairs, but slight coning or variations in the fat on the plug or even slight lipping probably do not greatly affect the outcome. We performed hair transplantation for many years with good results before the development of motor-driven punches and internal bevel punch, and before saline swelling of the donor area.

Size. A punch with a diameter of 4 mm is most frequently used to harvest. In patients with poor density (fewer hairs per square area), 4.5-mm plugs are harvested and pushed into 4.0-mm openings. In younger patients and patients with thick, vascular scalps, 4.5-mm plants grow well but do not do well when planted too close together, crowded into one area, or planted in the center of the crown. More hairs per plug are moved with larger plants, but as proven by Unger, produce no greater increase than the measured increase in area.[32] The larger number of hairs transplanted with the 4.5-mm plants makes a difference when trying to move as many hairs as possible. The larger plants are suited for the side the part is on, or just behind the front two or three rows. They are less well-suited for the frontal line or the crown, where they tend to accentuate the plugging effect.

Morbidity is surprisingly less when 4.0-mm punches are used. There is less bleeding, and donor-site healing by second intention is quicker. Also, the larger plugs waste more of the donor area because the diamond-shaped scalp that remains between plugs is larger (this is not a factor when total harvesting is performed). Except when using a 4.5-mm punch, we start out with a 4.0-mm punch. For subsequent sets, we adjust the size based on the results. If the plugs grow well, we repeat with a 4.0-mm punch, or may try a 4.5. If the plugs grow poorly, we may spread them out farther, do fewer in an area, or try a smaller punch.

Very rarely are 3.5-mm punches used, except to transplant miniplugs for fill-ins or hairlines. These techniques are discussed below. Unfortunately, some physicians use the smaller punches to increase the fee. Plugs made with punches larger than 4.5-mm have a poor growth history, with few hairs growing in the entire plug, or only the peripheral hairs growing.

Sharpness. Sharpness is the most important factor for the punches—hand-held or motor-driven. Transplants cut with a dull or nicked punch are irregularly shaped and have more lipping. On average, the punches should be sharpened after each 25 plugs. The experienced operator can easily tell whether or not a punch is sharp—even motor-driven punches. A punch should be replaced as soon as dullness becomes apparent, whether after only 1 or 2 grafts have been cut, or after more than 25. Scalp turgor also affects the speed at which a punch will become dull. The saline injections seem to soften the skin. Therefore, have many punches available so that dull ones can be exchanged frequently for sharp ones.

Chair Vs. Table

We differ with Walter Unger (someone we greatly respect, and from whom we have learned a great deal about hair transplantation) on the preferred patient position.[21] We have always liked to have the patient sit. Dr. Unger and others like the patient supine for harvesting, and prone or semiprone for planting, arguing that when the patient is seated, the operator's hand is necessarily in an uncomfortable position and that it is hard to see and cut the plugs at the proper angle. Because we use a barber chair that elevates and turns, and because we steady the patient's head while tipping it forward (which reduces the necessary dorsiflexion of the hand), the visibility of the field and the position of the dominant hand seems quite good (Fig 6–4).

The only drawback to using the chair is that when a patient develops syncope, we stop the operation and lay the patient back. Syncope is not a problem when the patient is prone. Otherwise, we have stayed with the barber chair for several reasons: the patient stays in the same position for harvesting, planting, wrapping, and discussions; also, the patient is comfortable and

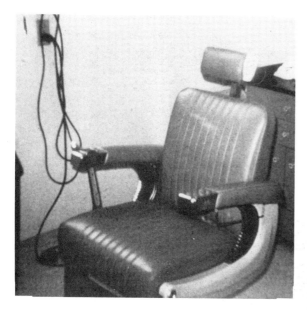

FIG 6–4.
Barber or hair stylist's chair used for hair transplant surgery.

does not fatigue as easily and can read or watch TV if desired. And, patients do not spend hours facing the floor with their faces buried in some special pillow. The physician and office staff can easily move around the room and have access to all sides of the patient. And, most important, if the patient is able to sit and converse with the doctor and staff and look around, the procedure is much more enjoyable and less frightening.

Having the patient sit or lie down is the physician's prerogative and makes a difference only if the physician is not comfortable. We know excellent transplanters from both schools.

Instruments

The types of needle holders, scissors, forceps, and other instruments used are the physician's choice. Easy access to the instrument tray is helpful, and once in a while during the procedure the instruments need to be wiped off and arranged in an orderly fashion. The only instrument we like that is not routinely used is the Coverse (Wilmer) scissors which bends 45 degrees at the proximal end of the blades so they can be inserted under a plug to cut the fat attachment (Fig 6–5). These scissors reduce operator fatigue because they keep the hand and

wrist down rather than the whole arm held up as it is when pushing a straight scissors under the plug.

We have never felt the need for the many gadgets developed for hair transplantation. Pneumatic tourniquets, marking grids and chains, chin rests, and the like have never seemed necessary. We used the cooled gel-filled holders for the petri dishes for a while, but they, like other toys, soon fell out of use as we drifted back to making the procedure as simple as possible.

Nowadays there is clearly a greater need for doctor and staff protection from blood and tissue debris. Particles of a size that can be inhaled are generated by motor-driven punches, in addition to the obvious splatter. Therefore, face shields, masks, gloves, and gowns are strongly recommended (Fig 6–6).

Patient Selection

The irony of hair transplantation is that if they are seen or detected there is often a negative connotation, while good results go unnoticed. Also, the gradual, stepwise procedure necessarily exposes incomplete work to the public. Will we ever really know the thousands of men who did not even get as far as the consultation before they were turned off by the procedure because they "have seen transplants and don't want any part of it." We must keep these unknown potential patients in mind when we accept patients for surgery and when we plan the course of treatment. Otherwise, we will drive

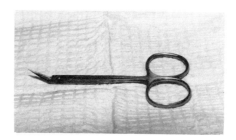

FIG 6–5.
Biro dermal naevus scissors with angled blades, which makes harvesting plugs easier.

Surgical Management of Alopecia

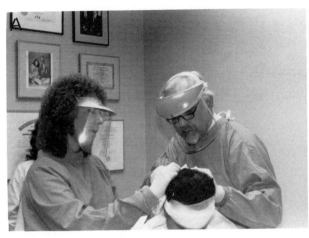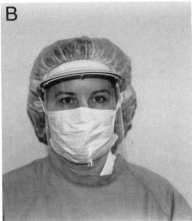

FIG 6–6.
A and **B**, gowns, gloves, masks, and shields are recommended.

away many, many potential candidates. Sticking a row or two of plugs on the front of a completely bald head may make one person happy, but how many who see that will ever again consider a transplant?

Of the many considerations discussed below, two stand out: the quality of the donor hair and the willingness of the patient to *complete* the procedure. It is impossible to create thick, transplanted hair from donor hair that is sparse, irregularly spaced, or of limited area. This is not to say that many patients with sparse and limited donors are not acceptable candidates for transplants—many are—but rather that a thick hairline and a full crown cannot be made from poor donors.

The assessment of the donor area and sharing that assessment with the patient are some of the first activities of a transplantation consultation. Record your findings and the results of discussion.

The second helpful patient characteristic is willingness and ability to complete the process. This includes the willingness to come back and be inconvienced by multiple procedures over several years, the ability to pay for several operations, and the unwillingness to become satisfied too soon. Bosley spoke at the annual meeting of the American Academy of Cosmetic Surgery in January 1989 and advanced the concept of patients being "too early happy." When

one or two sets of plugs are growing, they become satisfied, leaving the orchard on the crown and the cornstocks on the frontal row exposed for all to see. Again, this is not to say that patients with lesser financial means cannot be successfully transplanted—many can—but they require a different treatment plan than the patient who can have many surgeries as fast as safely possible.

A poor candidate for transplants is the young man just starting to lose his hair. Whether a man is 18 or 22 years old, at the beginning of the balding process *no one* can predict what his pattern of loss will be. Until some idea about the total loss area, and equally important, the size of the remaining donor area, can be determined, an orderly plan cannot be formulated. Do not let a young man talk you into filling in a few plugs to cover his temporal recession. There is nothing more difficult than to try later to build a normal hairline with even consistency around 20 or so plugs put in when that patient was 21. Also, when some of these men mature they are not as concerned with their appearance as they were when young. They retain those frontal transplants and lose the hair behind them. This leaves your work out there like a hairy island for all to see and for others to decide "what transplants really look like."

There are some cases in which the family history supports the *guess* that there will not be extensive hair loss; in these cases, frontal fill-ins are acceptable. Even then it is a treacherous undertaking because the quality and texture of the hair from the donor area may age differently than the hairs near the front.

How the patient grooms his thinning pate tells something about his aesthetic awareness and thus his capacity to understand what you say and why your recommendations are appropriate. The man who wears his thinning hair cut moderately short and combed over and down usually has some aesthetic insight, while the fellow who has let his remaining hairs grow long and tortured, teased them all around his head, and sprayed them solid will require some education. These men are used to the illusion—although poorly created—that they have lots of hair up front. What can be done for them through transplantation will be better-looking hair but much less of it in height and volume. Get out the comb and break that straw. Comb the hair down and over, or side to side, and indicate how much should be cut off and how transplants kept 2 to 4 inches long will blend in, be manageable, and will not tend to "fly away." Have the patient try the style you recommend before you start the surgeries. (We are aware of newer techniques that attempt to build such a natural frontal hairline that patients need not comb the hair down, or down and over, to hide the plugging effect. This will be addressed below.)

On the other hand, nothing hides the slow process of hair transplantation as well as the sprayed-down long combover. Patients can camouflage the surgery until several sets are done and growing, and then make the big switch. For some patients, the clinically apparent process of a transplant is traumatic either way.

A slightly less desirable patient is the one who combs his hair straight back because he is losing all of it over the front and crown, and has dark-colored hair and a white scalp. It is only rarely that transplants can build a frontal line that looks natural enough to allow this man to continue his pretransplant style. Remember that although you may make one man happy by acceding to his wishes, you may ultimately drive many others away.

The patient with curly or kinky hair is often a good transplant candidate because of the nat-

ural camouflage. Fewer curved than straight hairs are needed to cover the scalp, and the plugging effect is not as easily seen. Some transplanted patients may get a "perm" to help hide the plugging effect. Technically, the curly or kinky hairs are harvested in the same manner. The follicles are often curved as well, and a few may be transsected, but with close observation, the operator can adjust to the curved roots and harvest them without damage. Blacks do well with transplants, and even though slightly fewer hairs per plug survive the cutting, the overall effect is good.

There is a large population of adult men aged 40 to 60 years who would benefit from having only the central crown transplanted. These men do not have enough donors to build a good frontal hairline *and* cover the rest of the crown. They have a narrow fringe over the occiput. A marked aesthetic improvement is possible, however, by using their limited numbers of donors across the center of the head. They end up with a high forehead, open crown, and thin hair, but are not bald (Fig 6–7). These features are normal in many men their age. The fact that the transplants are high on the head and not exposed, as they are on the crown or frontal line, and that the hair is combed over the central scalp, nicely hides the plugging effect, even though there is a total of only about 100 plugs.

Age and gray hair are not contraindications for transplantation. It is the health and density of the hair and scalp that are critical. Actually, salt-and-pepper hair produces good transplants because the color differential helps hide the plugging effect. How long someone has been bald is not important, but how thin his scalp has become is important. In patients with thin scalps, plugs may be planted somewhat horizontally in a pocket made under the thin scalp skin. The plugs will grow, but seldom can enough be placed to produce a superior cosmetic result. This technique is best reserved for reconstruction after trauma, such as burns or scalp avulsions covered with split-thickness skin grafts.

Test Plants

We differ on the regularity that we offer test plants. T.A.T. and R.G.G. nearly always do; S.J.S. seldom does. An important reason for a test plant is that there is no better tool for in-

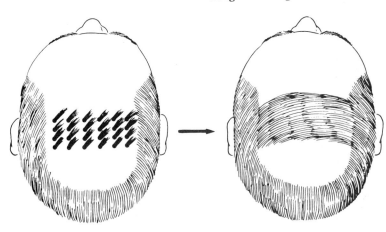

FIG 6–7.
Design to plant the center of the crown and to comb hair over for those men who do not have enough donor hairs for the entire bald area.

formed consent than going through the entire procedure. A test plant also teaches patients how to care for plugs and what postoperative healing and appearance really involve. And, there is no better way to convince the patient about the limitations of transplantation. If the goal of test plants is to walk the patient through the procedure for education and to allay his fears about the operation, test plants work, but if the goal is to demonstrate the "plugging effect," then six months must elapse before the process continues.

The reasons not to test include delay in a process already too long for many. In reality, little is gained that is not covered in a proper consultation. And it is wrong to set in four plugs randomly: the master plan must be determined and those four plugs placed in line with the plants that will follow. With a test, a lot of time and inconvenience are invested for little gain.

On the other hand, if the physician wants or needs to truly *test* whether or not plants will grow, trial plants are recommended. Sparse donors, thin scalp, scar tissue, severe skin disease like psoriasis, scarring potential, and other factors suggest that test plants are helpful. In these cases, four to ten plants near the existing hair fringe just above the parietal scalp can be hidden, do not require more work, and serve as a good test for growth.

Plan

Each patient should rightfully expect a plan that includes an estimate of the number of plants and other surgeries (i.e., the cost), the time se-

quence, and the expected outcome. Because most patients do not realize how difficult it is to propose such a plan until the results of surgery are actually seen, point out that your proposed plan may change as the process evolves. It is difficult to encourage the patient to complete the process on the one hand and, on the other, not be able to tell him exactly what will happen. Therefore, this aspect of hair replacement surgery requires a certain amount of patient trust from the beginning.

The treatment plan is the one area where we differ the most from our colleagues. A four-session, geometrical pattern to achieve a full head of hair has been the standard approach published and presented for many years, and is still the primary technique discussed, as evidenced by its inclusion in the latest texts on hair transplantation and cutaneous surgery.[21, 22] At the first of the four sessions, the frontal hairline is established and plants are placed with slightly less than one-plug diameter between plugs and also one-plug diameter between rows (Fig 6–8). At the second session, plants are placed between the previous plugs and should fit closely because just enough room was left at session one. At visits three and four, the space between the rows is filled in similarly. There are variations on this basic plan: planting between the rows on session two, leaving two-punch diameters between plugs. Also, not all areas require four sessions; the frontal line, the anterior portion of the side of the part, and the center of the crown require the greatest density. The side opposite the part and any areas scheduled to be removed during scalp reduction procedures—large or small—receive fewer plants.

We have used this technique because it works. We have seen beautiful results from other physicians who use it. We trust the reports and respect the authors who stress that this is the best way to arrange the plants. However, in our practice, far less than one-half of the transplant patients can afford so many plants or afford the time or money to have four sets done sequentially. It appears that far less than one-half of our patients have the wonderful, dense donor hairs we see almost exclusively in publications and at meetings. Some of our patients develop scar tissue around their plants, and subsequent plants that abut those scars do not grow well. Some of our patients do not grow plants well posterior to the first two rows, no matter what we do. The purpose of these comments is to point out that frequently the presented and published results we see are from ideal candidates who have thick donors, unlimited funds, and the ability and inclination to have surgery frequently. Unfortunately for us, and we suspect for most, such patients are a small minority.

Other considerations in planning are (1) the patient's need and ability to cover the healing and healed, but not yet growing, plants; (2) how to get some growth in the center of the head where the results are the poorest and growth may not occur at all if the frontal blood supply

has been inderdicted by rows of plants; (3) whether or not scalp reductions will be used; and (4) the frequency with which the patient can have the surgeries.

On many patients, we begin in the center of the head or the center and the side of the part. In these areas the new plants are easiest to hide—they can be combed over from the side and on top—and are the least visible (Fig 6–9). The area of poorest growth is treated before the blood supply is interrupted peripherally. Plants grow best the closer they are to the forehead; plants placed farther forward can always be put in later. The "new" hairs on the top will be able to be combed over future transplants, especially in the frontal area where the surgery shows the most and looks the worst.

One or two sets behind what will be the final front line also serve as the best possible test plants. If there is poor growth, adjustments are possible before those critical frontal rows are put in. We like it when the patient is not in such a hurry that we have to put in more plants before the previous set(s) are growing. Several hundred plants may turn out to be less than optimal, but we will not know that before the first ones grow and demonstrate how well or poorly they are doing.

We do not recommend the much-maligned "scattershot" technique.[23] Each area transplanted should be done with careful attention

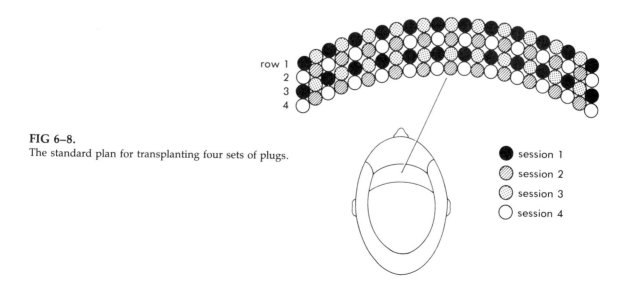

FIG 6–8.
The standard plan for transplanting four sets of plugs.

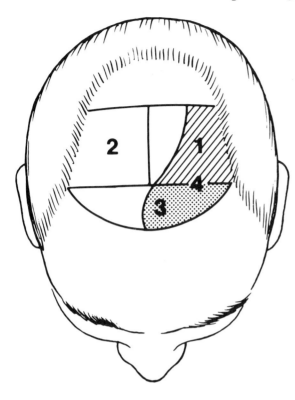

FIG 6–9.
Suggested plan for obtaining good coverage when there is less than an optimal number of donors available.

to spacing so subsequent plants will fit closely between existing plants and according to an overall plan. We also believe that not all—indeed not most—should begin with a four-session frontal half-circle program.

Planning for scalp reductions and mini- and microtransplants will be discussed here, and the actual designs and techniques of these procedures covered below. It has taken us 20 years of experience to realize that the normal frontal hairline is not a line at all but a gradual gradation of miniaturizing hairs that are most anterior to the terminal hairs behind it. The "line" varies: it may be only 5 mm wide in some but 1 to $1\frac{1}{2}$ cm in others. Although transplanters were pleased with creating dense hairlines, a degree of artificiality existed, and the cause of that unnatural appearance was not fully appreciated until scalp flaps were invented. Flaps create a sharp frontal line of dense hair and varying amounts of scar that further accentuate the line. This problem was addressed by burying the an-

terior suture line, cutting the leading edge of the flap irregularly, and by hair styling. Eventually, tiny plants were placed anterior to the flap line to break up the sharpness of the line. This technique soon grew into what we now call micro- and miniplants and focused our attention on what was aesthetically wrong with a full and tightly transplanted frontal hairline.

Micro- and miniplants, known by other names, especially for eyebrow reconstruction, are not new.[24, 25] The concept of recreating the true natural frontal line with small transplants has been appreciated by most transplanters only in the past five years. This truth spread rapidly, the instrument manufacturers became involved, and the aesthetic quality of hair transplantation jumped another quantum.

For the already transplanted patient who wants a better frontline, micro- or miniplants can be put in at any time. Now, when discussing the initial plan, we include the possibility of "completing" the frontal line with small plugs. In some patients who we *guess* will achieve a good front line, we recommend putting in a few microplants with each session. It is easy to harvest 10 to 30 microplants from a regular set of transplants when the area is already anesthesized. Because both types of plugs grow, the patient skips the artificial look and advances to a natural-appearing hairline.

Technique

Again, we encourage viewing videotapes and visiting colleagues to learn technique. Not only are basic methodology and variations learned, but it is possible to observe those subtle tricks that frequently even the operator does not realize are part of the procedure.

Preoperative Preparation

Any laboratory work ordered is based on the history. If the patient has no trouble clotting a shaving cut, it is not likely that routine laboratory studies will uncover any defects in clotting. It would be good to know if the patient is Hepatitis Ag positive or human immunodeficiency virus (HIV) Ab+ so proper precautions can be enforced. HIV-positive patients may need counseling and often do not heal as well as HIV-negative patients. CBC, SMA, and UA screening are indicated only if something in the history or physical warrants it.

Aspirin and nonsteroidal anti-inflammatory drugs must be stopped 10 to 14 days prior to surgery. We instruct the patient to wash his hair normally the night before or the morning of surgery. Infections are so rare with transplants (and most likely not from the patient himself) that we do not feel a need to upset the balance of the flora on the healthy patient with surgical preparations of the scalp. Comfortable, loose-fitting, front-buttoning clothing is preferred. We cover the patient with drapes, but not heavy surgical drapes, which are too warm to sit under for one and one-half to two hours. The patient is advised to let the hair in the donor area grow long so that it will completely cover the donor area in the first weeks postop. Occasionally, a patient will come in with a freshly cut, short haircut, thinking that it will be several weeks before he can get another one.

Preoperative antibiotic use is another option. More and more physicians admit to regular prophylactic antibiotic administration. There are so many different agents that the fear of sensitizing someone to the one or two medicines they may later need is gone. Broad-spectrum antibiotics are so commonplace and prescribed for such minor problems that trying to prevent an infection in a surgery that involves making 100- to 150 holes in the head seems relatively reasonable. Having said all of that, we rarely use antibiotics unless there is something in the patient's history, such as heart valve disease, or orthopedic prosthetic implant, or past transplant experience, that warrants it.

Prophylactic steroids are a different matter. Some transplanters use them routinely, especially when working in the frontal area which can produce forehead edema later. We are not aware of any problems from a pulse of steroids and use them if the patient has experienced swelling with past sets or has had them from another physician and requests them again. Intramuscular Celestone and oral prednisone or prenisolone seem to be the drugs used most frequently.

At the first session, we suggest that the patient have someone drive him home and that he take one or two days off work. After the first set, he can decide whether or not he wants to drive himself home and when he can go back to work. It is best if the patient comes back to our office the next morning so that our nurses can remove the wrap and clean the scalp. Cleaning the scalp on postop day one has proven to be a worthwhile effort. We are assured of the patient's recovery and that the plants are cleaned and not sitting in a bed of clots. On the first day, it is difficult for patients and even their family members to clean the plants. We can also reinforce postop instructions at a time when the patient is more likely to remember them.

Anesthesia and Analgesia

Analgesia is given according to the preference of the patient and physician. Most of the time, we do not give preoperative analgesia. The injection of anesthetic hurts a minute or so for local anesthesia, but then is painless. When analgesia is given, it often has the side effect of reducing the patients' inhibitions and they may behave poorly for the rest of the procedure. This is especially a problem when the patient is sitting. Sublingual diazepam (Valium) 5 mg quickly and smoothly relaxes the patient slightly. Heavier oral intramuscular, or intravenous medications are seldom indicated for simple hair transplantation. Except after the first session, we want the patient to be able to stand up and drive himself home as soon as the wrap is on.

In our office, T.A.T. will occasionally use Penthrane, an analgesic that historically has commonly been used during labor and delivery. R.G.G. uses it nearly 50% of the time, and S.J.S. does not like it. It is delivered through a "whistle," a long plastic device about the size of a cigar. The liquid Penthrane is poured in and absorbed by a cotton plug. The patient sucks air through the mouthpiece, which is shaped like the mouthpiece of a clarinet. The concentration of the aerosolized anesthetic can be increased when the patient holds a finger over an opening proximal to the cotton reservoir, which causes all of the air drawn in to pass over the agent. The patient holds the whistle and administers as much analgesic as he wants. This method is safe because if a patient loses enough control or consciousness, the whistle drops away from the

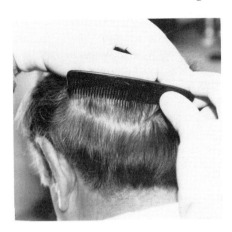

FIG 6–10.
A comb is used to inspect the donor area for density, evenness, and scalp condition.

mouth long before any toxicity can develop. It induces analgesia for 5 to 10 minutes, which is more than enough to numb the donor and recipient areas. S.J.S. does not use this because of the added time, the smell of the gas which permeates the room, and the patient's drugged behavior, and because he has had transplants, does not think the minimal pain is worth the effort. We have had patients who have had transplants with and without Penthrane and some definitely prefer having it.

The Donor Site

The examination and evaluation of the donor site is critical at the initial visit and before each session (Fig 6–10). Place your nondominant hand over the donor areas and use the wooden end of a long cotton-tipped applicator to pull down a few hairs at a time as you move your hand upward. This will provide a good look at the density and regularity of the donor hair. Before any hairs are trimmed, the features of the entire donor area must be known: (1) Where does the whisker hair start anterior to the ears? (2) How high does the fringe hair extend (remember to consider that any miniaturizing hairs will eventually be lost)? (3) How regular and dense are the hair follicles? (4) Where are the best hairs for each proposed recipient site (fine hairs for the front, thick hairs for the center)? (5) How did the last set heal? (6) Was there scarring or hypopigmentation and was it detectable?

The answers to these questions will determine where the donors are to be harvested, what is the pattern of harvesting, and how many and where the plugs will be placed.

The donor area is that area of fringe *not* genetically programmed to go bald. It is impossible to know for sure where that area is, but if the balding pattern is well-established, a good guess can be based on where the hairs are miniaturized. Even if these hairs do not stop growing completely, they are not good for transplantation and in time usually are lost. The midocciput is where the fringe often dips the deepest and may become as narrow as two inches. Do not be fooled by assuming that the edge of a bald crown is the limit of hair loss. The eventual loss may be considerably more. At the midvertical line of the ears and anteriorly, the hair begins to change, both in density and quality. In some patients, the hair anterior to the ear is much like the rest of the donor hair except that it is more sparse. In others it becomes stiffer and has different waves and colors. In still others, it is like whiskers—and is in fact whisker hair. These hairs are not good for transplantation. The scalp also changes in this area to a thinner dermis with less subcutaneous fat, and the follicles are at an angle more acute to the scalp.

Several patterns of harvesting have evolved over the years, and all are still used with good results. The original Orentreich method is to take plugs from a rectangular area, leaving bridges between each plug about two to three mm wide. As the holes contract during healing, the surrounding skin is stretched, resulting in adequate coverage of the fringe area. The hairs point downward and overlie each other to camouflage the donor area. For 50 plugs of 4.0 mm diameter, in 10 vertical rows of 5 each, the rectangle of donor scalp used is approximately 8 cm horizontally and 4 cm vertically. It is larger for 4.5-mm plugs and when the hair density is sparse or irregular.

With the rectangular harvest pattern, we usually do not suture. Only those plugs that actively bleed are closed. Over the years, the closing vs. the second-intention healing battles remain unresolved.[26] We have seen little scarring and occasionally significant scarring from both methods. Certainly, sewing takes longer and definitely hurts more from about postop day 4 to day 7 or 8.

The contracted scars are usually about 2- to 3-mm wide and hypopigmented. Sometimes they are firm and dome-shaped, but even then are hard to detect unless the hair is lifted up and closely inspected. In some patients, the sutured donor site heals better; in others there is no visible difference. With the total harvest method or the Pierce method discussed below, suturing increases the total number of donors available.

When the vertical row has more than five donor holes, the hairs tend to fall away from that row, making it slightly detectable. Also, in most men, the donor fringe is not wide enough to leave hairs above the site long enough to completely cover it when more than five plugs are taken from one vertical row. Although this is a temporary problem, the holes do not look good to the layman, and this problem limits how soon the patient can return to work. Also, it is more difficult to close the area when more than three 4.5-mm or four 4.0-mm holes are made.

Another harvesting pattern is the "total harvest." In this pattern, as many plants as possible are taken from an area (the fusiform area), leaving little remaining tissue (Fig 6–11, A). It is infinitely easier to obtain these plants while the scalp tissue is attached to the head. (Removing a similar-sized piece of scalp and trying to punch out the plugs like biscuits from dough does not work.) The remaining tissue is excised completely with scissors down to the fascia or galea

(Fig 6–11, B). The base of the fusiform wound is smooth and even but the edges are scalloped—hence the name "shark bite" harvest pattern. This opening closes easily. We often use the rectangular harvest pattern around the middle part of the donor fringe, and the total harvest around the lower part (the inferior but not the lowest fringe hairs, which are fine and irregular). The closure recruits the needed laxity from the neck skin. A 4- to 5-cm-wide opening closes without much difficulty and patients usually mention only a tightness in the neck for a few days at most.

A third donor harvest pattern consists of two rows of plugs separated by enough donor scalp for two more rows.[27–29] Usually two *sets* of rows are used in a given session. These rows are easily camouflaged by the surrounding hairs and close easily, either by placing a running suture through both rows, causing them to collapse together as the suture is cinched up, or by what is called the Pierce method, in which the thin strip of tissue between the rows is cut between the upper and lower hole.[30] As the running suture is placed, the upper hole is pulled slightly in one direction and the lower hole is pulled in the opposite direction (Fig 6–12). The little tabs interdigitate and the closure line nearly vanishes. The results of either technique are excellent, making the two rows of two rows each a popular harvest pattern. During ensuing sessions, the scalp between the sets is used.

After careful inspection of the donor area

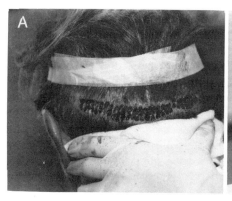
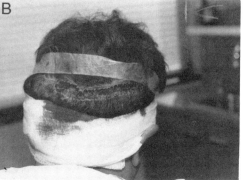

FIG 6–11.
A, total harvest just after plugs have been lifted out. **B,** total harvest just after the intervening stands of tissue have been excised.

Surgical Management of Alopecia

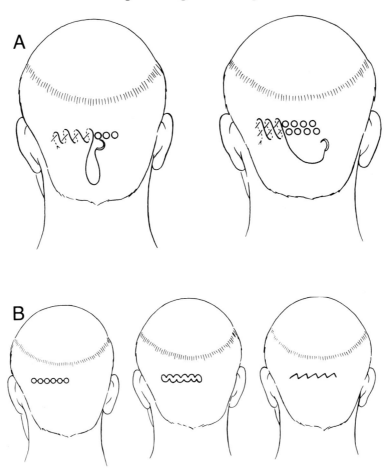

FIG 6–12.
Running suture to close the donor site. **A**, method used to close a single or double row of donors. Three rows can be closed with the same technique although a large needle is needed. **B**, Pierce suture closure. Donor holes show proposed tiny incision lines to make one single wound (*left*); resultant wound after cutting into the adjacent holes (*middle*); end scar line after suturing each inferior tip to superior concavity (*right*).

and after deciding which harvest technique will be used, the hair is trimmed to a 2-mm stubble. With experience an area just large enough will be cut, and the hairs above will completely cover it. The stubble is most important because it signals the direction of the follicles below the surface. The long axis of the punch is oriented exactly parallel to the follicular axis. Any deviation from that axis results in needless transsection of hair roots, reducing the number of viable hairs transplanted. The hairs surrounding the trimmed area are kept out of the field with paper tape, terry

cloth sweat bands of the kind used by tennis players, hair clips, or setting gels (Fig 6–13).

The area is cleansed with alcohol or chlorhexidine (Hibiclens) followed by alcohol. Lidocaine 1% with epinephrine 1:100,000 is the mainstay anesthesia. Mixing the epinephrine with plain lidocaine at the time of the surgery may reduce the stinging slightly because it primarily is the result of the low pH necessary to stabilize the epinephrine for a long shelf-life. The addition of sodium bicarbonate to further buffer the acid solution reduces pain but also

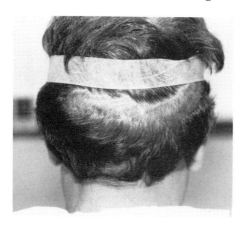

FIG 6–13.
Hair taped to expose donor area.

lowers the effectiveness of the lidocaine and epinephrine to a point where it is inadequate for this procedure. We had a few unhappy days when we tried it—hurting, complaining patients and growling doctors when the bleeding was profuse. If the bicarbonate and epinephrine are added to plain lidocaine just prior to use, it seems to work better.

The donor area is anesthetized by infiltrating the *entire* area (Fig 6–14). A block only along the inferior edge to catch the nuchal nerves as they progress upward numbs the area but does not provide the hemostasis necessary for easy harvesting. We start by putting the anesthesia in across the lower edge of the area and then stick into that numbed line to infiltrate the area above it. Patients are told they will feel stinging for 30 seconds; they grit their teeth and in 30 seconds it is over.

Keep track of the amount of lidocaine used. We count syringefuls. A fresh 25-ml or 50-ml bottle for each patient also allows monitoring of the amount used. When large numbers of transplants are performed in one session, the toxicity level may be approached. When that happens, dilute any needed remaining local. The lidocaine may be 1% or .5%; it is the epinephrine that needs to be 1:100,000.

Wait a full 15 to 20 minutes for the epinephrine to take effect. Some patients will experience an epinephrine rush that includes tremor, jitters, a strong heartbeat, and a feeling of panic. This comes on five minutes after in-

jection and lasts about 3 to 4 minutes. When patients are warned, they tolerate it well; if surprised, they will react in various ways, causing one more distraction that will need physician attention.

After waiting, we check to be sure patients are numbed in the *entire* donor area. One of the most common causes of syncope in this operation is hurting the patients after they are numb and not expecting to feel pain. Do not wander out of that sacred numbed area! Next, the recipient site(s) is anesthetized. This can be done with a ring or peripheral block around the entire area to be planted. The frontal line is the most difficult to block because of the many decussating nerve fibers from the supraorbital and supratrochlear nerve groups. The nerves spread to all levels of the skin and also fan from their foramina. Repeated infiltration intradermally helps; using 2% lidocaine does not help; but reinjecting with a second agent such as mepivacaine (Carbocaine) has amazing numbing effects across the frontal line. At this point the patient can safely be told that there will be no more pain for the remainder of the operation. The patient will then relax and the operation will proceed with the potential of good communication between doctor and patient. We can honestly say that we have frequently learned interesting things from visiting with our transplant patients during the

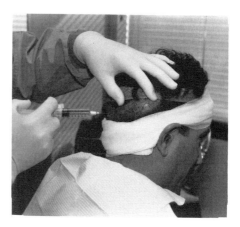

FIG 6–14.
Local anesthesia is injected into the donor area. Tape holds hair out of the way (see Fig 6–13) and roller gauze band below donor area helps with sponging.

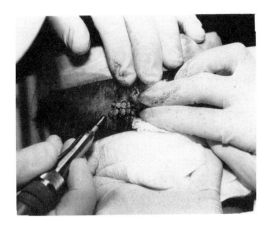

FIG 6–15.
Harvesting plugs using an American power punch on a Bell international hand engine. The doctor steadies the patient's head with one hand and cuts the plugs with the other; the assistant uses both hands for sponging.

hour of doctor time it takes to complete most sets. It is this same conversation that cements a good professional relationship and creates future trust.

Thomas Alt, M.D., has made several valuable contributions to the surgical management of alopecia, one of which is the use of saline to firm up the donor area.[31] *Immediately* before harvesting, inject saline into the site until the tissue is firm. Inject only an area large enough to harvest up to 10 plants, unless you work very fast; in that case, inject an area for 20. Cut those plugs and inject saline in the next area, and so on until the procedure is completed. It is of little value to inject saline and let some absorb before cutting.

The soft scalp skin will distort when it is pushed down, even with a sharp instrument like the punch. It is much less distorted by sharp and motor-driven punches. This distortion angles the follicles so that some are transected by the punch; the resulting plug is conical. Theoretically, the effects of the saline-induced tumescence prevent the distortion of the skin, producing a plug that has no lipping and is cylindrical, and with all of the follicles intact. Regardless of the validity of this theory, we can attest to the superior quality of grafts taken from saline-swollen skin. Certainly, the plugs look better, as is so well demonstrated by Alt's macrolens photography.[31]

The actual cutting of the grafts is the most critical part of the entire technique. Everything must be right: lighting, position of the patient and doctor, and magnification. Close observation of the stubble direction for each plug is necessary for making the fine adjustments in the angle that the punch touches where it cuts the scalp (Fig 6–15). Inspect the first few grafts cut in their entirety and inspect others frequently. Inspect more frequently if the density is uneven or if the follicle direction is variable. Look for the following: (1) conical-shaped plugs, which may indicate not enough saline or a dull punch; (2) transected roots, indicating an improper angle of attack or curved follicles; (3) uneven, nonsmooth and nonglistening plug walls, possibly the result of a dull punch or an unsteady hand; and (4) lipping, which suggests a dull punch or the wrong angle of punch when it first touches the skin.

It makes no difference whether all the plugs or only a few are cut before they are pulled up and the fatty base cut, lifted out, and placed in cold (refrigerator cold—approximately 20°C) saline. We cut all of them before we start to lift them out unless there is an arterial bleeder that requires a ligature. The saline tumescence and attention to the cutting angle are the crucial factors.

The donor area is cleaned with benzalkonium chloride (Zephiran) (Fig 6–16, A and B). We found it is easiest to spray it on with the kind of pump-spray bottle designed and sold for misting houseplants. It is covered with several layers of dry, folded gauze held in place temporarily until the end of the procedure by gauze that is rolled around the head. The best pressure and the most patient comfort are achieved by placing the roller gauze around the forehead in front and directly on the donor area at the sides or back. A loop just under the lambdoid ridge locks the gauze in place. This wrap does not cover the recipient site and can be stuffed with gauze squares at the temples to assist sponging while cutting the recipient holes. When the donor area is completely sutured, this temporary wrap is not necessary.

Hemorrhage

Arteriole and capillary hemorrhage are primarily controlled by the epinephrine and hand-pressure by the assistants. As the cutting progresses across the donor area, the assistant(s) cover the freshly cut grafts with folded cotton gauze. By the time all have been cut, most of the bleeding will have stopped.

Artery bleeders are stopped with a suture. Our favorite is 3/0 braided Dacron (Mersiline), which is soft, strong, and washes white, making it easier to see for removal. It is swagged onto a large curved needle and passed through the skin one or two holes distant from the bleeding opening and exits one or two holes on the opposite side. The ligature is most often effective if it is located slightly superior to the bleeding hole rather than right across it. Sometimes, however, the bleeder is elsewhere and several sutures in various directions are necessary before it can be caught.

Cleaning and Trimming the Plants

As the plants are transferred to the cool saline in a petri dish, they can be sorted for quality, density of hairs, color, size, and thickness of hair shaft. This triage can also be done by the assistant while the plants are being cleaned. Each team needs to establish its own conventions so the plant characteristics are best utilized in the recipient area. Lighter-density plants go behind the front rows; color and shaft size are matched to the existing recipient holes; smaller plants go for fill-ins, front rows, and the crown; and larger plants go where bulk is needed.

Although a few physicians prefer to clean and trim the plants, we and most other transplanters assign this task to assistants while we move on to cut the recipient sites (Fig 6–17). Two important steps are part of the plug preparation. Although any excess fat should be trimmed off, *do not trim off all of the fat.* The mesodermal portion of the follicle essential for growth is located in the immediate subdermal fat, and is almost transparent. The dermal portion of the follicular root is black and often mistaken for the lowest portion of the root. Therefore, some portion of fat must be left on the graft; about 2 mm is considered adequate in most cases. This is an essential part of training for the staff that trims the plants.

The second step is to clean off any clots, hair spicules, transected follicles, tissue debris, and epidermal lipping. Some transplanters are emphatic about removing absolutely every tiny hair spicule and cutting off any hint of protruding follicle. The merit of such an approach has not been demonstrated, neither by a lower incidence of "transplant folliculitis" (see below under complications), nor by a higher incidence of infection

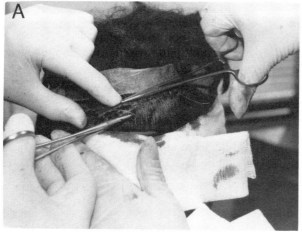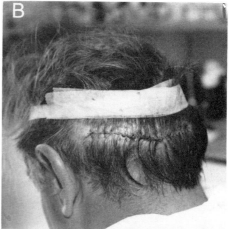

FIG 6–16.
A, the donor site is sutured with a 3/0 Mersiline locked running stitch. **B,** the donor site has been closed and cleaned.

Surgical Management of Alopecia

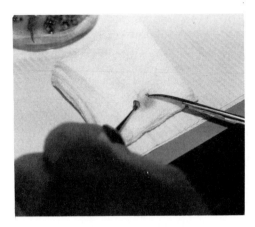

FIG 6–17.
An assistant trims plugs of excess fat and cleans them of hair spicules and debris.

that microplants can be harvested from the edges of the regular grafts, or full-sized grafts can be divided into miniplants.

For cleaning and trimming, a well-lighted countertop where the assistant can sit is necessary. Some like to use magnification. Basically, the plant is picked up with a small-toothed forceps at the epidermal edge to reduce any damage to the follicles. The blood, hair spicules, and debris are brushed away with the closed blades of a small scissors and the fat is trimmed. This plant is then placed on clean gauze in another petri dish with cool saline and in the appropriate group by size and quality. The plants are taken back to the operatory and given to us about the time the recipient holes are completed.

The Recipient Area

The second important function for the physician is the planning and location of the plants. This "strategic" planning involves planning generally where the plants will go, the location of the hairline, scalp reductions, and the spacing of operations. The "tactical" planning is determining exactly what is going to be done during

or foreign body reactions. Although the plugs certainly look better cleaned and lined up in an orderly fashion in the petri dish when they are returned to the operatory for planting, and segregating them makes it much easier to select which plugs go where, there is no evidence that they grow better (Fig 6–18). It is at this juncture

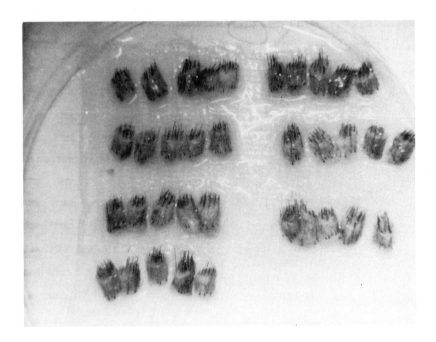

FIG 6–18.
After cleaning, the plugs are lined up in groups of five for easy counting and are triaged by quality.

each procedure. The first of every surgical visit should begin with a quick review of the strategic plan, followed by careful attention to the immediate task.

The patient's greatest concern is usually the frontal area. He confronts it daily in the mirror, it is seen most by others and by cameras, and the location and pattern of the receding hairline is a hallmark of aging. When establishing the frontal line (drawing on the patient with a marking pen), project what the patient will look like when he has reached full male-pattern baldness. Ignore the slowly miniaturizing tufts of hair which the patient so carefully husbands. Overlook the teased, overworked hairs pulled from the midscalp. Design the replacement based on the estimated number of donors and how they should be designed to cover the entire problem. As mentioned above, we are loath to transplant the thinning temples of someone in his 20s and then spend the next 20 years chasing a receding hairline, and trying to match the previous plants. Also, it will be embarrassing or worse if all the donors are used up on the anterior one-third of the head, with none left to cover the later-appearing posterior baldness. Even worse is to use all of the donors on a crown bald spot and have none left to fill in the advancing peripheral baldness. Soon there will be an island of transplanted hair. Therefore, keep in mind the strategic plan for the whole life of the patient.

The location and shape of the frontal line are the next consideration. The adult hairline is fairly high (Fig 6–19). It is not at the junction of the forehead and the scalp, but above it. The hair is combed over and down, creating a hairline at the forehead junction; the hairs themselves, however, start $1^{1}/_{2}$ to 2 cm above that visual line. The center of the hairline is the nose. Although most faces are asymmetrical, the nose is thought of as the center. Therefore, center the hairline on the nose and using a pen, mark with a dot where the center of the hairline will be and how high it will be.

How curved or V-shaped to draw the line is determined partly by the patient's anatomy and partly by the physician's aesthetic judgment. For the starting points on each side, study the direction of the hairs remaining. There is a point at which the hairs change direction: the top hairs

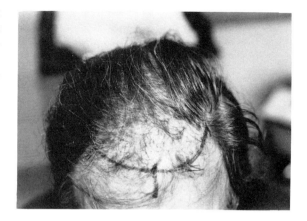

FIG 6–19.
The proposed frontal hairline is drawn on the patient, with the center mark based on the nose. The patient is shown this line before the procedure begins.

point forward and the side hairs point down. We mark that point on each side with the pen. Hair loss is uneven; one side may have lost more than the other, so be careful to place the two lateral dots at about the same place on each side. Then connect the three dots with a gradual arc, with a V, with sharp Vs at the sides and a gentle arc in the center—whatever looks best. The natural curve of the existing hairline may guide you, and the patient's combing pattern may help. The location of the lateral edges of the front line will be pulled in or toward the middle if anterior scalp reduction surgery is anticipated. Therefore the line is designed a little straighter than it is expected to be when reductions and plants are finally combined.

Having established the front line, choose the pattern for the plants. For the actual front line, few variations are acceptable. The plants should be 3.5 or 4.0 mm in diameter; larger ones show too much and smaller ones go anterior to soften the look. The space between plugs should be slightly smaller than the width of one plug. (One variation is to leave space for two more plugs between each one. This plan would apply to patients in whom poor growth is expected—something very rare in the frontal area.) Most front lines use up 20 to 30 plugs per row. Remember to plant as if there are no existing hairs there, because it is only a matter of time until that is true. Do not build the hairline around existing hairs. Those present will help camouflage your work and make the hairline thicker, but they will soon be gone, leaving only the transplants. The second row should be placed one plug width behind the first, slightly offset (staggered like theater seating) and spaced with one or two plug spaces between (Fig 6–20). Do the same for the third and fourth rows.

The angle and direction of the plants is extremely important. For the frontal rows, the hair should be pointed straight forward or forward and slightly pointed to the side *away* from the part. In the past there were some recommendations to aim the frontal plug on a radius from the center of the scalp. This made for a bunch of men who looked like Nero or Friar Tuck, and it was impossible for them to comb the hairs from one side to the other. The correct angle of the plants is about 45 degrees, *not* 90 degrees, although this is something we unfortunately still see; these patients look like pin cushions (Fig 6–21, A and B). There was a time when we planted the front one or two rows with a more acute angle—30 degrees—but the 45-degree angle gives a higher, more natural look.

A few microplants may be put in just anterior to the main front row. Doing a few at each session creates a natural front line from the beginning. At the next session, the spaces left may be filled in or another site planted; the fill-ins can be placed on the third session, allowing time for the first set to grow so success can be evaluated.

On patients with limited donors, rows three and further posteriorly can be spread out more. The plugs are placed closer together on the part side and spread out from the midcrown to the other side. This same distribution is used in those patients, discussed above, who are older and have only enough donors to fill the middle portion of the head. For these men, first plant the center and the center to the side of the part. Place the plugs one diameter apart at the side of the part and gradually spread that distance as you progress across the scalp. Once the center scalp is planted, if there are more donors left at subsequent sessions, gradually plant in either direction; it is the patient's choice. Most will want you to move forward.

Transplanting the crown is what we call a "plug-eater." For a patient with only crown baldness, with a family history of older members who are bald only at the crown, with little loss on the downslope of the head, and with no signs of miniaturization around the patch, it is reasonable to invest the number of plugs necessary to build a full and natural replacement for that area. It is on the crown that most people have a whorl or cowlick. (Some people have one on each side and some have none.) If most of the hair is gone, the new whorl or turning point can be replaced to the crown on the side opposite the part and just above (anterior) to where the head curves downward posteriorly. If the whorl is still present, build around the existing pattern. Design long curving lines of plants, starting at the center of the whorl with a tight curve, then straightening out to join the lines of transplants at the mid or anterior scalp. As before, place the plugs closer on the part side. Also place them close together at the whorl. The hairs are directed outward from the center of the whorl, which means that those to the left of the center will point left, those anterior will point forward, and those posterior will point backward. Use 4.0-mm plugs or smaller and plan to use 100 to 150 plugs for this one area alone. Scalp reductions are often a part of the management for crown baldness.

If the crown baldness is part of a more generalized pattern, it is not wise to use so many

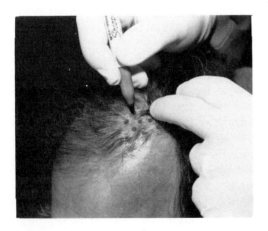

FIG 6–20.
The recipient sites are marked. This is helpful because once the operation is under way, hemorrhage and sponging obscure the field.

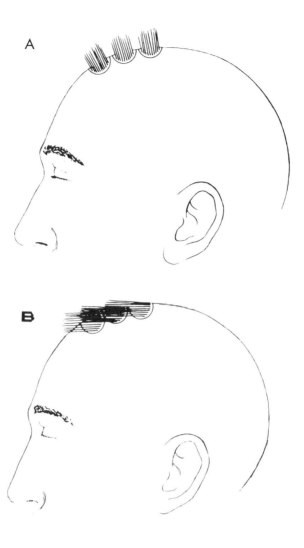

FIG 6–21.
A, B, simplistic schematic drawings that emphasize the value of acutely
angling the anteriorly placed plugs.

plants in this one area, nor is it necessary. Most
of the time the plants are designed to build hair
that sweeps from the part over the head and
around the front. The plugs are planted more
densely on the part side. This same pattern is
simply extended posteriorly, so the hair can be
combed from the part over the crown baldness.
The previously existing whorl is forgotten because only a few miniaturized hairs remain which
point in the circular directions.

Except when planting an entire crown and
building a whorl, it is doubtful that plants should

ever be placed pointing backward and downward. When the alopecia extends over the slope of the head and down onto the occiput, it is difficult to make transplants look normal or to camouflage them. It is better to leave the baldness on the downward slope untreated. It is one of the normal patterns to have only crown baldness, especially for older men, and scalp reduction scars or visible transplants seldom if ever look better and certainly look unnatural.

The technique for creating the openings is fairly straightforward once the tactical plan has been decided upon and the sites to be planted have been marked. With experience, less complete marking is necessary, but it is recommended for beginners and when the plants are being placed in between previous plugs or must follow exact patterns. We use hand rather than motor-driven punches, which range from .25 to .75 mm smaller than the punches used for harvesting. We also may use a different bevel to achieve a better fit. Until the plug is harvested and the opening cut, it is impossible to assess shrinkage and gaping, which critically affect the fit. We cut one opening and test a plug to see how it fits. Further tests with different sized punches are carried until we find the best fit. That size and type of punch is used for the remaining openings. This test is repeated for each size of plug we harvest.

After the punch is cut, it is lifted out. Because this tissue is thrown away, this is a less delicate procedure. Stand *behind* the patient, lift the plug up with a forceps in one hand, and slip the Biro Dermal Naevus scissors in from the back. Because the openings are cut at an angle, the tethering tail of fat is posterior to the surface opening. This position makes it much easier to cut that tail.

There are several myths about placing the plants. Some day, evidence may arise to disprove them. We have heard that plugs put in too tightly cause the dome-shaped elevations that some plants develop with healing. Nevertheless, we used to put them in very tightly and notice no more or less dome results than before, although it happens occasionally. We suspect it is a function of scar contraction much like the forces that make a "trap door" out of some curved incisions. We have also read that plugs put in

too loosely scar more, but this is not something we have observed.

Placing the plants is literally putting round cylinders into round holes (Fig 6–22). It can be done by one person or two. Our nurses do the planting and one of them, who is very experienced, can plant faster than any two others. It is helpful, if working between existing hairs, to have one person clear the hole and the other pop in the plug. Some plugs will need additional trimming if they do not set down well. And the doctor may need to come back and make a different-sized opening for a few others. But usually they fit in nicely, and with a minute or two of pressure, conform to the new location.

Actually, the plugs are not cylinders but truncated cylinders. Inherently, the truncated plane (epidermis end—hair stubble end) is angled at a fixed angle determined by the direction of the donor follicles. The openings have been cut at a bias at least 45 degrees above the skin surface. These two angled planes fit together well: the angle of the recipient hole brings the plug surface to the same plane as the surface. There is only one way to put in the plugs. But we have seen other doctors and certainly our own assistants get them in some other way. If the openings are cut properly, the stubble hairs will point in the desired direction and the plug surface will match the scalp surface.

When all of the plugs are in (actually while the planting process is under way), firm, steady

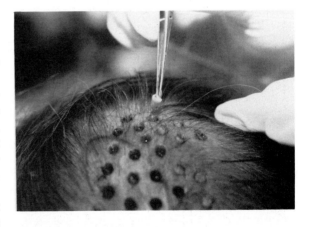

FIG 6–22.
Planting the plugs, a step often performed by assistants.

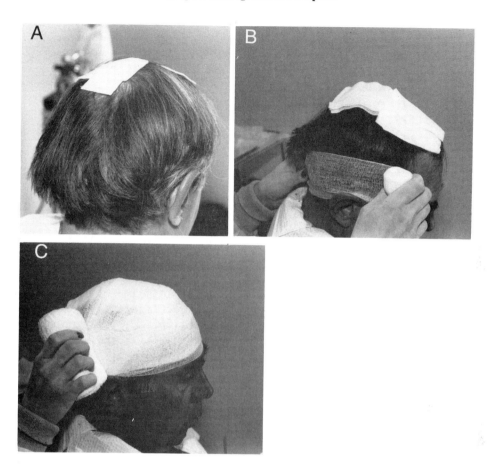

FIG 6–23.
Dressings. **A**, the donor and recipient sites are covered with an antibacterial ointment and a nonstick dressing such as Telfa. **B**, the sites are reinforced with gauze squares and roller gauze is wrapped around the entire head. **C**, Kerlix gauze is placed around the head as a final covering.

pressure is applied to the plugs already in place. Place one or two gauze squares on the planted plugs and apply gentle pressure with the palm of the hand. Sometimes, the patient can do this himself. It gets him involved, and more importantly, teaches him what he is to do if he experiences bleeding later. Over the phone when you tell him to apply pressure, he will know exactly what you mean. This step varies in length because some plugs swell in the saline and it takes a while to force the water out. Sometimes the plugs with the necessary tip of fat are longer than the scalp is thick. This is particularly true when the top of the head has been bald for a few years and has thinned but the donor areas remain full thickness. Making a little space with

closed scissors or a mosquito hemostat for the plant to sit in will speed its accommodation.

Dressings

The recipient area is cleansed, again with benzalkonium chloride from the plant mister, and the donor is checked for oozing and recleansed. We use an antibacterial ointment on Telfa and lay the pads over both donor and recipient areas, followed by gauze squares, followed by several turns of roller gauze, followed by a complete turban with Kling gauze (Fig 6–23, A to C). The turban actually looks better than just a circumferential wrap covering the donor site, and protects the plants from accident. Years ago we sent patients home with just a circumferential wrap around the donor area and simply combed the hair over the recipient area. The results seemed the same, but a neurosurgeon patient convinced us that the patient will feel better, look better, and be less likely to bump the plants if he wears a full head wrap. We agree.

Do not attempt to hold the plants in place with the dressing or be misled that any dressing can put enough pressure on the plants to hold them down. They must be well-seated and flat *before* any dressing is applied. Occasionally, as mentioned above, the plugs will sit up and sometimes it takes 30 to 40 minutes for an assistant to work them down. No dressing will accomplish this task.

Patients are given a sack of gauze squares, some roller gauze, and pain medication. If there is bleeding—almost the only problem that ever arises in the first 24 hours—and the patient calls, tell him, "Use the gauze we gave you in the following way . . . " This is infinitely easier than telling the patient to try to make a towel or T-shirt work as a pressure dressing. The pain medicine sent home also prevents night phone calls and the mad search for an all-night pharmacy. Patients usually feel euphoric when they leave the office and do not want to be seen with the head wrap on, so they often will not fill a prescription for pain medicine.

Patients are instructed to come back the next day for a dressing change. The wrap is removed, the plants and hair are cleansed, and the hair is combed. Patients are reinstructed on further home care, which includes instructions on avoiding strenuous activity and open-mouth sneezing and coughing, daily cleansing of both sites with hydrogen peroxide, replacing a fallen plant, and the signs of infection. We ask to see patients in a week for inspection and suture removal if sutures were randomly placed. If there was a running closure of some type, we leave the stitches in longer—for ten days or so. Further follow-up depends on the long-range plan (Fig 6–24, A and B).

Complications

Even though this list is long, complications are infrequent. In the 30-year history of hair transplantation, however, probably all possible problems have occurred.

Bleeding

Intraoperative bleeding is best managed with epinephrine in the local anesthesia, pressure by hand or dressing, and sutures. Gelfoam and Oxycel cotton stuffed into a bleeding donor site help, but we want that area dry and we want it to stay dry all night. That is why we suture, suture, suture until the donor site is dry. If a patient is

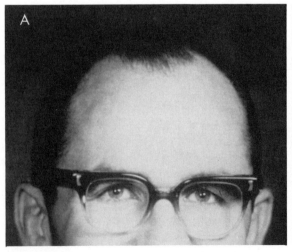
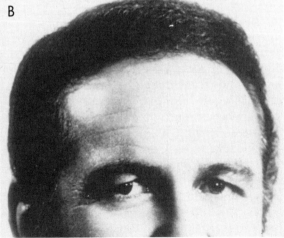

FIG 6–24.
A, patient before transplants. **B,** patient after transplants.

an "oozer" (from aspirin or occult von Willebrand's), it is better to completely suture the donor area than to try hemostatic agents. Also plan a long, mandatory, clean-up visit the next day and the day after that. Also expect oozers to heal more slowly. Bleeding from the recipient site usually stops when the plants are put in. Only rarely will you need a suture.

Delayed-onset bleeding that occurs when the epinephrine wears off occurs rarely but is an inherent problem. A good Valsalva may also pop off a clot and start an arteriole bleeder. Patients are instructed to take off the wrap, sponge up any blood, and look for the bleeder. When they locate it, they should hold firm pressure over the bleeder only for 5 to 10 minutes. This will usually stop the bleeder. If not, they should call and we will meet them at the office for a suture. Make it easy on yourself: when a patient cannot stop a bleeder, go right in. Do not send him to an emergency room.

Infection

The three or four serious infections we have seen in our practice in the past 20 years were most likely the result of a staff member's pharyngitis. Of course, at the time, the staff members did not know they were sick. We would have an infected patient return two days after surgery and, simultaneously, a staff member calling in sick. The infections responded to antibiotics and daily in-office cleaning. Most of the transplants survived and grew reasonably well.

An isolated localized infection is more common but also responds to antibiotics.

Scarring

Donor-site scars, discussed above, are a problem if the area is overharvested. Recipient-site scars are inherent and sometimes a problem. The transplant is a composite graft (hair and skin) and has the same features as a graft. The circumferential scar is nearly always imperceptible, but can be exaggerated in some patients. Our bias is that circumferential scarring is an individual patient factor rather than the result of something we did. The "cobblestone" effect is also a scarring function. The plug draws up—contracts—and forms a firm mound. This can happen to some or all of a set of grafts, but

not to every set. These scars settle naturally in a few months in some patients, but others require treatment. The hairs can be trimmed and the area lightly dermabraded, although this is reserved for the most severe cases. Light electrodesiccation with an epilating needle turned on its side is the best method.

As is true with many grafts, the melanocytes sometimes do not survive the transplantation, leaving a hypopigmented plant. The white dots are a problem in the frontal area, and it is has been recommended that these plants should be exposed to the sun. It is not that they did not tan in their former location, but that they are now a hypopigmented scar.

Telogen Effluvium

After surgery, the transplanted hairs go into a resting phase, the stubble falls out when the scabs fall off, and the hair begins to grow at three months. The trauma of surgery on both donor and recipient areas may trigger a telogen effluvium in the adjacent hairs. In the donor area, the hairs surrounding the donor sites fall out, and in the recipient area earlier plugs may also again go into a resting phase. This is upsetting to the patient and causes some cosmetic difficulty, but corrects itself in time.

Altered Sensation

It is not uncommon for patients to develop partial numbness and paresthesias above the donor site. This usually but not always resolves spontaneously in three to four months. The same effect rarely occurs in the recipient area. Occasionally, a patient will perceive this numbness as pain. Support and good rapport with the patient are the only helpful treatments.

Edema

Certain men notice forehead swelling on the second or third postoperative day. This happens more frequently when the surgery was performed near the front of the head. This swelling is painless and unrelated to physical activity, but can be quite large and disquieting. The patient will awake on the third day, look in the mirror, and gasp. The forehead is truly Neanderthal. This edema resolves or is absorbed in two or three days without treatment. As mentioned above, some physicians treat this edema pro-phylactically or actively with a pulse of steroids. The Nordströms' series of 44 patients found a 20% lower incidence of edema in those patients treated with methylprednisolone.[33]

The edema fluid is blood-tinged and passes under the eyebrows and into the upper and lower lids. This may produce massive black eyes, which understandably distress the patient.

Folliculitis

There is a very low incidence of "folliculitis" in a few of the transplants. This condition ap-pears to be a folliculitis in that there is a little crust and erythema at the hair-shaft opening. This is accompanied with pruritis in some, and in others it is a great nidus for picking. Tetra-cycline works well, but this is a chronic condition that sometimes lasts for 12 to 14 months. Hair growth is unaffected, and further transplants may or may not produce the condition.

One paper appeared in the literature re-porting multiple pyogenic granulomalike lesions following hair transplantation.[34] The patient de-veloped these lesions two to three weeks after his third session of transplants. They responded to shave-excision, followed by silver nitrate cau-tery. The histopathology was unrevealing and no historical reason for the event was discovered.

Arteriovenous Fistula

Rarely, when multiple plugs are cut out from a rectangular area, the veins and arteries will fuse. Most likely this is the result of cutting in-juries to proximal arteries and veins, which is entirely possible with punch transplants. How-ever, we are aware of only one study of these "A-V fistulas" designed to prove the true nature of this finding. Nordström and Tötterman stud-ied two patients with "fistulas" by angiography and found that the "fistula" was only a traumatic pseudoaneurysm in an artery.[35] Because the an-giography study was so limited and because this event has been called an A-V fistula for so long, we will continue to call it so; however, it may be only a pseudoaneurysm.

We have not seen a fistula develop when a total harvest or two-row harvest technique are used. The fistula appears from 18 to 60 days after the surgery as a pulsatile, fluctuant, bluish nod-ule in the donor area, and may be painful. The early lesions are less identifiable because the pulse is not detectable and because they appear to be delayed healing sites.

Management of this condition is surgical. Excise the entire nodule, identify the vessels and ligate them, and close primarily. A vertically ori-ented excision often provides the best visualiz-ation of the afferent (artery) and efferent (vein) vessels. If a pulsatile vessel can be palpated at one edge of the nodule, a large percutaneous suture will sometimes shut off the afferent loop and the fistula will resorb. If the percutaneous technique does not work, excision is indicated.

Poor Hair Growth

Some patients have a resting phase longer than 3 months and the new hairs do not emerge for 4 or 5 months. Be sure to wait long enough before deciding they are not going to grow. Lack of central or peripheral growth from the plants may indicate an error in technique. Scarring may be excessive for one set, and hamper hair growth. Planting between previous grafts increases the degree of scarring. For reasons we do not fully understand, the central part of the scalp has the poorest record for growth and the edges have the best. This must be related to the proximity of the blood supply.

Sparse donor hair naturally produces sparse plugs. This finding must be considered in the physician's overall strategic plan, and shared with the patient. Also, blond, thin, shaft hairs seem not to survive the operation as well as thicker, darker hairs. On balance, blonds with fine hair shafts do not need as many hairs per centimeter in order not to look bald. Thin recip-ient scalp skin will support a fewer number of plants, and the growth from these plugs is some-times sparse—not always, however.

No Hair Growth

It is only rarely that we have patients who show no growth from punch transplants. One of our patients whose hair did not grow was a woman we transplanted twice with zero results. (She got her money back, bought a fine wig, and accepted her fate.) We have no explanation for this event.

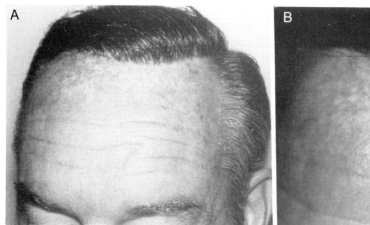
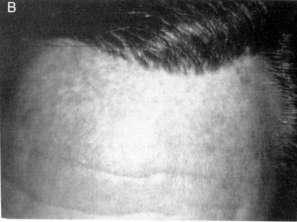

FIG 6–25.
A, a good hairline created with transplants. **B,** close-up of the same hairline. Mini- and microplugs can be placed in between and in front of this line to improve it if the patient desires.

Micrografts

In this text minigraft is defined as a regular punch graft taken with a punch smaller in diameter than 3.0 mm; a micrograft is a specially cut strand of scalp tissue containing one to five hairs. In 1977, Ayers published a discussion recommending that smaller (mini) grafts be used to soften the frontal hairline.[36] Discussing this indication and others, Nordström published several papers on mini- and micrografts.[37–40] The subject was also popular and frequently discussed at meetings throughout the 1980s.

Below Bradshaw lists eight uses for minigrafts, which in this article he called "quarter-grafts," because they were obtained by quartering a regular 4.5 mm-diameter graft.[41]

1. To design and fill in whole frontal hair lines; to give a quick moderately dense and more natural appearance than that usually seen with 4 to 4.5 mm grafts.
2. To fill between 4.5 mm (or other) grafts in the frontal hairline in order to finish off the transplanting with a smooth, more natural looking hairline.
3. To fill between any grafts more posteriorly on a punch-transplanted scalp, thereby softening an "orchardlike" appearance when there is insufficient donor area available to produce good hair density.
4. To grow hair on scalps that for any reason seem to accept grafts poorly.
5. To grow hair on scars secondary to trauma, infection, disease, or radiation.
6. To treat a large bald area with a "sprinkling" of hair when a very poor donor-recipient site ratio exists.
7. To construct eyebrows.
8. To transplant temporal hairlines or thicken sparse temporal hair.

The most useful indication for the minigrafts is the second point above: to fill in and make a more natural-looking hairline or crown (Fig 6–25). In South America, transplanting the whole head with minigrafts is more common; it takes two doctors five hours at each session. The few patients we have seen who have had this technique have very natural although sparse-looking hair. Other uses are for compromised recipient areas, and the method is worth the effort for trauma patients and postrhytidectomy temporal alopecia.

The quarter-graft plug is created by cutting a regular plug with a #11 or #15 blade, a small scissors, or a razor blade segment in a blade holder. (Each doctor or staff member has an individual preference: moist gauze squares, metal plates, etc.) This procedure is easier to accomplish if the plug is cut on the surface of a wooden tongue blade. Magnification is usually necessary. Place a drop of cool saline on the blade, hold the plug with jeweler's forceps, and divide it in the direction of the hair follicles. Smaller micrografts of only one or two hairs can be obtained by further division of a regular plug, or by cutting a few hairs off the edge of a regular plug. Another source is the hairs between plants when the total harvesting method is used. Plants taken specifically to be divided into minigrafts for the frontal hairline are best harvested from the lower fringe just above the neck. These hairs are naturally smaller and softer, and will blend well up front. The plants are lined up on moist gauze and taken to the operatory the same as regular ones.

The openings are deep incisions (slashes) with a #15 or #11 blade oriented vertically and perpendicularly to the scalp. Twist the blade a little to make a larger opening and be sure it goes all the way through the scalp to the galea. Wait 10 to 15 minutes before planting so the fibrin clot has time to form. Gently grasp the graft with tiny forceps (toothed or nontoothed) and push the graft down into the slit. The graft should be pulled all the way into the slit, with the graft epidermis sunk below the epidermis of the recipient area. This is tedious work and takes a lot longer to do than inserting regular plugs. Some recommended that the hairs and epidermis be cut off and the remaining graft sunk entirely into the recipient opening.

Merritt designed stainless-steel mandril-like dilators to help with minigraft planting.[42] There are two designs at the time of this writing: a sharp-tipped model, and a spatula-shaped tip. The latter is for larger grafts (three to five hairs). These are inserted into the scalpel slit and left for several minutes. You will need 10 to 20 of these because they all are stuck in at once. Working along the row of dilators, gently twist and lift one out and immediately be ready to shove in the graft. The twist serves to keep the hole open for a fraction of a second, whereas pulling it out tugs on the fibrin plug and it snaps shut. With practice, the technique goes fast and the assistants become skilled as well.

Mini- and micrografts can be incorporated into a session for routine transplants or done separately. Patients transplanted and "finished" years ago may benefit from hairline or crown softening, and have a high rate of growth and little morbidity.

Finally, try not to get caught up in the "contest" of who can create the most natural hairlines. You will go crazy. Some transplanters now maintain that the job is good and complete only if the patient can comb his hair straight back or directly to the side rather than forward and swept around to hide the plugging effect. Mini- and micrografts represent a major improvement for hair transplantation, but we are still operating on patients who have a wide range of needs and responses. Keep a sense of balance.

Scalp Reduction

History

For surgical management of alopecia, the technique of scalp reduction burst upon the scene at the International Hair Transplant Symposium in Lucerne in February 1978. At that meeting, Blanchard and Blanchard presented their work on "hair lifting" and distributed copies of their paper (which had a publication date of 1977).[43] Sparkuhl presented a videotape of his method, which he called scalp reduction. This name has persisted even though alopecia reduction is a more accurate term. His videotape and presentation are less well remembered, primarily because he did not publish his methods and findings elsewhere. The co-directors of the meeting, Webster and Stough[44] presented their work, which involved midline fusiform excisions of bald scalp with M-plasties on the occipital end.

The Ungers gave a paper at the meeting of the American Society for Dermatologic Surgery in April 1978 discussing 60 patients who had had bald scalp removed in sections measuring 2 to 4 cm in width and 10 to 15 cm in length. They estimated that this area of scalp removed saved the need for 180 to 360 3.5-mm plugs, depending on the density of coverage desired. Walter and Martin Unger have stated that they had accomplished this study a year earlier and submitted it to the Plastic and Reconstructive Surgery Journal, only to have it rejected as "nothing new or important."[45] Their paper was then submitted to and published by the *Journal of Dermatologic*

Surgery and Oncology in September 1978,[46] but they had lost the opportunity to claim primacy for the technique and could only share it with the Blanchards, Sparkuhl, Webster, and Stough.

In February 1979, Bosley et al. published a large series of scalp reduction cases[47] with Bosley claiming to have originated a technique of excision of bald scalp that was so new and original that it was protected with the title of "Male-Pattern Reduction" (M.P.R.). He was also present at the International Hair Transplant Symposium in Switzerland the year before. Later that year he was able to publish a report of 749 cases of scalp reduction.[48]

Schultz and Roenigk discussed the use of a reduction technique for removing scarring alopecia.[49] Roenigk later listed the many other medical indications for this procedure: aplasia cutis congenita, burn scars, cutis verticis gyrata, discoid lupus erythematosus, pseudopelade, lichen planopilaris, traction alopecia, nevus sebaceus of Jadassohn, localized morphea, and scleroderma.[50]

A variation of the technique was popularized by Thomas Alt in 1980 in which, with use of a paramedian incision and very wide undermining, more scalp was removed.[51] He also recommended serial relaxing incisions in the galea, closure with layered sutures, and postoperative administration of steroids.

Over the years, several others have modified, improved, and advanced scalp reduction techniques: Norwood and Shiell,[52] Nordström,[53] Marzola,[54] and Brandy.[55]

Indications and Patient Selection

When we first started performing scalp reductions, we thought that nearly 80% of the patients undergoing surgical treatment for alopecia would benefit from one form of reduction or another. With time, this figure has become considerably lower—probably around 25% to 30%. Even though the techniques have improved and there are several variations of reductions, experience has taught us a few lessons that must be factored into the total planning for alopecia management.

Most important is the fact that there will be a scar. Reduction design and layered closures have reduced the visibility of the scars in some patients, *but not in all.* To avoid an unnatural appearance, the scar must be covered by transplants, comb-overs, or other hair styles (Fig 6–26). Little is gained if 2 to 3 cm of bald scalp is excised from the crown, leaving an area of crown baldness with a scar across it. A reduction should not be planned if there are not enough donor hairs to transplant a coverage for the full length of the reduction scar.

Often, it is not the sight of the scar itself that is objectionable, since in many patients it fades out well and is flat—but, rather, how the hair falls away from the scar. The reduction, even midline, moves hairs pointing in different or slightly different directions closer together and creates a new part. There is a technique for trimming the wound edges of both sides of the reduction that allows the hairs to grow through the scar,[50] which sometimes helps hide the scar, but does not correct the more severe problem of the new pseduo-part. If the reduction includes the whorl, the whorl will be lost, necessitating a planned new pattern for the entire crown.

Both problems—scar visibility and pseudo-part formation—are especially troublesome for the man with the crown balding extending over the flat plane of the top of the head onto the occipital region. As mentioned earlier, transplants oriented downward over a sloping crown do not look natural, and the pseudo-part from a midline reduction makes a notch in the otherwise round fringe of the occipital alopecia. Recently, most physicians have learned to design the midline reduction so the posterior pole is kept well on top of the head and is not extended over the slope onto the lambdoid area. The Y and the crescent patterns of reductions also minimize this problem.

This lesson was painfully learned by some physicians when they saw an attorney's advertisement in the Los Angeles newspapers advising any patient who looked like the picture in the ad to call for legal counseling. The photograph showed the back of a head with a scar running down the center of the crown baldness and extending into the lambdoid area, with the hairs falling away from both sides of the scar.

The single most important factor for the appropriate use of reduction is scalp looseness.

Surgical Management of Alopecia

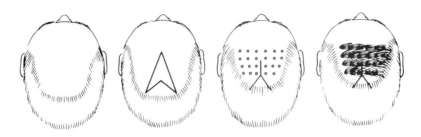

FIG 6–26.
Scalp reductions and transplants should be designed so the reduction scar is covered either by natural hair or transplanted hair.

Proponents of this procedure say that a 2-cm wide strip of scalp can be removed from everyone, no matter how tight their scalp feels. This is probably true, but says nothing about the cosmetic value of the surgery. If only a small portion of the alopecia is removed in exchange for a scar, a potential problem with hair direction, and increases in the total time of restoration, cost, and morbidity, then the procedure is not worth it. Hair transplant patients worry about the wind blowing their hair and exposing the transplants. They are worried doubly when there is a scar *and* transplants to camouflage.

The right candidate for a reduction has a loose scalp—preferably a "three-wrinkle scalp." The clinical test to assess the looseness of the scalp is to place the pads of the fingers on both sides of the crown and push medially. If two or three wrinkles of bunched-up scalp develop, the patient is a good candidate. If little or no scalp bunches-up, it is unlikely that reductions will help much. We have heard that not all clinically tight scalps yield little redundant tissue; some "one-wrinkle" heads, after wide undermining and galeotomies, yield 2- or 3-cm wide strips of excess tissue. This, however is not common and is unpredictable.

Scalp reduction is useful and beneficial in the following circumstances: (1) a wider recipient area may be covered or a denser recipient area may be created from the same donor area; (2) it makes transplants possible in some patients with too few donor areas; (3) it allows complete correction in some patients with only crown or central loss; (4) it can raise a part line, moving it to a cosmetically more pleasing position and allowing the comb-over hairs to be shorter, better managed, and more natural looking; and (5) specially designed reductions can remove bald scalp between flaps and transplants, between rows of transplants, in over-harvested donor areas, and between transplants and receding hairlines.

Timing of Scalp Reductions

Ideally it is best to perform all of the major scalp reductions first. (Small reductions between transplant rows and removal of advancing fringe lines are performed later.) Since it is impossible to predict how much scalp will come out and how existing hairlines will be affected, some guesswork must be used in planning the location of transplants, especially on the frontal line, if transplants are started before all of the reductions are completed. The wings of the frontal lines are placed farther forward than their intended final location because when the closure of the reduction(s) pulls the scalp toward the midline it elevates the frontal line laterally. Next, scarring from existing transplants makes reductions technically more difficult to undermine and reduces scalp stretch. Also, the reduction must be designed around the existing transplants and the surgical trauma may cause a telogen effluvium of the transplants.

After loose skin is removed, the closure is accomplished by stretching both the adjacent bald and hair-bearing skin. When the hair-bearing skin is stretched, the hair density is diminished, which means that this future donor site will yield less dense (less desirable) plugs. Reducing potential donor density is not much of a problem with the first reduction, in which mostly loose skin is removed, but becomes real when subsequent reductions utilize galeotomies and closure under tension. A first reduction could be pulled tightly and stretched with galeotomies and would also stretch and thin the potential donor areas.

Since the incision line and scar from properly designed reductions are not as noticeable as healing transplants, in some patients the reduction is better hidden and moves the part hair closer to the midline, which makes the comb-over more efficient.

The most troublesome drawback to performing the reduction(s) first is the increased waiting period for the patient before new hair growth occurs. It is probably this pressure for "results" that makes most physicians start transplants soon after or in conjunction with reductions. With experience, it is not too difficult to plan where transplants will be needed, and to design compatible transplants and reductions.

A midline or Y reduction and transplants around the frontal area can be done on the same day, or the reduction can be performed first and the transplants 1 or 2 days later. The only real problem with the latter plan is the edema resulting from the first operation, which can be partially controlled with steroids. Another plan is to reduce as much as possible without stretching the lateral donor areas; this type of reduction essentially consists of taking out all of the loose skin, not performing galeotomies or a closure under tension, and performing one or two sets of transplants using the lateral scalp as the donor area. This is followed by another reduction if needed.

We have come to believe that reductions are best performed when there is loose scalp skin in or near the balding areas. The problems with scarring, hair direction, and other complications (discussed below—stretch-back, pain, etc.) so significantly reduce the value of removing just a portion of the alopecia that we select only loose-scalped patients who would gain a lot from the procedure.

Scalp Reduction Designs

The midline fusiform, the Y, and the para-median designs have become the most popular. Several other patterns have been used, but not as often (Fig 6–27). The midline is popular because it is the easiest to do technically, removes large areas of baldness due to the looseness of the scalp laterally, and does not interrupt nerves or vessels. The design sets up a simple side-to-side closure without any three-point corners, which is less troublesome to suture because the tensions are only one direction (across the

Scalp reduction designs

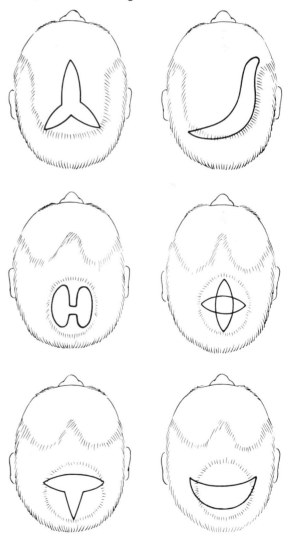

FIG 6–27.
Various designs of scalp reductions. The top two and the bottom left are the most commonly used.

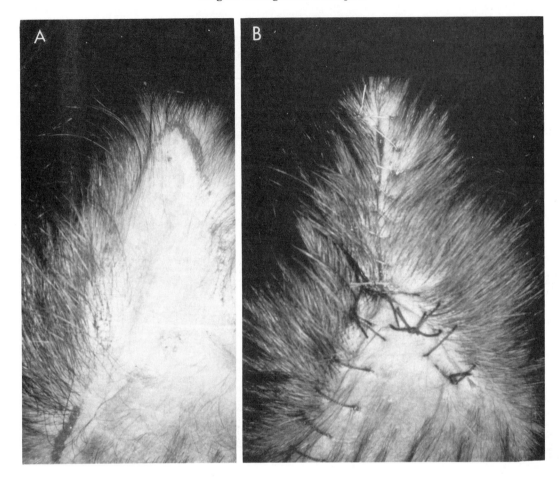

FIG 6–28.
The Mercedes or "Y" design for a scalp reduction. **A**, before surgery. **B**, after surgery.

wound) and the wound walls are the same thickness. With the Y or Mercedes patterns, the three-point junction is difficult to approximate exactly because of the tensions and the difference in flap thickness. The simple ellipse is the easiest to combine with transplants.

Both poles of the suture line can become problematic. Anteriorly, the scar must not extend onto the forehead and posteriorly it should not drop over the slope of the head into the vertical side of the occiput. M and Y designs help correct this problem, and the posterior pole of the ellipse can also be curved into a gentle C toward either side.

The Y pattern has the advantage of removing more tissue in the posterior half of the scalp where the balding pattern often widens out at the crown (Fig 6–28). Tissue is recruited from the sides and the occipital regions. This pattern leaves a scar that does not extend too far posteriorly; such scars are easier to hide because they are multidirectional and diverge closer to the natural hairline. The same caveat applies; do not design the incision so the scar shows, and plan to cover the scar with hair. The Y design variations conform more easily to individual patterns of baldness. The limbs of the Y do not have to be of equal length nor do the angles at the junction of the flaps need to be similar. The Y could also be called an ellipse with two dog-ear repairs, with those dog ears designed to best fit the patient's hair pattern. Also, the hair direction on the occipital scalp when recruited and moved upward points downward, which is the best way to cover the posterior, sloping crown.

Second reductions after the Y present more of a problem. Midline or paramedian reductions cross one of the limbs of the Y, leaving an island of scalp that is nearly devoid of blood supply near the junction. Repeat reductions not in exactly the same pattern increase the number of final scars, which are harder to camouflage.

The disadvantage hardest to solve is the technical closure of the flaps at the three-point corner. On paper a three-point closure is easily achieved, but on the scalp—where the flaps are of different thickness and the tensions can be considerable—it is difficult to get a tight closure at the junction. Problems with this three-point closure area include a wider and noticeable scar, suture splitting because a big knot often resides there, and possible necrosis of the tip of the posterior flap.

For the inexperienced surgeon there is a tendency to want to undermine the scalp over the occiput. The undermining laterally is so straightforward that it seems logical to carry the dissection to the same level posteriorly. Herein lies a big set of problems: the occipital arteries and the ligamentous attachments of the galea to the lambdoid ridge. Dissection in that area requires that the physician be ready to isolate and ligate the occipital arteries. This requires good directional lighting, good and experienced assistants, and the mettle to open the occiput widely to find the vessels by direct visualization. Suddenly it is much more complex surgery. Ligation of the occipital arteries may affect future donor site wound healing or the fullness of crown transplants. The planned ligation of these vessels is part of an operation described below (Major Flaps and Reductions).

A second difficulty is the "undermining" of the galea where it attaches to the lambdoid ridge. This requires heavy instruments, good anesthesia, and, again, the ability to open it up and continue under direct visualization for hemostasis or complete dissection. It is not something that should be attempted with the patient sitting up and lightly numbed. We have heard the dissection of the occipital ridge described as being like "cutting chicken bones." It certainly sounds like that. All of this is not to say that the un-

dermining should not be carried as far as can be accomplished *easily*. Some patients have a loose occiput and the simple undermining with almost closed scissors will free it up, yielding a lot of hair-bearing scalp for the posterior crown. But if it does not free up easily, do not proceed with the attempt unless you are fully prepared for a different level of surgery.

The Y design and the attempts at undermining in the occiput increase the incidence of numbness postoperatively. The Y shape also creates a flap that has a reduced blood supply, and transplants on that flap must be performed cautiously.

Alt is properly credited with designing and popularizing the paramedian technique.[51] He, too, started performing reductions in 1978 and 1979, but found that a special design and additional surgical techniques made it possible to remove a larger area of bald scalp. The design was a gentle S or C on one side of the crown, with the anterior pole extending about to the plane of the external ear and the posterior pole curving around the crown well past the midline. The center of the ellipse is designed wide because it is located at one side of the crown where there is the most laxity on the postauricular area of the sides of the head. He also performs galeotomies routinely, undermines widely—down to the level of the ears—closes under tension, and prescribes steroids perioperatively to keep edema to a minimum. There is not reason that this pattern cannot be used without galeotomies and wide undermining. The tradeoff for less tissue excised is less operative morbidity.

If the patient has hair-bearing scalp high posteriorly—i.e., does not have a low, sloping bald crown—the paramedian C pattern is excellent. It is designed on the non-part side and easily covered by the parted hair, the scar is at the natural junction of the top and side hairs (minimizing the pseudo-part effect), and technically it is a side-to-side closure with dog-ear repair built into the design.

Other patterns such as the J, H, and U are usually presented by the Ungers.[56, 57] These patterns are basically individualized reduction designs for given patients. Patterns of existing hair and already growing transplants require originality and planning, which are probably commonplace in the offices of many experienced hair replacement physicians.

Technique

Anesthesia

The kind and amount of preoperative medication needed is related to how much difficult undermining and how much closure tension is anticipated. A simple midline fusiform reduction taking essentially just the loose scalp engenders little morbidity, whereas a large, tightly closed, widely undermined reduction is more stressful and the preoperative sedatives will be helpful.

Local infiltration with 1% lidocaine with epinephrine is the mainstay for reductions. There are several patterns of administration. We like to first place a ring of anesthesia just inferior to the level that we anticipate to be the extent of undermining (Fig 6–29). After the ring of anesthesia has numbed the head and the patient has recovered from the epinephrine rush, the edges of the proposed incisions are injected with 1% lidocaine with epinephrine to ensure total numbness and the epinephrine effect as well.

Excision

The scalpel is the one of choice for the physician. We have used no. 15 or 10 blades, but also like the Shaw scalpel, which is an electronically controlled heated blade that seals the small vessels as it cuts (Fig 6–30). Unless one is very sure of being able to close, only one side of the proposed reduction should be incised (Fig 6–31). Our technique is to cut through the scalp down to the galea-periostial plane all along one side. We quickly follow with partial undermining of both sides of the incision (under the bald island to be removed and under the lateral edge) (Fig 6–32). If the epinephrine effect is active or the Shaw scalpel was used, the only bleeding is from small arteries in the dermis. The assistant slips her index fingers under the scalp and grasps with her thumbs outside, one hand at each pole of the incision, and everts the edge. (If the patient has some hairs at the edge of the incision, they can be grasped by the assistant to help evert the wound edge.) The physician or second as-

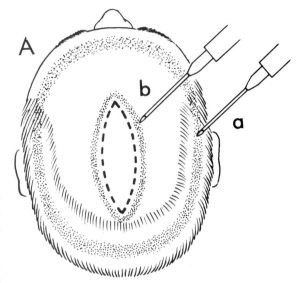

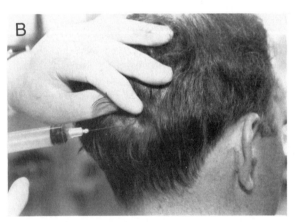

FIG 6–29.
A, local infiltration as a ring block and around the incision sites. **B,** clinical example of ring block being injected.

sistant sponges the wound edge and exposes only a few centimeters. The physician then cauterizes the obvious bleeders (Fig 6–33). Again, the Shaw scalpel will work for cauterizing vessels but it builds up char and is slow and awkward. The fastest and most limited wound comes from the electrodesiccator. As mentioned in other chapters, we like the Birtcher hyphrecator. It is quick and simple to have one assistant evert the wound edge, a second assistant sponge the wound, and the doctor hold the hyphrecator in the dominant hand and a cotton-tipped applicator in the other, and start at the anterior pole of the wound and move posteriorly. The assistant who is sponging the wound keeps just ahead of the doctor, and, as the assistant uncovers a bleeder, the doctor desiccates it. With this technique, the bleeding from one entire side of the reduction is controlled in 30 seconds, with no need for clamps, ligatures, or involved procedures.

When we first started reductions, we tried to use Rainey clamps, which are commonly used by neurosurgeons to stop the bleeding at the scalp wound edge (Fig 6–34). They are disposable plastic clamps 2 cm long, and are snapped over the wound edge by a special instrument.

Like other innovations we tried, they produced added work with minimal help. It is hard to improve on the simplicity and speed of the above-described technique.

The next step is to undermine (Fig 6–35). Again, physicians develop their preferences. Many tools will work since the subgaleal-periosteal plane on the scalp is almost bloodless and filled with only a wispy stroma, which is easily separated by almost any instrument, including the human fingers. We have seen bent (curved) scalpel handles with a no. 15 tip used to sweep around the curve of the cranium and periosteal

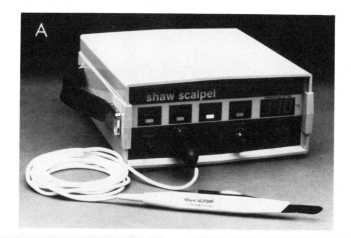

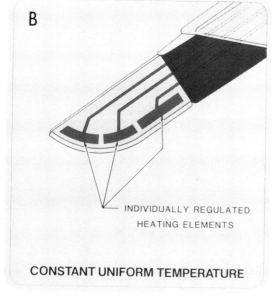

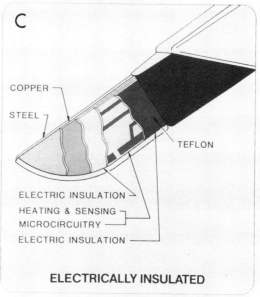

FIG 6–30.
A, the Shaw scalpel. **B,** the heating elements in each blade. **C,** the insulation and coating steel layers.

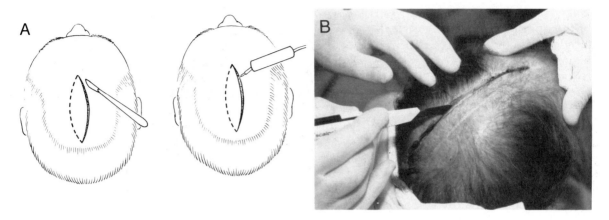

FIG 6–31.
A, the incision is made with the Shaw scalpel or a regular blade. The wound edges are electrodesiccated. **B,** a clinical example of the incision.

elevators slid over the periosteum; the Luikart Iconoclast, straight or curved, works, but so do straight or curved scissors of many types, such as Webster face-lift scissors, Castanares scissors, and thoracotomy scissors. The only decision is how far to undermine. Obviously the extent of the anesthesia will practically limit the dissection. The location of the first incision dictates how far the undermining can go, because the curve of the cranium is limiting. If it is a midline design, about the same length from the wound edges is possible on both sides. If it is paramediun, it will be easier to undermine further down the side of the reduction since the opposite side would require an instrument properly curved and long enough to reach across the top of the head and then down the opposite side. Generally, for our reductions we undermine with scissors under the entire top of the head and down the sides to just above the ears. We undermine the occiput until we encounter firm resistance.

Only rarely does undermining set off a brisk bleeder, but when it does it must be stopped. First try suction and visualization through the reduction opening. Again, the assistants lifting up the wound edges with their fingers provides a good look for several centimeters under the flap. If the bleeder cannot be seen, try a percutaneous suture ligature with something large on a large curved needle, such as 0 silk or 1–0 Dexon on a CU-6 needle (Fig 6–36). As a final

trial, incise toward where you think the bleeder may be and ligate it under direct observation.

This is the time for a "trial closure." One side of the opening is pulled over the other to estimate how much can be trimmed off (Fig 6–37). The maneuver is accomplished by using the hands on both sides to push the scalp toward the opening, or by fastening towel clips on the edge to be excised pulling it up and over the opposite side, or it has been suggested that an instrument originally designed for face-lift surgery, the D-Assumpco Marking Tool, works the same way for scalp reductions.[59] One blade of a forceps-like instrument hooks onto one edge of the reduction and the other edge is pulled over it, and the second blade clamps down and marks off how much tissue can be removed without taking too much. Such instruments are helpful, but there is still considerable surgical judgment about how much to take: How tight should the closure be? How much more can be gained with undermining and galeotomies? Should the scalp be trimmed off just at the proposed junction of the two flaps, or should a little more be removed to maximize the reduction or a little less to reduce the tension?

If the trial closure reveals too little scalp to be removed, further undermining is the first maneuver to try. Rotating the two flaps a few degrees so they do not move directly toward each other (this creates an "S" closure) may pull from

A

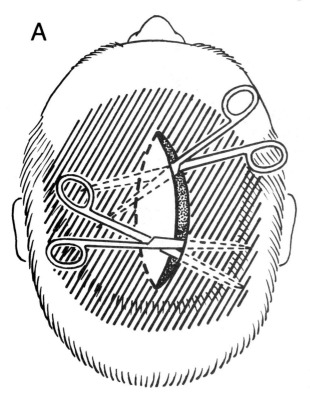

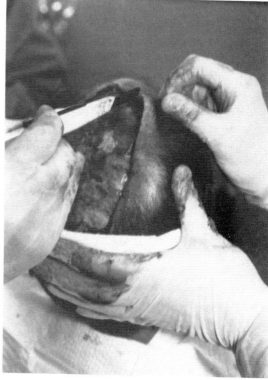

FIG 6–33.
A technique for electrodesiccating or electrocoagulating the edge bleeders is to have the assistant raise the edge by pulling on the hair.

B

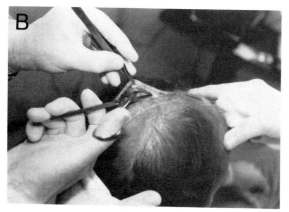

FIG 6–32.
A, undermining on both sides of the incision can be performed with scissors, scalpel, or especially designed instruments. **B,** a clinical example of undermining.

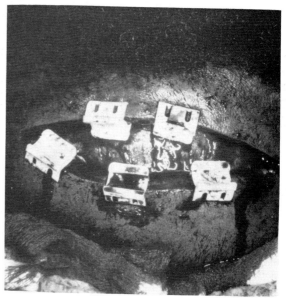

a slightly different angle and utilize a looser part of the scalp. Whether or not to cut galeotomies is the next option (Fig 6–38). We are not aware of any long-term difficulties from galeotomies; they can be a little awkward to cut and occasionally a vessel will be transsected and require

FIG 6–34.
Rainey clamps used to stop edge bleeders. We do not now believe they are necessary.

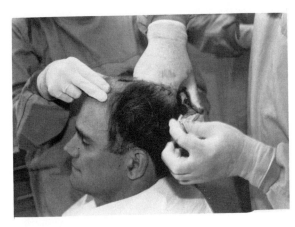

FIG 6–35.
Blunt, atraumatic undermining with the hand is most effective.

suture ligature, which is quite awkward to place. The edge of the opening is lifted and everted as much as possible. Under direct visualization, a scalpel is used to cut just through the galea in a line parallel to the wound edge. As the galea is cut through, it will begin to gap. It is not necessary—it is actually contraindicated—to cut deeper than just through the galea. The incision should be several centimeters long at the location of the most tension. Conceivably, the galea cut could be as long as the skin incision. If there is a little edge bleeding, it can be desiccated; larger bleeders require sutures.

Again, attempt a trial closure. If it is still the case that too little skin is available for removal or the closure will be too tight, go back and cut a second galeotomy parallel to the first or cut one on the opposite side in the same fashion. Three parallel cuts is the most that should be made for either side.

After wide undermining and galeotomies, the amount that can be removed is limited only by how much tension across the wound is acceptable. The scalp will tolerate a great deal of tension, especially with two-layer closures starting with the galeal approximation, but there is also more immediate postoperative pain and swelling. Both are managed with postoperative medications. The important and unanswered

question is: Does tension across the wound affect the amount of stretch-back (discussed below) or actual scar spreading? We like to say we design a "snug" scalp reduction, trading a millimeter or two of scalp for less morbidity.

The prescribed amount of scalp excised again with the Shaw scalpel and the few bleeding arteries are cauterized under direct visualization as the assistants evert the wound edges (Fig 6–39). No matter how carefully estimates are made, we always cut about 3 mm less tissue that we estimated would be the maximum. It is a safety step, and more tissue can always be taken off of one or several sections if the edges still have extra skin. Another technique is to pull the scalp flap over the opposite side and cut 2 to 3 incisions toward the opposite side. This allows precise observation of the amount to cut off. A stay suture or staple there holds it in place until the other sites are checked.

Suturing

Nearly all we have seen or read indicates that two-layer closures are preferable; the two layers are the galea and the skin. There is some

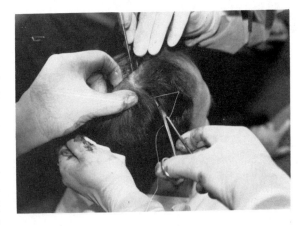

FIG 6–36.
If a bleeder is discovered on the flap a long distance from the wound edge which makes it difficult to desiccate, a percutaneous stitch will stop the bleeding.

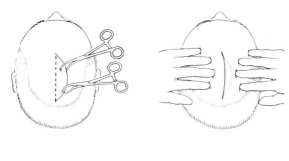

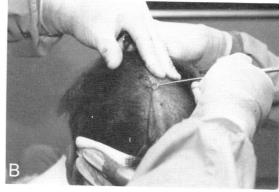

FIG 6–37.
A, a test closure is tried to see how much scalp can be cut off. Towel clamps or digital pressure both work for this maneuver.
B, a clinical example of pulling one edge over the other with fingers and a hook.

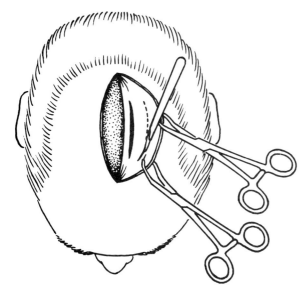

FIG 6–38.
If little looseness develops, the amount of scalp that can be sacrificed can be increased by cutting galeotomies on one or both sides of the wound.

controversy, however, about which suture material is best for the galea closure. Nordstrom et al. proved that the scar itself is a few millimeters wider at 3 months if absorbable (Dexon) suture is compared with nonabsorbable (Prolene) suture.[60]

We have not measured or compared the width of scars in our patients but most of the

time have been happy that there is little true scar widening. We use 1–0 Dexon on a CU-6 needle or 2–0 nylon for the running galea closure. After the first loop and knot, approximately 3 mm of galea on each side is caught up in the needle using a simple running or locked stitch, with the second knot at the opposite end. One long suture is usually adequate for a fusiform reduction, and second or even third sutures are needed for the Y or Mercedes designs. The skin can be closed with the physician's suture of choice: 3–0 Mer-

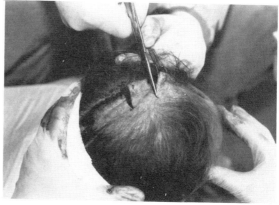

FIG 6–39.
A second way to measure how much should be cut off is to cut perpendicular incisions in order to visualize exactly where the two edges will come together.

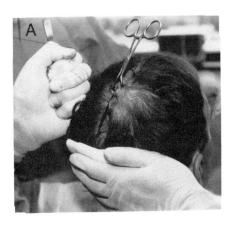
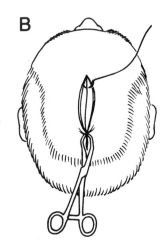
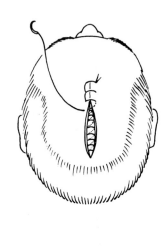

FIG 6–40.
A and B, towel clamps or other clips hold the wound edges together while the buried sutures are placed in the galea.

siline (braided Dacron) nylon, Prolene, or staples. Staples on the scalp look like they might be troublesome, but they are not and patients tolerate them well.

A temporary closure of the gaping reduction defect is extremely helpful—actually probably necessary to getting the galeal suture in tightly and evenly. We use towel clamps to pull the edges together and remove them as we close the galea. It usually requires only two or three clamps to hold the whole wound together (Fig 6–40). The clamps are unsightly, but do not seem to leave scars and are easy to use. Temporary sutures or assistant's hands could all serve the same function (Fig 6–41).

Dressing

After reduction, a dressing is optional; a full head wrap is protective and comfortable, and can be taken off the next day. But just as often, we simply comb the hair over the suture line and send the patient home. Sutures and staples come out in 10 to 14 days. Steroids, antibiotics, and analgesics have been discussed above and are given at the physician's discretion.

Complications

Stretch-Back

Although stretch-back is not truly a complication it certainly is a phenomenon that diminishes the value of reductions. Nordstrom is the

only researcher to carefully study and report this event.[60] He states that all of the stretch-back occurs in the 12 weeks following surgery; most of it happens in the first 8 weeks. His measurement of 13 patients revealed that between 30% and 50% of the reduction is lost. Unfortunately, most of the stretching is in the scalp tissue adjacent to the excision—not the hair-bearing scalp but the bald scalp—the very skin the procedure was trying to eliminate. Subsequent reductions are not followed with as much stretch-back, although it is still a significant amount.[62] Also, since the stretching is adjacent to the area of the reduction under the most tension, the poles of the reduction stay much the same as immediately after surgery. With a fusiform design, the posterior crown is actually slightly compressed.

There seem to be no other ill effects from the stretching, but multiple reductions may thin the scalp. Also, not all doctors report the occurrence of stretch-back. Martin Unger believes that the tension on the closure directly affects how much stretch-back develops.[61] He has little trouble with this because he removes only enough tissue so that the galea closes easily and without undue tension.

We close under moderate tension, but have come to avoid the high-tension designs. The postoperative pain and swelling are also reasons we have stopped "cutting out the last bit of scalp."

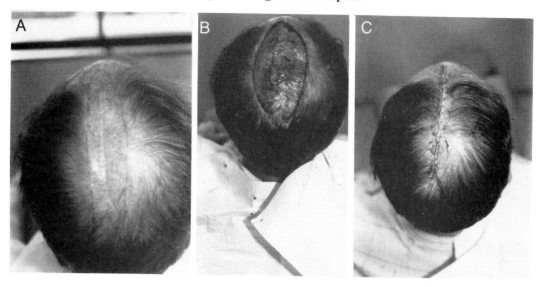

FIG 6–41.
A, patient before reduction. B, patient as loose scalp is being excised. C, patient scalp closed.

Scarring

As discussed above with the midline, fusiform reduction there is a potential problem of development of a visible scar and alteration of the occipital hair pattern. Either or both can be significant cosmetic liabilities (Figs 6–42 to 6–44). If one or several reductions will nearly completely remove crown or midline baldness, there will be little problem with the scar, but if the reduction only removes part of the alopecia—as is true for most patients—the patient is left with baldness and a scar across the baldness. A bald spot is natural; a bald spot with a hatchet mark across it is not. The correction of scar visibility is prevention and planning. The reduction scars must be located where they will be covered with hair—either natural hair combed over or transplanted hair around the scar.

Hair falling away from the reduction scar is also a problem that is difficult to correct. The scar is around 2 mm wide and the hair growing up on either side of the scar at a 30 degree angle creates a false part 4 to 5 mm wide. When that "part" is running directly down the lambdoid ridge, it is most difficult to cover. There is no way to comb the hairs on the back of the head sideways over the scar and false part. When the S- or C-shaped scar of a paramedian reduction lies on the posterolateral crown opposite the part, hairs—natural or transplanted—must be present to comb over it. Even the paramedian scars draw attention because of the false part composed of the scar width itself and the hair direction growing away from that scar.

With the Y or Mercedes pattern there is a three-corner suture line. It is not unusual for the junction of the three flaps to heal with a widened or depressed scar. Such a depression can be revised by cutting it out at a later date.

Miscellaneous

Infection is extremely rare with reductions. As with transplants, forehead swelling may develop on the third or fourth postoperative day, especially if the work was more anterior. This is self-limiting, but may be limited with systemic steroids given preoperatively. Pain is probably related to tension, which can be considerable for several days. Analgesics are prescribed as needed. Numbness is not a problem with midline reductions but can develop superior to C- or S-shaped designs. It usually is gone within 5 to 6 months and is self-limiting (Figs 6–45 and 6–46).

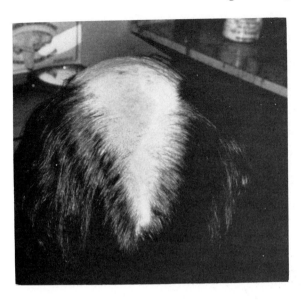

FIG 6–42.
A complication of the midline reduction when the incision is carried too far posteriorly.

the frontal hairline, it may be more successful to remove a narrow island of scalp than to transplant it with closely spaced plants. There are times when, after several frontal rows have been planted close together, more plants will not do as well because of the scarring. Yet there is a bald strip close enough to the front to show. Cutting that strip out is the treatment of choice.

The design is to remove a long, narrow strip of scalp and close primarily. Or multiple 4- to 6-mm diameter contiguous holes can be cut with punches. The scalloped edges interdigitate when closed side to side.

The same technique is workable on a donor area from which too many plugs were taken or, for some reason, healing was poor.

Maxi-Reductions

This refers to the series of procedures that remove great amounts of bald scalp and undermine extremely widely. Brandy has popularized

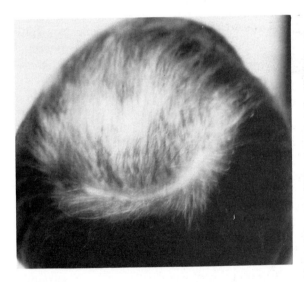

FIG 6–43.
The scar is visible when it is placed so far posteriorly that the hairs comb away from it.

Mini-Reductions

Cutting out bald scalp between rows of transplants or between flaps and transplants is straightforward and helpful.[63] Particularly near

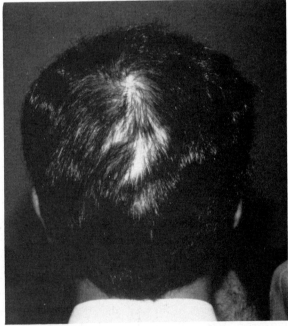

FIG 6–44.
A patient who had a scalp reduction with the midline incision extending too far posteriorly; this patient has had Z-plasties that attempt to camouflage the scar and are only partially successful.

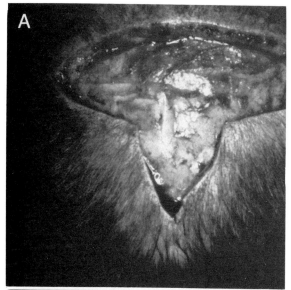

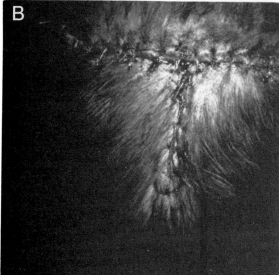

FIG 6–45.
A T-shaped reduction. **A,** after skin is excised. **B,** after closure.

the whole series in the United States.[62, 63] It has been reported at meetings and by Unger[64] that the concept of wide undermining was introduced by an Australian physician, Dr. Marzola, and a concomitant use of bilateral flaps by a compatriot, Dr. Bradshaw. It was the Australians who taught the procedure to Brandy, who added all the parts together under the heading of "Extensive Scalp-Lifting."

For bilateral occipitoparietal flap (BOP), a long U-shaped incision starts just posterior to the temporal hairline; extends along the fringe hairs of the parietal region, the occiput, the opposite parietal region; and ends on the opposite temple (Fig 6–47). The undermining extends under the entire hair-bearing scalp: to and behind the ears, to and beyond the lambdoid galea at-

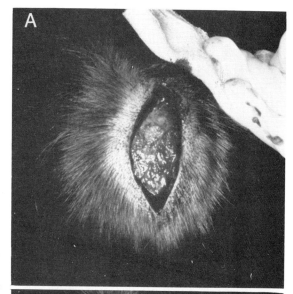

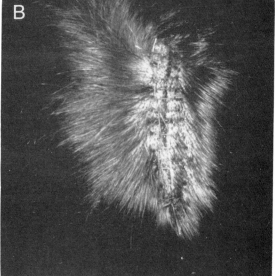

FIG 6–46.
A midline reduction. **A,** after skin is excised. **B,** after closure.

Surgical Management of Alopecia

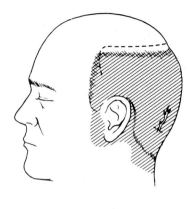

FIG 6–47.
For a maxi-lift, the incision is a long U-shape that extends around the edge of the fringe hairs.

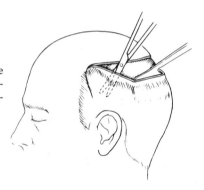
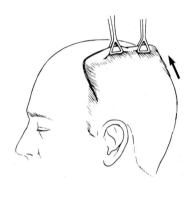

FIG 6–48.
Undermining is wide and extensive. The occipital arteries are identified, transected, and ligated. The scalp is dissected from the lambdoid ridge.

ommends that the operation be staged by locating and ligating the occipital arteries. Others who do extensive lifting will ligate both occipitals several weeks before the BOP flap.

The extensive undermining and the U-shaped incision necessitate the transection of the greater occipital nerve, the postauricular artery and vein, the occipital arteries bilaterally, and the superficial temporal artery and vein. The posterior scalp dissection extends inferior to the hair-bearing scalp onto the neck. Work in this area requires the proper retractors, lights, and assistants, to operate safely and effectively.

After the undermining, the hair-bearing scalp is advanced anteriorly and medially (Fig 6–48). The usual movement is 3.5 to 4.0 cm forward. Since this is a bilateral advancement, great amounts of baldness are eliminated. The patient retains a normal U-shaped baldness and the hairline at the posterior neck may be slightly

elevated.

Some months later—3 to 4—the remaining central baldness is excised again by an extremely widely undermining procedure. The incisions are made on both sides at the fringe and down the center of the head with a dog-ear hook posteriorly to take out redundancy that develops there (Fig 6–49). The incisions start anteriorly at the temporal hairline, curve medially and posteriorly, join midline, and cut to the crown where the dog-ear is placed (Fig 6–50). The intervening bald scalp is excised and the two sides are closed together. Drains, heavy dressings, vital sign monitoring, and IVs, are integral for both operations.

These giant reductions/flaps need to be combined with regular transplants to build a normal frontal hairline. Brandy starts with transplants in the frontal area before doing the BOP. He adds more plants—regular and micro—at var-

Surgical Management of Alopecia

A

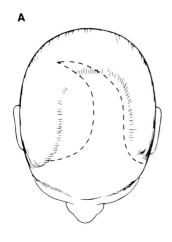

B

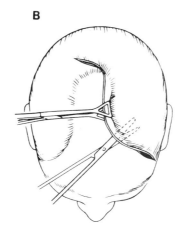

FIG 6–49.
A, the incisions for a maxi scalp reduction (after a maxi lift) are first made down the center of the baldness and along the edge of the fringe on one side. **B,** after wide undermining, that side is pulled upward.

A

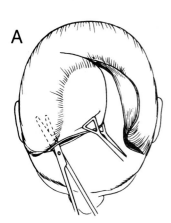

B

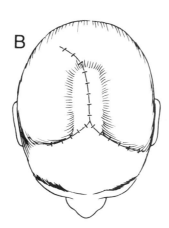

FIG 6–50.
A, the other side is widely undermined and pulled upward. **B,** the overlapping skin is excised and the two flaps sutured together. A frontal hairline must be built with transplants or flaps.

ious times around the larger procedures.

These procedures are major with extensive disruption of the vascular and nerve supplies to the scalp. Proper experience and equipment are essential and the patient needs much more and deeper anesthesia and more medical support than with regular reductions.

The advantages lie in the amounts of bald scalp removed. With the regular and mini-transplants used to build a frontal area, and these reductions used to remove nearly all of the remaining baldness, the patients do truly benefit. But the "cost" is high and the disadvantages are so many that Martin Unger, many Australian physicians, and some of the originators have abandoned the procedure.[67, 68] As mentioned above, the posterior hairline may be raised and

the hairless space above the ears is increased. The scars along the temple and frontal areas do not always camouflage well. The frontal line may be artificial, since just behind the transplant lies the sideward-directed hairs sewn side to side. There is commonly widespread numbness. Postoperative telogen effluvium is extensive over much of the scalp in some patients, and take several months to resolve.

The most disturbing complication—the one that has persuaded several to stop the procedure—is the high incidence of necrosis. Some surgeons reported necrosis in as many as 50% of patients, which was extensive in a few.[68] However, other surgeons have an acceptably low complication rate.

When the procedure is totally successful,

some patients can gain dramatic correction of baldness, but the total morbidity, risk, and somewhat unnatural results make only a few good candidates for this kind of surgery. Most patients who come in for the surgical management of alopecia seek and welcome coverage of their baldness, but, appropriately, do not expect to be subjected to major surgery and major risks.

Scalp Flaps

When the subject of flaps for alopecia arises, the old saw, "If you're so smart, why ain't you rich?" pops into mind. Another version is, "If flaps are so good, why aren't more done?" We hear the virtues of flaps discussed at meetings, followed by many pictures of befores and excellent afters. Yet there is nagging doubt. We hear other experts decry the inherent problems with flaps. All surgical treatments for alopecia have inherent problems, so why choose transplants over flaps?

From our own experience, our exposure to others' work, and extensive reading, we conclude that there are two primary limiting factors in scalp flap surgery for alopecia: (1) the size, extent, morbidity, and cost of the procedure, and (2) the unnaturalness of the resulting hair pattern. Nearly all experienced flap surgeons who write and speak about it state that one or two delays are necessary to reduce the incidence of necrosis. Most recommend general anesthesia or heavy twilight anesthesia for the procedure. There is considerable morbidity after the flap is rotated, requiring 6 to 10 days of convalescence. Then several scalp reductions are necessary to eliminate remaining baldness. All of this is traumatic and costly.

The appropriate euphemism for success is patient selection. That selection eliminates most bald men. The patient should not have much more than Norwood classification baldness II—loss of hair in the anterior one-half of the head. Although more extensive baldness has been treated with flaps, the recommended third flap is difficult to do because of the scars, the tight scalp, the compromised blood supply, and other factors. And the *multiple* scalp reductions needed to eliminate any intervening baldness and future baldness are not easy to perform,

either. The patient must be able to tolerate the unevenness of the thick hair of the flap in juxtaposition to the balding miniaturizing hairs on the rest of the crown. The patient will need to style the backward direction of the flap hair growth. There is a big difference in the "need" to style hair after transplants, where the requirement is that the patient comb down and to one side—a common and natural pattern—vs. the "need" to comb the frontal hair up, back, and over in a giant wave to accommodate the direction of the flap hair and to cover the wispy balding hairs behind.

There is controversy about whether or not the frontal hairline of a flap looks artificial. If the patient has only frontal baldness and dense, coarse hair behind, a similar frontal line looks fine. If the patient has thinning hair behind the flap, the flap stands out as an island of hair. The techniques discussed below to ameliorate the sharpness of the frontal line are helpful, but do not eliminate for all patients this major drawback with the flaps. We have often wondered if the popularity of the Juri flap was in part the result of the dense, thick coarse hairs and the sharp frontal hairlines of Argentine men.

History

Modern-day flaps used for baldness began with a temporoparietal design described by Lamont.[69] The Juri brothers worked with flaps for years, gradually extending the length, adding delays, and experimenting with the width. What was known as the Juri flap in 1969 when it was first invented and as it is still known today is a temporoparietal-occipital (TPO) flap. It was reported at the First International Congress of Aesthetic Plastic Surgery in 1972 and in the literature in 1975.[70, 71] Elliott designed a flap that was random, shorter, and narrower than the Juri, or TPO, flap.[72]

Over the years, the designs have been refined and certain operators have developed their own variations.[73–76] Basically, the designs fall into two groups: short, random, narrow, nondelayed flaps that cover only one-half of the frontal line, and long (TPO) axial (based on a branch of the superficial temporal artery) wide flaps, usually delayed once or twice, that recreate a full frontal line. Second flaps are used to cover mid and posterior baldness. There is controversy about the delays; some use them and some do not. But certainly flaps wider than 2 to 3 cm need a delay, and if a branch of the superficial temporal artery can be included in the design, the chance of some necrosis is greatly reduced.

The history of flaps includes some widely divergent attitudes about the indications. Flemming and Mayer believe flaps to be excellent for extensive baldness if the donor areas are good and the scalp is loose.[78] Nordström uses flaps only if the baldness is in the anterior one-third to one-half of the head.[77] And Unger believes their use is precluded if the scalp flap is meant to rebuild a frontal line.[79]

With this much controversy and divergent opinion, it is hard to predict if scalp flaps will survive as a surgical treatment for baldness. As stated above, morbidity and cost are factors that limit their popularity. It may be that only a few physicians will do them. This is not a bad circumstance, because those physicians will become quite skilled with whatever technique they prefer and the few patients who are motivated and have the financial means for a flap will be referred to these experienced specialists.

Technique
Juri or TPO Flap

The flap is designed so that it begins directly over the posterior branch of the superficial temporal artery, which can be located by palpation or by a Doppler flowmeter. The inferior edge is located about 3 cm above the anterior aspect of the helix, and the superior edge 4 cm beyond that. Some physicians make the anterior one-third of the flap 3 cm wide to reduce the size of the rotation dog-ear and thus make closure of the donor defect easier. The flap angles 30 to 45 degrees upward and then curves gently over the ear, down onto the parietal scalp postauricularly, and onto the occiput. It may even go past the center of the back of the head. The shape of the flap is dictated by the shape of the new frontal hairline. If there are to be deep temporal recessions, the flap will need to be longer and curve appropriately at its mid and distal sections. About 3 to 4 cm will be used for the rotation so the actual hairline will start somewhere on the flap above the ear. Be careful that the flap

does not curve too far superiorly, because the superior edge, which will become the leading edge and thus the very front of the hairline, is not in the part of the scalp programmed to go bald.

In general, those who design a 2- to 3-cm-wide flap do not delay, and those who mark out wider flaps do. There is worry about the incidence of necrosis with the nondelayed flaps, and examples of this complication have appeared in the literature. However, we are not aware of any studies that prove to what degree the delay is necessary.

Nevertheless, the flap design needs to be marked on the scalp with pen or small tattoos, or a template can be constructed with plastic, foam rubber, or adhesive tape folded upon itself for stiffness. The more flexible materials allow the proximal end of the template to be held down and the distal end to be rotated to the desired position. This helps anticipate the dog-ear and makes it possible to design the frontal line properly.

The delayed sections are incised under local anesthesia (Fig 6–51, A). The incisions go to the level of the periosteum—completely through the galea. The first delay is both sides of the middle one-third of the flap. These incisions are closed with sutures or staples.

One week later, the second delay is performed, again under local anesthesia. The distal one-third of the flap is cut and raised to transsect any perforators. It too is sutured back in place.

One week later, or two weeks after the first delay, the flap is completely elevated and transposed (Fig 6–51, B). This operation is usually done under general anesthesia but can be performed with a local only, or with twilight anesthesia. The patient is placed on his side and the hair within the flap is moistened and pulled into little tufts with rubber bands. There is no reason to cut any hairs; doing so only delays the immediate benefit of this procedure. The area around the flap but not the flap itself or the base of the flap are anesthetized with lidocaine 1% or ½% with epinephrine 1:100,000 or 1:200,000. The flap is elevated entirely, and kept moist with normal saline. Bleeders are lightly coagulated or ligated on the flap, and the bleeders on the wound edges are treated more vigorously. Ex-

Surgical Management of Alopecia

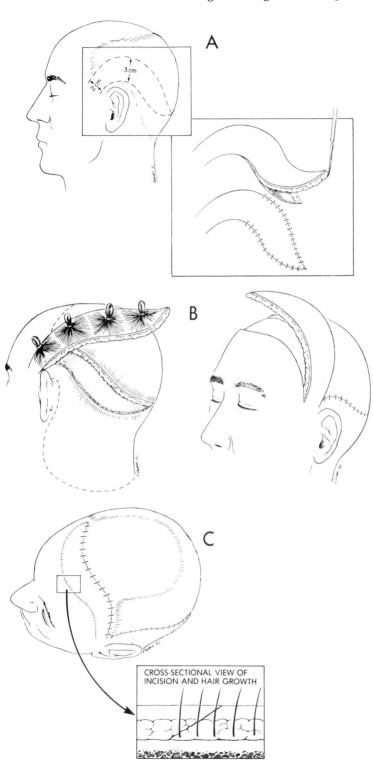

FIG 6–51.
The Juri-type of scalp flap. **A,** the design of the flap and the second-delay tip elevation and replacement. **B,** the rotation of the twice-delayed flap. **C,** the flap sutured in place in the new location with de-epithelialization of the anterior edge to reduce scarring.

tensive undermining is performed on both sides of the wound. Inferiorly, the scalp is dissected in the subgaleal plane to under the hair margin, then further dissection is made just subcutaneously down onto the neck, behind the ears, and around the occiput. The other side of the wound is undermined in the subgaleal plane over most of the crown and to the proposed frontal hair line. We sometimes put in a Jackson-Pratt-type drain in the postauricular area, but not if the area is dry.

The frontal incision is made and the posterior edge of that wound undermined, with the dissection joining the earlier undermining of the scalp. The donor defect is closed. This is a critical step in the operation and one of the most difficult. Once the donor defect is closed, the rest of the procedure is meticulous and artistic but not demanding. There are two keys to getting the donor area closed without undue tension: wide undermining over the scalp and neck, and a posterior and lateral rotation (toward the donor side) of the scalp on top of the head. This is possible because incision for the new hairline recipient site has been cut. The posterior and lateral movement of the top scalp helps close the donor defect and creates some of the recipient site for the flap. It is important that there be enough movement from both sides of the defect so it will close easily. The problems of scar-spreading and traction alopecia in the donor area were some of the worst that we encountered when we first started doing this flap. The closure is two-layered: galeal with 0 Dexon, and skin with suture or staples of choice.

The leading edge of the flap is sometimes de-epithelialized so that the flap edge will slip a little under the forehead skin (Fig 6–51, C). The hairs in that de-epithelialized lip grow up through the scar and help camouflage it. When this process works, enough hairs grow through the scar to help reduce the sharpness of the flap hairline (one of the major drawbacks with flaps) and hide the scar. But it does not always work and then the scar is visible and sharp.

The flap should be handled carefully and gently draped over and into the recipient site. There are two ways to suture it in. One is to start sewing on the leading edge at the proximal end of the flap just anterior to the dog-ear at the depth of the temporal recession and to move distally on the flap. Small sutures such as 5/0 nylon, either simple running or interrupted, are all that are required here. The flap is gently pulled longer as the suturing advances across the forehead. The flap contracts somewhat when elevated, and the one or two delays produce some edema. Therefore it is neither unwise nor dangerous to tug it out a little while placing it in the new location. A second method, particularly if the flap is not edematous, is to lay it in the desired new location and tack the leading edge with interrupted sutures and go back and fill in once the placement has been properly made. If for some reason the flap is too short, do not pull too hard. It is better to do a small flap from the opposite side than to lose some of the major flap.

When the leading edge is in place, the rest of the recipient site is cut. If the scalp was moved posterior-laterally to close the donor defect, there might be little or no more scalp that needs to be excised. Whatever it takes to lay the flap in easily is what should be cut. The trailing edge of the flap is sewn in with the suture or staples of choice. Sometimes a Penrose drain under the trailing edge of the flap is indicated.

A full-head dressing is necessary, as well as careful postoperative monitoring for vital signs and excessive bleeding or swelling. Steroids, antibiotics, and analgesics are used according to the physician's choice. Insist that the patient take several days—up to six—for convalescence. Plan to see the patient several times in the first postoperative week (Fig 6–52).

Additional Procedures

The dog-ear at the base of the flap rotation site almost always requires later removal. It is usually removed six weeks afterwards. A second flap can be done in 3 or 4 months if the scalp has regained its softness and mobility. The second flap is designed like the first, except that it is usually laid straight across the scalp and does not need to be curved for a frontal hairline and thus does not need to be as long. It can begin a little higher and more posteriorly because it will be placed more posteriorly on the head. Even with these two factors making it easier, this can be a more difficult flap because of the closure of

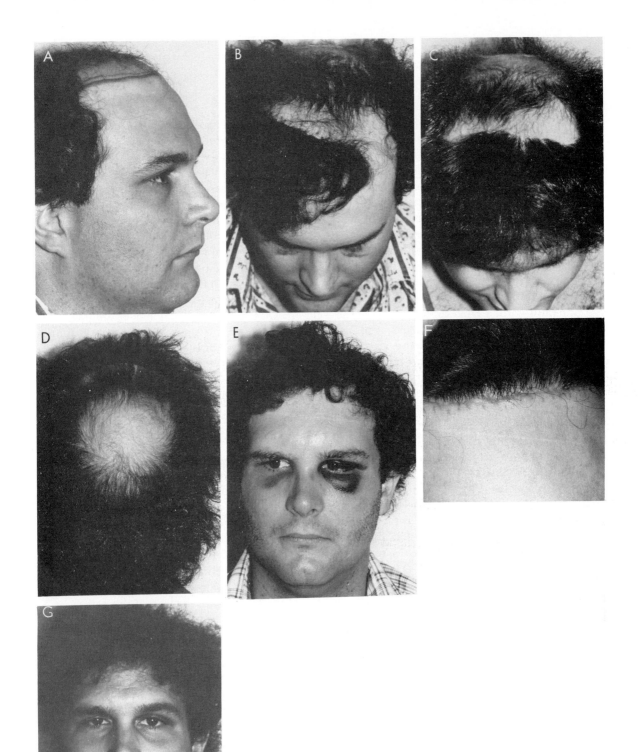

FIG 6–52.
Man, 38 years old, having a Juri-type flap procedure. **A**, marking for the location of the anterior edge of the flap, which is the new frontal hair line. **B**, after the flap is in place. **C**, after a second flap is in place, covering the rest of the frontal line and thickening the anterior hair replacement. **D**, a posterior view with both flaps in place. **E**, 1 week after the second flap has been rotated. **F**, close-up of the hairline showing the hairs starting to grow through the scar. **G**, 6 months after the second flap.

the donor area. Much of the looseness has already been used up and the scalp cannot be shifted as easily to the donor side to facilitate closure. Undermining must tunnel down onto the neck and all around the ear, even onto the posterior pinna.

The third flap, as described by Juri, is seldom done. Most of the time the patient can satisfactorily cover the baldness and the doctor does not really want to try to close still another large defect. The location of the flap is more difficult than portrayed in idealized schematic drawings because of scarring, narrow posterior donor fringe areas, and the shape of many men's lambdoid ridge.

Reductions to remove bald scalp between flaps or between a flap and further balding should be planned at 6 to 8 weeks. Often these reductions are mentioned as though they were easy surgeries. If the patient does not have a loose scalp and one that becomes loose again after the flap surgery, the reduction(s) may need to proceed in several stages to "remove" all of the intervening baldness.

Transplants also are used in conjunction with flaps. If the flap produces the frontal hairline, the plants may be placed anywhere posterior to the flap. If the flap is used on the center crown, plants complete the process either anteriorly or posteriorly. Micro- or miniplants in front of a frontal flap help disguise the sharp line of hair. These plants, however, must be oriented in the direction of the hair on the flap, which is usually posteriorly.

Complications

Two major surgical complications make this flap a procedure that involves major risk. Necrosis of any or all of the flap has occurred. If it happens, there is little recourse but to wait until the necrotic area has defined itself and separated. After that, wait three to four months for growth of any adjacent hairs which may only be in traumatic shock (resting phase). Then start reparations in the form of transplants, scar removal, or a short flap from the opposite side to fill in the hairless part of the flap.

For flaps as long as the TPO, the patient should not have any compromising factors: be a smoker, have diabetes mellitus, previous scar-

ring in the donor area, or collagen vascular disease, or be on any medications that might negatively affect circulation. If there is any doubt about the scalp blood supply, delays must be part of the planning.

Scarring in the donor area is another major complication that fortunately is now uncommon. (Fig 6–53). Not only will some patients' donor scar spread, but they may also develop alopecia—assumed to be traction or traumatic—around that scar. Sometimes the spread scar and alopecia are out of proportion to the tension on the closure because some scalps are more sensitive to the tension. If there is excessive tension on the closure, these events are more common.

A true design error is to make the front line too straight without temporal recessions. It might be placed unevenly, with the donor side lower (more anterior) than the opposite side. Some believe that transposing a thick, hair-bearing flap across the front of a totally bald crown is also an error. With reductions and transplants, the head posterior to the flap can never have hair as thick as the frontal flap, meaning that the patient will always have a markedly unnatural appearance.

Other complications are more cosmetic but nevertheless annoying. One complication is a frontal line that is sharp and full. Normal frontal hairlines are a graduation of vellus to miniaturizing to terminal hairs for 5 to 10 mm. This natural gradation is what is partly addressed by the micro- and minitransplants. With flaps, the abrupt start of fully dense and fully terminal hairs produces a look which in some is more artificial than a hairpiece.

There are several techniques that can be used to try to soften this line. De-epithelialization of the leading edge of the flap helps in some patients. Actually cutting the leading edge of the flap in an irregular line—a geometric broken line—helps a little but is a great deal of work. Plants placed anterior to the flap, in cases where the flap was purposely placed about 1 cm higher than the final line, are very helpful.

The scar at the leading edge of the flap always shows for a while but in most patients fades within 6 to 12 months. A few patients will have permanently visible scars. Dermabrasion

Surgical Management of Alopecia

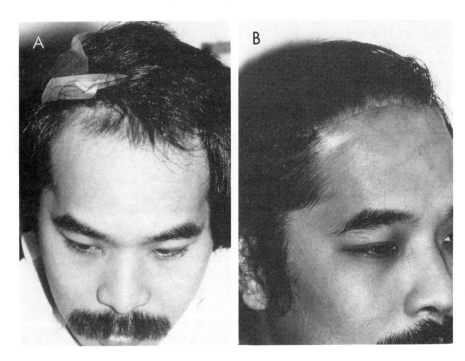

FIG 6–53.
A, man, 23 years old, before two Juri-type flaps were performed. **B**, the scar is visible when the man combs his hair back four months after the last surgery.

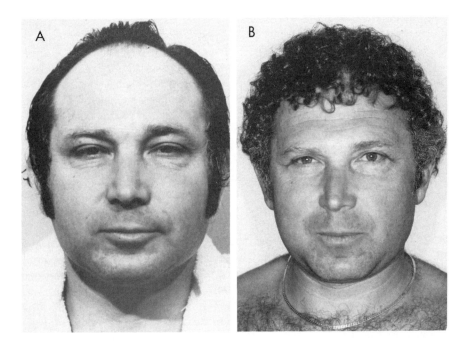

FIG 6–54.
A, man, age 40, before two short temporal flaps are performed. **B**, after the flaps and with a hair permanent. (Courtesy of Drs. Toby Mayer and Richard Flemming, Beverly Hills, Calif.)

and scar revision can be used with moderate success. Some patients will develop telogen effluvium on parts or all of the flap. This too diminishes one of the advantages of flap surgery—instant results—but hair will regrow after the two- to four-month resting phase.

Infections have occurred but are rare and have responded to appropriate antibiotics.

Advantages

The results of scalp flaps are immediate except when complications develop. The results from transplants, however, are minimal at six months, and full hairlines can take years. The transposed hair is thicker than can be achieved with transplants, so thick that the hair can be parted through the flap (Fig 6–54). On heads that have dense, natural hair behind the flap, the dense hairline is completely appropriate and could not be accompanied by any other technique. A single transposition flap into a bald crown also covers with a density not achievable with transplants and creates a styling problem that is not as difficult to manage as those that occur following some scalp reductions.

Short Flaps

We define short flaps as those flaps that cover no more than one-half of the frontal hairline, are not delayed, and may be based inferiorly or superiorly. By definition, these flaps are random rather than axial. Their use is for patients with deeply receding temples or for men who particularly hate the temple recession and otherwise have every indication of keeping most of the rest of their hair. The flaps provide a good, dense, and if aesthetically designed, natural hairline—natural if the rest of the scalp hair remains thick and dense (Fig 6–55). A flap across the temples in front of thin, sparse, and miniaturizing hair does not look good or natural.

The demands on the doctor and patient are less than for the long Juri or TPO flaps. The choice of superior or inferior basing depends on the height and shape of the temple hair pattern and the quality of hair anterior and posterior to the ear. If there is dense, thick, ample terminal hair (not whisker hair) anterior to the ear, the superiorly based flap is best. It has only a 60-degree rotation, transposes hairs that point forward rather than backward, and can be done with the patient seated and under local anesthesia.

If the hair anterior to the ears is not acceptable, the inferiorly based temporoparietal flap is necessary. This is designed as a gentle curve beginning at the root of the ear and curving over the ear. Thus, the donor hair is from above and just posterior to the ear. This flap needs to be longer than the superiorly based flap, and the hair points posteriorly. It is still short enough to perform without delay, using only local anesthesia.

The technique for the short flap is similar to that for the long flap, except that each step is shorter, easier, and quicker. The biggest problem is aesthetics. The flap may blunt the temple recession, which is often a normal adult characteristic. Another problem is the difference in the color and quality of the temporal or temporoparietal hair compared with the frontal hair.

Tissue Expansion

History

Tissue expansion has been apparent since woman first became pregnant and hydrocephalics were born. Tissue expansion was not recognized possible until certain tribes were discovered who expanded their lips, necks, and noses. Readers in the occult know that genitalia have been expanded for years, and advertisements in sex magazines commonly display suction devices for "tissue expansion."

Although he did it only once in 1956, Neuman placed a type of expander in the postauricular region to gain tissue for a subtotal ear reconstruction.[80] He reported that it expanded by 50%. That expander was designed with an external filling port, something that has already come full circle. Most filling ports are buried with or distal to the expander, but some newer designs have external ports.

Twenty years after Neuman's experiment, Radovan expanded the skin near a tattoo to stretch up the skin so that removal could be a one-step procedure.[81] He then applied this prin-

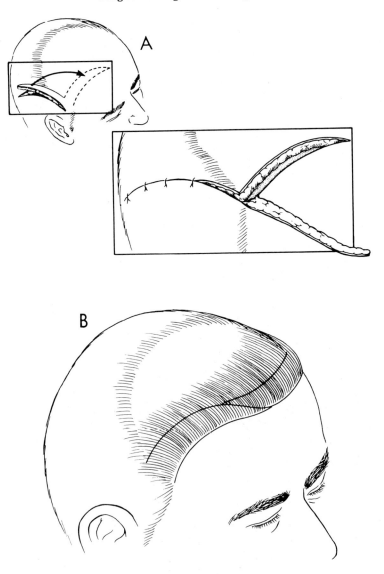

FIG 6–55.
A, short temporal flap. **B**, two short temporal flaps interconnecting at the midline.

ciple to breast expansion and used it in this way for several years before others began using this obviously successful technique in other areas.[82] Several doctors added their own innovations, the industry responded, and in ten years, tissue expansion has become controlled, reproducible, and scientific.

The Radovan design contributed several features that are still used. He used a silicone silastic elastomer envelope and a self-sealing injection port. One side of the envelope is stiff-ened so that it is placed down and the expansion takes place above or over it. For example, for scalp expansion the stiff side lies next to the cranium. He also designed the filling port with a stainless-steel backing so that when the needle is inserted through the skin and the top of the port, moving it back and forth makes enough noise and resistance that both the doctor and patient can be sure it is in the right place. Many different sizes and shapes of expanders are now available, and custom designs for new uses are appearing all the time. The separated filling port connected by a silastic tube is giving way to ports built into the bag itself. Experience has shown that the filling port can be palpated through the expanded tissue so that locating it for filling is not difficult. Also, capsule formation around the bag is difficult enough to dissect off without also "digging" out the filler and connecting tube.

Manders applied the technique to the scalp to repair massive defects in children.[83] Not long later, it became obvious that scalp expansion could be used in the surgical management of alopecia. Expansion could increase the amount of area removed with scalp reductions, aid in closure of the donor defect with TPO flaps, and expand the donor areas of the large, bilateral advancement flaps.

Histology

Human and animal studies performed to date suggest that the result of expansion is not simple stretching and thus thinning of the expanded skin. Metabolic changes in the skin occur that imply new skin production. Austad et al. investigated expansion in 27 albino Dunklin-Hartley guinea pigs.[84] They developed the following conclusions: (1) the epidermis undergoes an increase in mitotic activity but does not thin; (2) the dermis does thin but most if not all of this thickness (volume) is replaced by the development of a fibrous capsule; even though thinner, there is an increase in collagen synthesis activity in the dermis; (3) the vascularity increases and fortunately there is no change in the morphology of the hair follicles nor are there any signs of dysplasia in the epidermis; and (4) there may be some telogen effluvium overlying the expander, but this is thought to be a pressure phenomenon and not the result of any intrinsic change in the follicles.

Others have also recorded the increased vascularity from expansion, and happily, flaps created by expansion have a greater vascularity and therefore greater survival.[85–87]

Indications

In those patients with total crown baldness but high fringes, for whom the giant (maxi) scalp reductions would be useful, the expanders are

a great help because they recruit skin from the hair-bearing fringe and not from the neck. Also, the occipital and postauricular nerves and vessels are spared. The trade-off is that the hair density is thinned by the stretching. The same artificial hair pattern, however, is created with the sides pulled together in the midline. Either procedure fails to create a frontal hairline, which must be constructed with transplants.

If a patient has only crown baldness, the expander may permit total removal and coverage in one operation. The fringe hair is expanded and drawn in from posterolateral areas and the occiput. The same is true for cases of central crown baldness; the fringe can be expanded on one or both sides, the bald center can be removed with any of the standard scalp reduction techniques, and the expanded hair-bearing sides can be pulled over the defect.

Large flaps benefit from expansion for several reasons. If the patient is otherwise a good candidate for a flap, expansion directly under the proposed flap allows the flap to be cut wider (4 to 6 cm), improves its blood supply, thins the hair density (one of the disadvantages of flaps is hair so dense it looks artificial), and makes it easier to close the flap donor defect.[88]

Technique

Having decided which hair-bearing scalp skin is to be expanded, the proper size and shape of expander is chosen. Usually, for large reductions, both lateral fringe areas are expanded with rectangular bags (Fig 6–56). Some bags have been designed to expand more on one end than the other in order to develop greater expansion of the middle and posterior parietal scalp than in the temple region. Sometimes a third bag is used in the occiput if the fringe hair is high enough.

Patients are carefully counseled about the discomfort, the side effects, the marked disfigurement, and the length of time necessary for expansion. We tell them three to four months will be necessary and that hurrying the process will only increase the complications. We try to talk to family members so they understand how strange these patients will look.

The patient is instructed to shampoo his hair the morning of surgery and to come in without having applied any hair-grooming agents. The scalp is cleansed with the surgical prep of choice and the incision lines are marked. The patient is draped and local anesthesia is administered. As usual, physicians have individual preferences. We use a .5% lidocaine and 1:200,000 epinephrine mixture for a ring block which starts with the brow line so the supratrochlear and supraorbital nerves are infiltrated. We work around the scalp to the ears, over them, and to the lambdoid ridge. When the patient has recovered from the epinephrine rush, we inject the incision lines with 1% lidocaine and 1:100,000 epinephrine.

The expanders are placed so that hair-bearing, not bald, skin is stretched. The incision lines should not be directly over the expanders if at all possible. For rectangular expanders in both sides, there are two workable locations for the incisions: a vertical line in the midocciput, or two lines just above the fringe hair on both sides. The incision is carried into the subgaleal plane and those few arteries that bleed are easily coagulated. The instrument of choice is used to create a subgaleal pocket for the expander. A Hegar dilator or Van Buren male urethral sound are popular for this task, but a long scalpel, a curved Luikhart iconoclast, or a broad Army/Navy retractor will work. When the pocket is made on one side, fill the expander with approximately 100 ml of saline; doing so will make it easier to slip the expander into place. The expander should be tested by filling it to tension to be sure the filling port—intrinsic to the bag or separate—is properly located for easy and successful filling. The first bag is deflated and the second one placed and tested in the same way. Other than the injection of local anesthesia, this procedure is not terribly painful or disturbing to the patient. The incisions are closed in two layers, with permanent sutures on both layers: galea and skin. Drains may be necessary if there is a lot of oozing.

There is seldom much morbidity with the placement of the expanders. Sutures come out in two weeks and then the filling begins. Some physicians will fill only one bag per visit and the second or third seven days later. The patient comes in weekly; only one expander is filled at each visit. Other physicians will see the patient every two weeks and fill both expanders. The rule of thumb is to fill the bags to slight tension or to a point where the patient experiences tense but not painful feeling. Generally 40 ml per visit is the average fill. Patients are a bit uncomfortable for the first night, and mild analgesics can be used. If there is persistent pain, a few ml of saline can be withdrawn and further expansion can proceed more slowly. A recent paper from Finland suggests that overfilling the bag at each visit will speed the expansion and produce a greater stretch.[89] Overfilling produces severe pain and skin that is white. A Doppler flowmeter monitoring the pressure will show that the dermal capillary flow is zero. Then just enough sa-

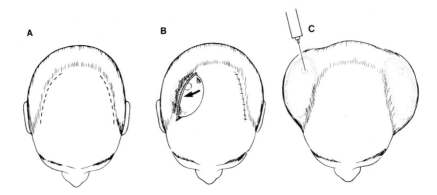

FIG 6–56.
A, for tissue expansion to treat alopecia, incisions are made at the junction of the bald and fringe hair. **B,** the bags are inserted under the galea. **C,** 2 weeks later, filling begins and progresses until the scalp is maximally expanded.

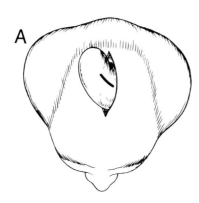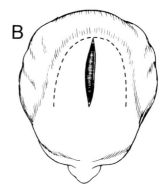

FIG 6–57.
A, after expansion, the bags are removed through a midline incision; sometimes a capsule is also removed. **B,** incisions for the removal of excess or stretched scalp are designed.

line can be removed until the symptoms abate and the Doppler shows capillary flow. This additional technique adds up to 59% more stretch.

We, as others, have learned to use a 23-gauge butterfly needle on a short tube. It is long enough to reach well into the filling port but not heavy enough to come out. The section of tubing makes the process much easier. Some patients can be trained to fill it themselves. Obviously patient motivation, intelligence, and reliability are factors, as well as where the expander is anatomically located and how difficult it is for the patient to come into the office. There must not be any hurry, and 8 to 12 weeks is average. Faster expansions have a higher rate of overlying skin atrophy and bag extrusion.

The endpoint is reached when there is enough stretched scalp to accomplish the goal. The scalp should be measured before and during expansion. Measurement can be circumferential or across the top from ear to ear. For example, if there is an area of central baldness 8 cm wide, the ear-to-ear measurement should be at least 8 cm longer before expansion is stopped.

When expansion is complete, the head is prepared again and anesthetized in the same way. If the insertion incisions have healed well, different incisions can be used at will (Fig 6–57). If the original scars have spread, incorporating them into the design of the flap advancement is valuable. As with all scalp surgery for alopecia, the incision line should be placed so it will be hidden by hair and not extend over the slope of

the scalp. There is definitely capsule formation. It may dissect out easily with little bleeding, but it may also be bound down so tightly that trying to get it out leaves a large oozing surface. In the latter case, leave it. It will not be visible and will not be palpable within a few weeks after the surgery. Capsule formation around distal filling ports has contributed to their decreasing use.

When the expanders have been removed, assess the amount of loose skin and how best to plan for its removal and closure of the defect. Each scalp will expand a little differently. While standard patterns to cut out the bald head are a good guideline, be sure that each operation is designed for that particular head (Fig 6–58). As in regular scalp reduction, do not cut both sides of the bald skin until it is certain that the defect will close. One side can be cut and the laxity checked, or the removal can begin at one or the other pole of the head and the wound closed as short segments are removed. Either method guarantees closure with minimal tension. Two layered closures are recommended, with permanent or absorbable sutures on the galea and sutures or staples on the skin.

Dressings and postoperative care are the same as those for reductions and flaps, discussed above.

Complications

The complication rate is still higher than desired. With the expanders in for 6 to 12 weeks,

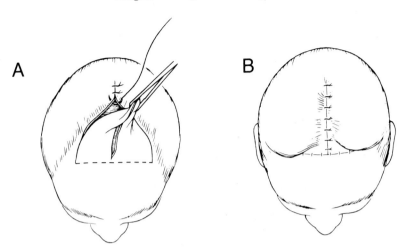

FIG 6–58.
A, the loose skin is excised and the sides are pulled together and sutured at the same time; this prevents gaping and makes the procedure more controlled. **B,** when the scalp is closed there is much less baldness, but a frontal hairline must be constructed with transplants or flaps.

and with the constant pressure and manipulation, there will probably always be a high incidence of troubles that are inherent to this technique. Mechanical problems such as bag breakage, filling-port leakage, and uneven expansion occur less frequently as the product improves and as doctors become more experienced.

Infection was as high as 5% in the first years the expansion technique was used, but it is assumed that rate will come down.[90] Bleeding under the galea, or even an organized hematoma, can release toxic substances that can jeopardize a flap or a reduction. Cases have been reported of the process eroding a major vessel and presenting a hemorrhagic emergency.[91] The most common problem is erosion of the bag through the skin. If only a small area of thinning is present over the bag, it can be reinforced with sutures and the expansion can continue. Most of the time, however, further expansion must stop and the surgeon must either go ahead with the proposed surgery or wait a few months and try again.

Future

It is difficult to predict how common a technique tissue expansion will become in the surgical management of alopecia. Transplants are still used the most because of the ease of the surgeries and the generally gratifying results. Flaps and reductions have a lot to offer patients with certain hair patterns and specific cosmetic needs, but the morbidity and cost are high. It is a very rare patient who would adequately benefit from an expansion and reduction only; most patients need additional procedures in combination with the expansion—flaps, frontal transplants, etc. The use of tissue expansion is a new and exciting part of cosmetic dermatologic surgery but it is too early to predict its final role.

References

1. Dieffenbach JF: Nonnulla de Regeneratione et transplantatione (dissertation inauguralis) 1822.
2. Orentreich D, Orentreich N: Androgenic alopecia and its treatment, in Unger WP, Nordström REA (eds): *Hair Transplantation,* ed 2. New York, Marcel Dekker, Inc, 1987.
3. Butcher EO: Hair growth in skin transplants in the immature albino rat. *Anat Record* 1936; 64:161–170.
4. Orentreich N: Autografts in alopecias and other selected dermatological conditions. *Annal New York Acad of Scien* 1959; 83:463–479.
5. Sasagawa M: Hair transplantation. *Jpn J Dermatol* 1930; 30:493.
6. Okuda S: Klinische und experimentelle Untersuchunger uber die Transplantation von lebenden Haaren. *Jpn J Dermatol* 1939; 40:537.
7. Okuda S: Clinical and experimental studies of transplantation of living hairs. *Jpn J Dermatol Urol* 1939; 46:135–138.
8. Kuster W, Happle R: The inheritance of common baldness: Two B or not two B. *J Am Acad Dermatol* 1984; 11:921–926.
9. Keenan BS, Meyer WJ III, Hadjian AJ, et al: Syndrome of androgen insensitivity in man: Absence of 5 α-dihydrotestosterone binding protein in skin fibroblasts. *J Clin Endocrinol Metab* 1974; 38:1143–1146.
10. Stough DB III, Berger RA, Orentreich N: Surgical improvement of cicatricial alopecia of diverse etiology. *Arch Dermatol* 1968; 97:331–334.
11. Rizer RL, Wheatly VR, Orentreich N: Androgens in human skin surface lipids: A radioimmunoassay analysis (abstracts). *J Invest Dermatol* 1981; 76:327.
12. Gummer CL: Diet and hair loss. *Semin Dermatol* 1985; 4:35–39.
13. Keyes EL: The cutaneous punch. *J Cutan Genitourin Dis* 1887; 5:98–101.
14. Parish LC: The Keyes Punch (letter). *Arch Dermatol* 1983; 119:791.
15. Urbach F, Shelley WB: A rapid and simple method for obtaining punch biopsies without anesthesia. *J Invest Dermatol* 1931; 17:131–134.
16. Orentreich N: Hair transplants, in Madden J (ed): *Current Dermatologic Management.* St. Louis, CV Mosby Co, 1970.
17. Stegman SJ: Commentary: The cutaneous punch. *Arch Dermatol* 1982; 118:943–944.
18. Unger W, Baran R: *Hair Transplantation,* New York, Marcel Dekker, Inc, 1979.
19. Hagerman D, Wilson JW: The skin biopsy punch: Evaluation and modification. *Cutis* 1970; 6:1139–1143.
20. Alt TH: Evaluation of donor harvesting techniques in hair transplantation. *J Dermatol Surg Oncol* 1984; 10:799–806.
21. Unger WP, Nordström REA: *Hair Transplantation,* ed 2. New York, Marcel Dekker, Inc, 1987.
22. Pinski JB: Hair transplantation, in Roenigk RK, Roenigk HH (eds): *Dermatologic Surgery.* New York, Marcel Dekker, Inc, 1988.
23. Merritt E: Scattershot hair transplant technique blasted. Cosmetology Seminar Highlights. New York, Beth Israel Medical Center, 1988.
24. Merritt E: Transplantation of single hairs from the scalp as eyelashes. *J Dermatol Surg Oncol* 1980; 6:271–273.
25. Arkawa I: Cosmetic evaluation of eyebrow surgery with transplants of single hairs. *Jpn J Plast Reconstr Surg* 1967; 10:1.
26. Sturm H: The benefit of donor site closure in hair transplantation. *J Dermatol Surg Oncol* 1984; 10:987.
27. Hill TG: Closure of the donor site in hair transplantation by a cluster technique. *J Dermatol Surg Oncol* 1980; 6:190.
28. Morrison ID: An improved method of suturing the donor site in hair transplantation surgery. *Plast Reconstr Surg* 1981; 67:378.
29. Carrierao S, Lessa S: New technique for closing punch graft donor sites. *Plast Reconstr Surg* 1978; 64:455.
30. Pierce HE: An improved method of closure of donor sites in hair transplantation. *J Dermatol Surg Oncol* 1979; 5:475.
31. Alt TH: The donor site, in Unger WP, Nordström REA (eds): *Hair Transplantation,* ed 2. New York, Marcel Dekker, Inc, 1987.
32. Unger WP: *Hair Transplantation* (appendix E). New York, Marcel Dekker, Inc, 1979.
33. Nordström REA, Nordström RM: The effect of corticosteroids on postoperative edema. *Plast Reconstr Surg* 1987; 80:85–87.
34. Sarnoff DS, Goldberg DJ, Greenspan AH, et al: Residents' corner: Multiple pyogenic granuloma-like lesions following hair transplantation. *J Dermatol Surg Oncol* 1985; 11:32–34.
35. Nordström REA, Tötterman SMS: Iatrogenic false aneurysms following punch hair grafting. *Plast Reconstr Surg* 1979; 64:563–565.
36. Ayers S: Prevention and correction of unaesthetic results of hair transplantation for male pattern baldness. *Cutis* 1977; 19:117.
37. Nordström REA: Eyebrow reconstruction by punch hair transplantation. *Plast Reconstr Surg* 1977; 60:74.
38. Nordström REA: Punch hair grafting under split-skin grafts on scalps. *Plast Reconstr Surg* 1979; 64:9.
39. Nordström REA: "Micrografts" for improvement of the frontal hairline after hair transplantation. *Aesth Plast Surg* 1981; 5:97.
40. Nordström REA: Special techniques in surgical hair replacement. *Fac Plast Surg* 1985; 2:78.
41. Bradshaw W: Quarter-grafts: A technique for

minigrafts, in Unger WP, Nordström REA (eds): *Hair Transplantation.* New York, Marcel Dekker, 1987.

42. Merritt E: Single hair transplantation for hairline refinement: A practical solution. *J Dermatol Surg Oncol* 1984; 10:962.

43. Blanchard G, Blanchard B: Obliteration of alopecia by hair-lifting: A new concept and technique. *J Natl Med Assoc* 1977; 69:639–641.

44. Stough DB, Webster RC: Esthetics and refinements in hair transplantation. International Hair Transplant Symposium, Lucerne, Switzerland, Feb 4, 1978.

45. Unger M: Alopecia reduction, in Unger M, Nordström REA (eds): *Hair Transplantation.* New York, Marcel Dekker, 1988.

46. Unger MG, Unger WP: Management of alopecia of the scalp by a combination of excision and transplantation. *J Dermatol Surg Oncol* 1978; 4:670–672.

47. Bosley LL, Hope CR, Montroy RE: Male pattern reduction (MPR) for surgical reduction of male pattern baldness. *Curr Ther Res* 1979; 25:281–287.

48. Bosley LL, Hope CR, Montroy RE, et al: Reduction of male pattern baldness in multiple stages: A retrospective study. *J Dermatol Surg Oncol* 1980; 6:498–503.

49. Schultz BC, Roenigk HH Jr: Scalp reduction for alopecia. *J Dermatol Surg Oncol* 1979; 5:808–811.

50. Roenigk HH Jr: Scalp reduction, in Roenigk RK, Roenigk HII (eds): *Dermatologic Surgery.* New York, Marcel Dekker, 1988.

51. Alt TH: Scalp reduction as an adjunct to hair transplantation: Review of relevant literature and presentation of an improved technique. *J Dermatol Surg Oncol* 1980; 6:1011–1018.

52. Norwood OT, Shiell RC: Scalp reductions, in Norwood OT (ed): *Hair Transplant Surgery,* ed 2. Springfield, Ill, Charles C Thomas, 1984, pp 163–200.

53. Nordström REA: Change of direction of hair growth. *J Dermatol Surg Oncol* 1983; 9:156–158.

54. Marzola M: An alternative hair replacement method, in Norwood OT (ed): *Hair Transplant Surgery,* ed 2. Springfield, Ill, Charles C Thomas, 1984, pp 315–324.

55. Brandy DA: The bilateral occipito-parietal flap. *J Dermatol Surg Oncol* 1986; 12:1062–1066.

56. Unger MG, Unger WP: Alopecia reductions, in Unger WP (ed): *Hair Transplantation, a Text.* New York, Marcel Dekker, Inc, 1979, pp 102–108.

57. Unger MG: The Y shaped pattern of alopecia reduction and its variations. *J Dermatol Surg Oncol* 1984; 10:980–986.

58. Puig CJ, Haenchen RJ, Sandham R, et al: New instrumentation for scalp reduction. *J Dermatol Surg Oncol* 1986; 12:730–733.

59. Nordström REA, Nordström RM: Absorbable versus nonabsorbable sutures to prevent postoper-

ative stretching of wound area. *Plast Reconstr Surg* 1986; 78:186–190.

60. Nordström REA: "Stretch-back" in scalp reductions for male pattern baldness. *Plast Reconstr Surg* 1984; 73:422–426.

61. Unger WP: Concomitant mini reductions in punch hair transplanting. *J Dermatol Surg Oncol* 1983; 9:388–392.

62. Brandy DA: A six-step approach for the treatment of extensive baldness. *J Dermatol Surg Oncol* 1987; 13:519–525.

63. Brandy DA: Pitfalls and pearls of extensive scalp-lifting. *Am J Cosmetic Surg* 1987; 4:217–223.

64. Unger WP, Nordström REA: *Hair Transplantation.* New York, Marcel Dekker, Inc, 1988, pp 435–518.

65. Norwood OT, Shiell RD, Morrison ID: Complications of scalp reductions. *J Dermatol Surg Oncol* 1983; 9:828–858.

66. Norwood OT: Treatment of extensive baldness. *J Dermatol Surg Oncol* 1987; 13:465–466.

67. Unger WP, Unger MG: Alopecia reduction, in Eystrom E (ed): *Controversies in Dermatologic Surgery.* Philadelphia, WB Saunders, 1984, pp 329–336.

68. Marzola M: An alternative hair replacement method, in Norwood OT (ed): *Hair Transplant Surgery,* ed 2. Springfield, Ill, Charles C. Thomas Publisher, 1984, pp 315–324.

69. Lamont ES: A plastic surgical transformation: Report of a case. *West J Surg Obstet Gynecol* 1957; 65:164.

70. Juri J: Use of parieto-occipital flaps in the surgical treatment of baldness. *Plast Reconstr Surg* 1975; 55:456.

71. Juri J, Juri C, Arufe HN: Use of rotation scalp flaps for treatment of occipital baldness. *Plast Reconstr Surg* 1978; 61:23.

72. Elliott RA: Lateral scalp flaps for instant results in male pattern baldness. *Plast Reconstr Surg* 1977; 60:699.

73. Flemming RW, Mayer TG: Short versus long flaps in the treatment of male pattern baldness. *Arch Otolaryngol* 1981; 107:403–408.

74. Kaboker SS: Juri flap in treatment of baldness 1979; 105:509–514.

75. Lauzon G: Transfer of a large, single, temporo-occipital flap for treatment of baldness. *Plast Reconstr Surg* 1979; 63:369.

76. Nataf J, Elbaz JS, Pollet J: Etude critique des transplantations de cuir chevelu et proposition d'une optique. *Ann Chir J Plast* 1976; 21:199.

77. Fleming RW, Mayer TG: Scalp flaps, in Roenigk, Roenigk (eds): *Dermatologic Surgery.* New York, Marcel Dekker, 1988, pp 1085–1121.

78. Nordström REA: The Nordström variety of a temporoparieto-occipital flap, in Unger, Nordström (eds): *Hair Transplantation.* New York, Marcel Dekker, 1987; pp 645–655.

79. Unger WA: Free temporo-parieto-occipital flaps

(editor's comment), in Unger, Nordström (eds): *Hair Transplantation*. New York, Marcel Dekker, 1987, p 645.

80. Neuman CG: The expansion of an area of skin by progressive distention of a subcutaneous balloon. *Plast Reconstr Surg* 1957; 19:124–130.

81. Radovan C: Adjacent flap development using expandable Silastic implant. Presented at the Annual Meeting of the American Society of Plastic and Reconstructive Surgeons, Boston, Mass, 1976.

82. Radovan C: Breast reconstruction after mastectomy using the temporary expander. *Plast Reconstr Surg* 1982; 69:195.

83. Manders EK, Friedman M: Scalp expansion for male pattern baldness, in Roenigk RK, Roenigk HH (eds), *Dermatologic Surgery*. New York, Marcel Dekker, 1987, pp 1123–1137.

84. Austad ED, Paysk KA, McClatchey KD, et al: Histomorphologic evaluation of guinea pig skin and soft tissue after controlled tissue expansion. *Plast Reconstr Surg* 1982; 70:705.

85. Pasyk K, Austad ED, McClatchey K, et al: Electron microscopic evaluation of guinea pig skin and soft tissues expanded with a self-inflating silicone implant. *Plast Reconstr Surg* 1982; 70:37.

86. Sasaki GH, Krizek TJ: Functional blood flow and skin viability in random skin flaps constructed on expanded skin: Delay phenomenon in action. Presented at Plastic Surgery Research Council, Durham, N.C. May 19, 1983.

87. Cherry GW, Austad E, Paysk K, et al: Increased survival and vascularity of random-patterned skin flaps elevated in controlled expanded skin. *Plast Reconstr Surg* 1983; 72:680.

88. Nordström REA: The Nordström system: A specially designed tissue expander combined with the Nordström variety of the temporoparieto-occipital flap and advancement flaps, in Unger WP, Nordström REA (eds), *Hair Transplantation*. New York, Marcel Dekker, Inc, 1987, pp 551–560.

89. Pietilä JP, Nordström REA, Virkkunen PJ, et al: Accelerated tissue expansion with the "overfilling" technique. *Plast Reconstr Surg* 1988; 81:204–207.

90. Sasaki GH. Tissue expansion. Presented at Annual Meeting of the American Academy of Dermatology, Washington, DC, December 1988.

91. Ashall G, Quaba A: A hemorrhagic hazard of tissue expansion. *Plast Reconstr Surg* 1987; 79:627–630.

Seven

Filling Agents

The need for and use of fillings agents in cosmetic medicine has long been appreciated. Many agents have been used over the years; some, such as paraffin, are bad, and some, such as silicone, are good. In spite of the knowledge that some agents were available, it was not until the Collagen Corporation received Food and Drug Administration (FDA) market approval in 1981 for Zyderm Collagen Implant (ZCI) that aesthetically oriented physicians realized how frequently they would use an approved filling agent.

The appearance of ZCI focused the attention of aesthetic surgeons on filling agents, and it soon became apparent that there are many, many uses for filling agents in the battle against aging as well as in reconstruction. Zyderm was tried for all of these perceived needs and, as could be predicted, failed in many. Like any new product, with time the best uses and techniques for ZCI have been identified; used within these parameters, it is a safe and successful product.

This new tool focused attention on existing products, of which silicone is the oldest, and stimulated the development of new products such as Fibrel®. Autologous fat transplantation once again became of interest because new techniques for harvesting large amounts of fat were developed in connection with liposuction, although the need for this type of implant had already been long appreciated.

Therefore in this chapter we will discuss Zyderm collagen, silicone, microlipoinjection, and Fibrel. In the 5 years since the first edition of this book was published, the discussion of filling agents has grown from a consideration of a "new" filler and mention of an old filler to descriptions of four important agents.

Zyderm Collagen Implants (ZCI)

Product

Bovine dermal collagen is solubilized and purified through a combination of pepsin digestion, filtration, and ion-exchange chromatography.[1] This collagen in solution (CIS) is reconstituted into an injectable form by neutralization from acid solution. Fibrils are harvested by centrifugation and resuspended at a collagen concentration of 35 mg/ml (ZCI I) or 65 mg/ml (ZCI II), in phosphate-buffered saline containing 0.4% lidocaine (without lidocaine in France). The addition of glutaraldehyde during processing causes cross-linking of the collagen fibrils and is called Zyplast (Zp).

The CIS is 95% type I collagen and the rest is type III. By SDS polyacrylamide gel electrophoresis, in conjunction with silver-staining techniques and bacterial collagenase digestion, CIS has been shown to be free of noncollagenous proteins (sensitivity less than 0.1%). Optical rotation has shown that CIS is more than 95% triple helical, and electron microscopy revealed it was 80% monomeric and 13% dimeric. CIS is sensitive to temperature, with the lower temperature (5° to 10° C) producing smaller fibrils and 37°C producing a much higher proportion of fibrils that are larger.

The persistence of ZCI and Zp has been evaluated using radio-labeled collagen in rat and guinea pig subcutaneous models.[2, 3] Zp lasts longer and is more resistant to bacterial collagenase. It is presumed that the more tightly bound Zp is more resilient under physical pressure and retains more water than ZCI. Clinically, Zp remains larger, shrinks less, and does not turn into the small microimplants seen with ZCI once the saline and lidocaine are absorbed from the implant.[4]

Persistence

The clinical history of the implant has turned out to be different from what was predicted from the laboratory studies. The correction does not last as long in humans as it does in animals nor does it persist subcutaneously in humans. A study done in human volunteers scheduled for rhytidectomy may have addressed the discrepancy between the clinical and laboratory studies on ZCI persistence.[5] The implant was injected monthly into skin normally sacrificed as part of the face-lift operation. Thus, the life of the implant could be followed.

Normal Histology and Dynamics

Histologically, a mild perivascular and peri-appendageal lymphohistiocytic infiltrate begins to appear as early as 7 days after implantation of ZCI and gradually disappears by three months (Fig 7–1). In 1 to 3 months, ZCI is interspersed between host collagen in the mid to deep dermis. There is no colonization of the implant by either connective tissue or blood vessels. At three to six months, a few scattered fibroblasts attach to the borders or within the clefts and crevices of the implant. Electronmicroscopic studies of these fibroblasts reveal them to be in a resting phase, with no evidence of collagen synthesis. There is no vascularization of the implant. After six to nine months, the implant loses some of its integrity and stains less intensely.

Zyplast has significantly different histologic characteristics. At 1 to 3 months, the implants are larger, rounder deposits that tend to displace the dermal host collagen rather than spread between and among the fibers. Early on, a sparse population of fibroblasts penetrates the periph-

ery of the implant within the dermis. These fibroblasts seem much more active and appear to lay down new collagen as soon as 60 days after implantation. This implant is not vascularized, either. By 3 to 6 months, the fibroblasts within the implant increase significantly, and electron-microscopy shows that many have dilated cisternae of rough endoplastic reticulum. New collagen appears adjacent to the implant. The amount of new collagen varies greatly; some implants acquire a lot of new collagen and others very little. However, ZCI almost never induces any, whereas Zp commonly does.

Both ZCI and Zp gradually migrate deeper into the dermis and are eventually extruded into the subcutaneous spaces. This "cutaneous elimination" phenomenon may be the most significant finding with regard to the longevity of clinical correction. It has been reported by several investigators that the correction gradually fades some with ZCI and little with Zp, but both quickly disappear between 6 to 9 months.[4, 6] Correction seems to persist longer over bony prominences, and there are a few patients who retain the correction longer than the average. The "migration" or "elimination" phenomenon could explain these findings. The implant persists, but when it is eliminated from the skin into the subcutaneous spaces, it loses its ability to push up or fill the dermis to effect a correction on whatever soft tissue depression it was filling, unless the implant is over a bony prominence where it can still exert some upward correction from the subcutaneous space.

The implant lasts longer in scars than in creases and furrows. Possible explanations are that the scar collagen is less active in eliminating the implant and thus it sits where it was placed, or that the elimination is much slower in scar dermis. Another factor may be that the movement of the skin at the crease or fold location forces the implant down and out sooner than a static location. As with any biological event, some individuals will have a slower than average elimination speed.

Immunogenicity

Patients tested prior to skin testing or treatment with ZCI have an 8.4% incidence of anti-

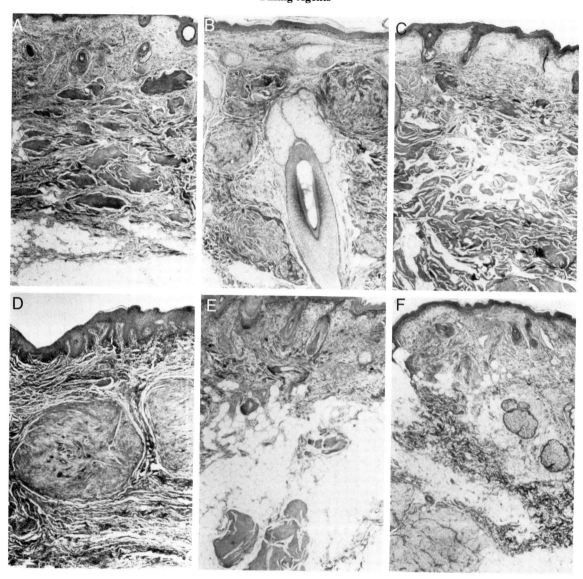

FIG 7–1.
A, C, and **E,** Zyderm II in human skin at 3, 6, and 9 months postinjection. **B, D,** and **F,** Zyplast in human skin at 3, 6, and 9 months postinjection. Note the differences in the morphology of the two types of implants and that both "migrate" deeper with time (Gomori's trichrome stain, ×20).

collagen antibodies as measured by an enzyme-linked immunoadsorbent assay (ELISA).[7] It is assumed that these patients have been sensitized to bovine collagen through their diet. Individuals with high pretreatment anticollagen antibodies have a six times greater chance of developing an adverse reaction if treated with ZCI. Most patients with a positive skin will have evidence of anticollagen antibodies. The rate of

localized hypersensitivity reactions to the initial test injection of ZCI ranges from 3.0% to 3.5% in the literature. Reactions to treatment, all in test-negative patients, range from 1.1% to 5.0% in the literature.[8] A workable statistic to give patients is that about 2% will develop allergy to the product sometime while using it if the skin test was negative.[9, 10] The greatest number of patients develop allergy after the first treatment exposure and with less than 5 ml total of collagen used.

The antibovine antibodies that form with test or treatment site reactions are predominantly immunoglobulin-G (IgG), but some patients develop IgA anticollagen antibodies as well. These antibodies react to both native and denatured bovine collagen. The response is species-specific to type I bovine collagen, and importantly, does not cross-react with human or other animal collagens.

Zyplast, with its gluteraldehyde cross-linking, has a lower incidence of hypersensitivity reactions than does ZCI.[8]

The Skin Test

A skin test is required becasue there is a pre-existing allergic rate of 3%. (This is the rate of clinical allergic reactions even though the rate of anticollagen antibodies is 8.4%, as mentioned above.) Nearly 90% of positive reactions occur within the first three days, but the other 10% manifest over the first four weeks.[8] Therefore, it is recommended that there be a four-week interval between testing and treating. A positive test remains reactive for weeks to months. It is not a transient phenomenon. After a negative skin test there is a 1.5% to 2.0% chance that the patient will aquire allergy to ZCI, which also tends to show up within the first few weeks after exposure.[11] These data have convinced several physicians to do some form of double skin-testing to reduce the number of times the first treatment exposure results in an allergic reaction. Double testing is carried out sequentially, with the first test given in the standard manner on the forearm. After four weeks, if this test is negative, a second-exposure dose (0.1 to 0.5 ml) is administered on the opposite forearm or the postauricular area or at the periphery of the face. Four more weeks should elapse before full treatments are given on the center of the face. Some physicians wait only two weeks after the first test and then wait four weeks after the second exposure, which shortens the double-testing to a total of six weeks. We do not routinely double-test unless something in the patient's history is worrisome or unless there is a question about the first skin test results.

Clinically and histologically, the test site and the treatment site reactions are the same, and will be discussed below. (Fig 7–2). There is no treatment for either, and only rarely has the test reaction been so violent that there was scarring.

We do not routinely retest a patient who has not had ZCI for over two or three years, nor do we routinely test new patients who tell us they have already had ZCI from another physician. We take complete ZCI history from these patients and test only if something is suspicious. Some patients will lie, but we see no reason to penalize all the rest of the patients to uncover a few who prevaricate. It only hurts them, and if we have a good history recorded on the chart, we are blameless.

Indications and Technique

These subjects will be discussed together because often the technique varies depending on what kind of lesion is being treated. A few general suggestions need to be made first, however.

Observation is the best way to learn how to inject ZCI. Watching experienced physicians treat a variety of patients is almost all that is necessary to learn technique, although learning which patients and lesions to treat takes longer. Videotapes in some circumstances are preferable to

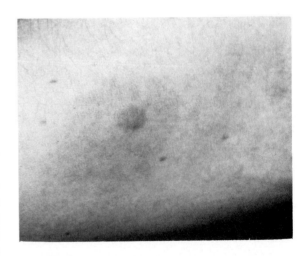

FIG 7–2.
A reactive (positive) skin test to Zyderm I shown 4 weeks after injection. This erythematous and indurated lesion faded spontaneously within 3 months.

live observation because the viewer, through video magnification, can see as well or better than when watching a treating physician. Many tapes are available, and often at meetings there will be live demonstrations with video enhancement and magnification.

Most wrinkles and soft scars are significantly altered when patients move from the vertical to the horizontal position. Therefore, treat only forehead creases with the patient supine. For all other locations on the face, the patient should sit or be nearly upright. We sometimes ask patients to lean forward, with an assistant helping to steady their heads, to accentuate the crease or depressed defect. The incidence of syncope is higher with the patient seated, especially on the first treatment visit, but implant placement is much more accurate.

Overhead or tangential lighting is essential. Some scars and wrinkles are visible only with side lighting. Even badly scarred or wrinkled faces are more easily treated when there is tangential lighting. Side lighting helps differentiate both depressed and pigmented scars.

This is one of several techniques for which we recommend using magnification. Although the lens can be the physician's choice, 2 to 3 diopters of magnification will focus and hold the physician's eye on the treatment site, which must be watched continuously to be sure the implant is flowing exactly where and at the level desired.

Two things that we always do when we have the Zyderm syringe in hand as we approach the patient is (1) remind the patient that he can *become* allergic to Zyderm at any time, and (2) tip the syringe up and push the plunger hard enough to force out any air in the syringe or needle. If the air is left in, the first Zyderm injected will be a poof of air that will distort the lesion being treated. It will then be necessary to wait a few minutes before the air is absorbed and the lesion returns to normal.

We believe pretreatment analgesia or topical anesthesia such as cooling packs are unnecessary. Most topical applications interfere with the true shape of the defect or how it will respond to ZCI and thus interfere with the treatment itself. The pain of the 30-gauge needle is minuscule; the pain from the ZCI is only that of lidocaine, which in certain areas like the lip can

be quite painful. Most of the time, however, a gentle hand and a well-motivated patient successfully counteract the pain of injection. If the topical anesthetic agent EMLA (eutectic mixture of local anesthetic) is eventually approved by the FDA, and if it works as well as the European literature suggests it will, we will probably use it on selected patients prior to injection. It requires 90 minutes application before the anesthesia is effective, so patients can apply it before coming to the office. Also, several instruments are being developed which can be applied with lidocaine to drive in the agent and achieve anesthesia without a pin prick. For certain areas such as those around the mouth, we will often do a field block, which makes some patients much happier.

The Collagen Corporation recommends a soap and water washing before treatment. We agree, and follow this advice if the patient uses makeup or has oily skin. However, if the face is clean, an alcohol wipe is all that we use, knowing that it probably does little for antisepsis but does a lot for the patient's state of mind. We prefer to wipe on the alcohol with a gauze square rather than a cotton pledget. We hold the gauze while injecting because invariably some Zyderm will extrude from the pores or from the needle as we try to inject superficially. The gauze will easily wipe up the Zyderm and the cotton will not.

The direction of the needle bevel probably does not make a great deal of difference. Every physician can determine what direction will provide the best chance of placing the implant where desired. Also, when we plan to treat a very superficial scar or crease, we bend the needle approximately 45 degrees at the hub. This does not impede the flow of the collagen, but the vector forces of the bent needle help keep the needle tip high as it advances forward in the skin. We always use the 30-gauge needle which comes with the syringe because it works as well or better than other needles we have tried over the years.

The following factors should be considered with each injection of ZCI: (1) the dermal compartment being filled with the implant; (2) the Zyderm product being used; and (3) the lesion being treated. ZCI and Zp do not last long in the subdermal spaces — 2 months at most on the average — and in that location the implant does little to elevate a depressed lesion. Putting great amounts (3 to 4 ml) of ZCI under a furrow may temporarily elevate it, but such use of the product is wasteful, expensive, and of very short-term benefit. Zyderm persists longest in the dermis. It should be placed as high as possible in the dermis because of the migration that naturally takes place.[5] If the dermis is thick and soft, as it often is on the cheek or paranasal area, greater amounts of thicker material (ZCI II or Zp) can be injected. If the dermal compartment is thin, as it is on the eyelids or lateral canthal area, a tiny amount of ZCI I is the most one should expect to use. Overfilling the dermis will cause extrusion below the dermis or into the epidermal-dermal junction: the former is wasteful and the latter will bead up and look like a milium.

Another quality of the dermis that must be considered is the sebaceous gland density. In highly sebaceous skin, ZCI often squirts out through the sebaceous ostia, which can be frustrating and wasteful. There is no way to prevent the pore extrusion; the needle is advanced or withdrawn a hair in hope of moving out of the gland. In densely sebaceous areas, it is sometimes hard to find an area that will accept the ZCI yet not be in a gland. We disagree with the recommendation that the pore ostia should be covered with something like colloidin. It is important to know when the needle tip is in a gland so it can be repositioned. Filling sebaceous glands with ZCI is not the goal of the implant.

The three Zyderm products behave in a similar fashion, but have very different physical characteristics. ZCI I and ZCI II become tiny droplets of implant in the dermis after the saline and lidocaine have been absorbed. With ZCI II it is possible to place so much so high in the dermis that it shows — it looks like a cream-colored plaque in the skin. Zp, however, sets up in larger drops within the dermis. If these are near the surface or very large, they show as lumps — cream-colored lumps. Eventually the visible or lumpy implants settle down, but the patient has to live through weeks to months with the deformity.

Finally, it is necessary to consider the lesion

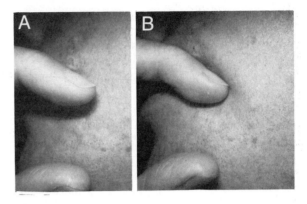

FIG 7–3.
A clinical maneuver to test whether or not a scar will respond to a filling agent. **A,** the fingers are placed on both sides of the lesion. **B,** the fingers are spread apart; if the floor of the lesion elevates and looks acceptable, the lesion will respond favorably.

being treated. Deep acne scars should be overcorrected so that they end up with as much implant as possible after the fluids are absorbed. On the other hand, fine creases need only microdroplets of implant to achieve correction and still not have the implant look like a string of beads. Massage immediately after injection will help smooth irregularities to a limited degree.

Each physician will develop a preferred technique and soon will choose a favorite material. The size and strength of the doctor's hand will also play a part in deciding which product is most often used. The half-filled syringes are easier for those with smaller hands because the plunger is less extended. Zp, with its more robust quality and deeper placement, is easier for some. We recommend that a plastic or lucite device be slipped over the tuberculin syringe to create a wider finger-grip and to increase leverage on the plunger. Without it, and after a few ZCI patients have been treated, the physician's fingers can become very sore.

Treating Acne Scars

The most responsive scars are those that are soft and that have sloping borders. These can be identified by placing the thumb and index finger on each side of the scar and spreading the skin (Fig 7–3). If the surface of the scar comes into a flat plane with the skin surface, the scar will probably respond well. Fibrotic perpendicular-walled scars are less successfully treated. Repeated injections into the center of the scar *may* somewhat soften the scar, and partial correction is achievable. When we first received Zyderm, we tried to cut under fibrotic scars with a goniotome (ophthalmalogic knife) blade. It was not a successful maneuver. It did create a pocket under the scar but that pocket had no side walls and would not hold the implant immediately below the scar as we intended. Also the site often became bloody, which prevented treating the scar at that session. And many scars were so fibrotic that placing an implant below them only raised the whole ugly scar and not just the depressed portion. Dermabrasion is usually the best treatment for these scars. Ice-pick scars are the least likely to respond and should be treated with punch elevation or punch transplantation. Attempts to elevate fibrotic ice-pick scars may cause a "donut" effect in which the entire scar, not just the depressed base, elevates. Also, examine the floor of the scar for color and texture before elevating it. There are times when the hyperpigmented, irregular scar floor is better left in the shadowy depressions.

The scar needs to be stabilized either by pinching it between the nondominant thumb and index finger or by pressing and slightly stretching the adjacent skin with the thumb and index finger (Fig 7–4). The needle enters the skin 3 to 5 mm from the scar edge and is advanced until the tip enters the scar, which is detected by increased resistance to advancement. The tip can be advanced to the opposite side of the scar with injection upon withdrawal, or injection with the initial push through the scar. Generally with ZCI I or II 50% to 100% overcorrection is recommended. When the fluids are absorbed only one-third to two-thirds of the volume remains, depending on whether ZCI I or II was used. With Zyplast, correction is to the plane of the surface with full filling but not overcorrection (Fig 7–5). Molding the implant is possible to a limited degree by gently pinching or massaging it. Overly aggressive molding may force the implant deeper or even into the subcutaneous space.

For small-diameter or round scars, insert the needle perpendicular to the skin at the center of the scar. As soon as the bevel has penetrated the skin, start injecting. Often the implant will flow evenly in all directions, perfectly filling the depression. Be especially vigilant when treating atrophic scars. There is little dermis and the needle can easily slip below the dermis, spilling the material where it has limited longevity.

Linear scars are filled by multiple punctures starting at one end and advancing as far as the implant will flow easily. Reinsert the needle in an area already treated to take advantage of the anesthetic effect. Scar consistency is variable. Soft areas will fill easily and fibrotic areas may take several treatments. When there are multiple

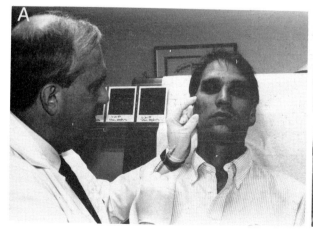
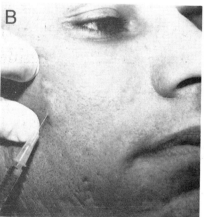

FIG 7–4.
A, use photographs of patient to help judge progress. **B,** stabilize skin and inject directly into scar.

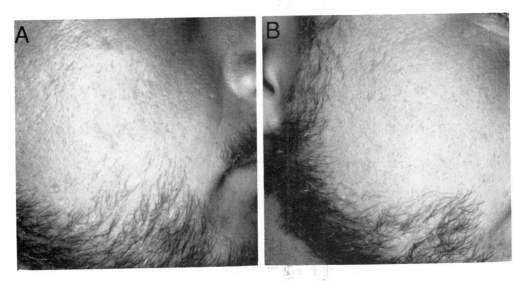

FIG 7–5.
Man, 24 years old, with acne scars. **A**, before treatment. **B**, 4 weeks after treatment with 1.5 ml Zyderm II.

scars, be sure to ask the patient which ones are the most bothersome. Usually they will have scars which they can see easily in the mirror but which may not be their worst scars. It is important to identify those and to treat them first before the material is all used up. Otherwise, the patient will leave unhappy or frustrated at the need to purchase another syringeful. A Polaroid photograph is helpful for those patients who have a multitude of depressed scars (Fig 7–6). As the treated scars are overfilled and a little edema develops, the adjacent scars become distorted and it is impossible to tell what needs treatment. Consulting the photograph will help you keep track of what has been treated or what needs further treatment.

Treating Other Scars

Postsurgical, posttraumatic, and postviral scars are often too fibrotic for implant treatment. That is not to say that many of these scars have not done well with filling agents[12] (Fig 7–7). ZCI has worked best on young scars and on those scars with a soft, gradual, depressed shape and with skin of normal color and texture. Fibrotic and sharp-walled scars do better with surgical treatment, although ZCI will soften them with repeated injections.

Treating Creases and Furrows

Because creases are shallow and soft everywhere, except sometimes on the forehead, ZCI I and occasionally ZCI II is placed high in the dermis. Although we have treated creases by inserting the needle perpendicularly to the line of the crease when trying to fill a difficult spot or avoid pore extrusion, we usually recommend the linear puncture technique. The skin is stabilized by pinching it up or by two- or three-point pressure with the other hand. The injections begin at either end of the line (usually the inferior or closer end) and multiple tiny injections are made along the long axis (Fig 7–8). The skin varies. Sometimes this technique will produce tiny bumps of implant which should be smoothed out and blended by gentle massage, and at other times the multiple injections will produce a smooth filling of the crease. Only tiny amounts are used, which means that many creases can be filled from one syringe.

We believe creases are the lesions most successfully treated by ZCI. If the patient has prominent, early, or multiple discrete creases around the mouth, on the cheeks, vertically on the glabella, or lateral to the orbital rim, Zyderm is usually the treatment of choice and often the *only* successful agent (Fig 7–9). For these creases,

Filling Agents

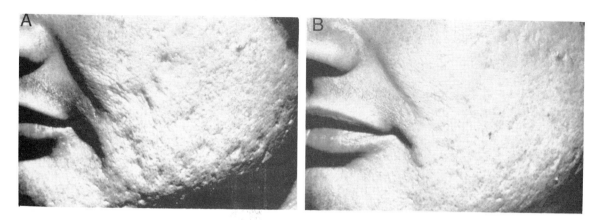

FIG 7–6.
Man, 20 years old, with severe acne scarring. **A,** before treatment. **B,** 6 weeks after treatment with 2 ml Zyderm II. This is the kind of case for which a pretreatment photograph is especially helpful.

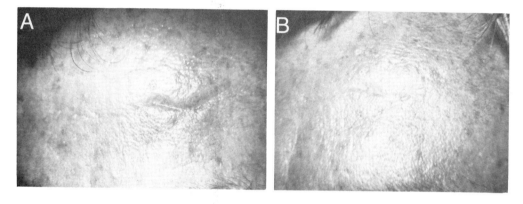

FIG 7–7.
Man, 42 years old, with a post-traumatic scar on the forehead. **A,** before treatment. **B,** four months after second treatment with Zyderm II, total 1.5 ml used.

Fibrel is too bulky, and silicone must be placed too deeply. Horizontal forehead creases sometimes respond, depending on how thick and firm the skin is. If the creases are in firm skin, the implant may only partially elevate them.

Furrows may be shallow or deep, requiring various amounts of implant to correct them. Some are treated by placing the implant in the middle of the trough, using the multiple puncture technique. Others require punctures at the middle of the trough where the most material is deposited, and punctures at each edge, where less material is deposited. Zyplast or at least ZCI II is needed to fill the volume for deep or wide furrows. It is not unusual for a furrow to have a crease in the center of the trough. The furrow is treated with Zp or ZCI II and the crease is treated concurrently with ZCI I. Also be aware that a line may look like a furrow when it is really a sharp but low fold that is easily pulled out. Obviously, folds are not treated with a filling agent.

Filling Agents

The Smile Line(s)

The line(s) generated by the smile are the long crease and/or furrow that begins below the nasal ali and extends obliquely toward the oral commissure. This is commonly called the nasolabial line. The extension of that line lateral to the oral commissure and onto the chin, and parallel lines on the cheek and chin, are sometimes called the secondary nasolabial lines. These lines are some of the first changes related to aging and certainly are the most common, thus there is a big demand for treatment. These lines are all passive, meaning they are caused by movement of underlying muscles, not by skin attachment to some underlying structure. The muscles that move the lateral commissure laterally and superiorly join into a pseudotendon called the modiolus which lies about 1 cm lateral to the commissure. When it is pulled laterally, or lat-

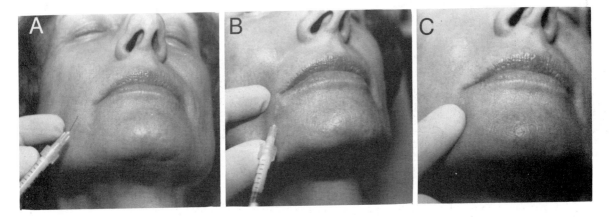

FIG 7–8.
A–C, technique for treating creases.

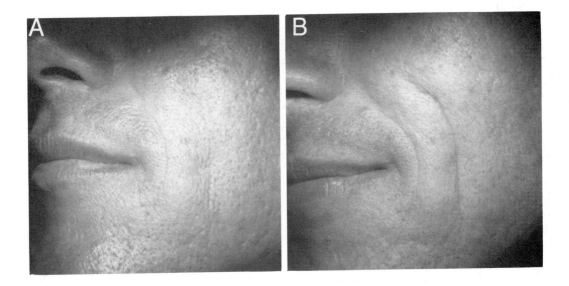

FIG 7–9.
Man, 31 years old, with a deep secondary smile line in the cheek. A, before treatment. B, 6 weeks after treatment with ZCI I, 1 ml on each side.

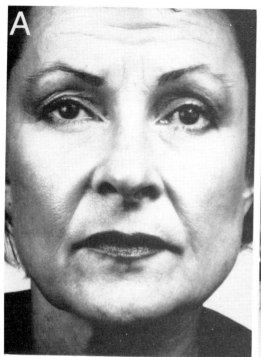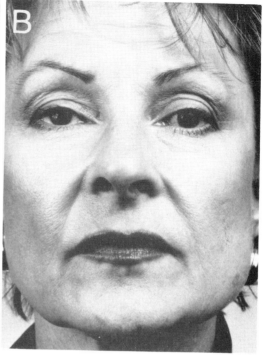

FIG 7–10.
Woman, 48 years old, with multiple creases and folds that make up the smile line. **A**, before treatment. **B**, 4 weeks after treatment with ZCI I and II, 1 and 0.75 ml used respectively. Note the improvement after obliterating small creases and building up skin medial to the fold.

erally and superiorly, the hanging curtain of the cheek can only fold on itself like a drape. The individual variations of the smile line that are created are functions of the thickness of the skin — thin skin pleats into many small lines, while thick skin drapes into one large furrow or fold. Variations are also created by the predominant movement of the smile. A broad smile creates a nasolabial line; a Mona Lisa smile creates only commissure parentheses. How much the mouth is opened determines the extension of the nasolabial line onto the chin, and hereditary and racial differences in the origin and insertion of the muscles, the size of the facial bones, and the size and presence of the teeth are also factors.

Although many of the lines created by the smiles are creases and furrows that are amenable to treatment with a filling agent, a common feature is a fold of cheek skin which is the entirety of the smile line or an additional nasolabial crease or fold. The fold is very prominent on some faces, and can be found on some young faces. On younger faces the fold is not long and is not

a cosmetic liability. But when the fold becomes prominent even when the face is not smiling, or when it lengthens to the level of the oral commissure or beyond, it places an unattractive line on the face. The extension of the nasolabial line to and beyond the oral commissure draws the focus of the viewing eye lower on the face and accentuates the mouth, producing what is called the bull-dog mouth. Ptosis of the mental fat pad and development of vertical, linear lines from the oral commissure to the chin, called marionette-mouth or hinge-mouth, also contribute to the unwanted accentuation of the lower face which is a hallmark of aging.

Needless to say, all of these changes cannot be corrected with a filling agent like ZCI. But the filling agents beautifully correct or fill early creases and furrows, putting off the accentuation of the lower face for years in some patients. It is astounding what cosmetic improvement can be gained by obliterating some or all of the negative parts of the smile line (Fig 7–10). Because the line is dynamic and a direct result of the smile, no correction will be permanent, but ZCI every six to nine months (on average) is a great benefit until many other aging changes make it unnecessary.

The fold which is a part of the smile line in many people is currently almost refractory to treatment.[13] The superficial musculoskeltal aponeurotic system (SMAS) seldom extends to the central face near the nasal ala, and therefore face-lift procedures are seldom successful at pulling out that portion of the smile-line fold. Because the fold is created just inferior to the fatty cheek, in those individuals with lots of subcutaneous fat the fold is a large mound of fat. Removal of that fat has not been a safe or wholly successful treatment. Liposuction has left fibrotic scarring, which is accentuated by the otherwise normal fluidity of the cheek in facial expression and mastication, and it has also converted an unsightly fat fold into an unsightly fold that is thin and slack. Special face-lifting techniques for that part of the line are difficult and dangerous and seldom work (face-lifts work well for that portion of the smile line that extends inferior to the oral commissure.) The excess folded skin can be cut out and that procedure is described in the plastic surgery literature, but the operation is seldom performed because of the scars left in prominent locations. Many times we have removed the entire nasal-labial fold as part of a nasal-labial fold flap used to repair deep and large nasal defects, but within a few months the action of the mouth in smiling and mastication regenerated a new fold.

Currently, the only cosmetic treatment for the fold is to decrease its prominence by filling the skin immediately medial to it. Often that area is a furrow, and filling it is indicated. If there is no furrow medial to the fold, placing a filler into that area to build a gradual slope up to the fold will reduce the fold's prominence to the viewing eye.

The techniques for building that plateau include the multiple puncture method followed by massage to smooth out the bumps, and a single-puncture linear or fanning method. The latter approach requires experience because the needle is threaded a long distance through the dermis and could easily drop into the subcutaneous plane where Zyderm is not wanted. The clini-

cian can be easily fooled because the surface of the skin continues to elevate. Actually, injecting in the subcutaneous plane is easier because the material flows out with less pressure on the plunger and the surface of the skin elevates more obviously, but it is false success because the implant is so much more quickly absorbed.

Treating the Glabellar Lines

The vertical glabellar lines are furrows, creases, sometimes folds, and sometimes all three. The creases and furrows respond well to ZCI and Zp, and if the folds are interspersed with furrows, treating the furrows will reduce their prominence (Fig 7–11). The linear puncture method is the best technique, with the patient semisupine and the physician at the head of the table leaning over the patient.

Pore extrusion will sometimes make the treatment more troublesome because the skin on the glabella is often thick and sebaceous, but persistence in trying to find a dermal plane that will accept the implant usually pays off. However, there have been a few patients we could not adequately treat because of pore extrusion. The one case of partial unilateral blindness occurred shortly after ZCI was injected deeply at the glabella.[14] This tragic event happened early in the history of Zyderm, and emphasis on placing the implant in the dermis had not yet been stressed.

Using ZCI, obliteration of the vertical glabellar lines is a simple and highly desirable procedure. These lines designate the frown or scowl and detract from the eyes. Their removal brightens the face and lets the viewer focus on the eyes and center of the face.

Treating the Crow's Feet

Several questions need to be answered by the patient and physician before treating the radiating, curved lines that emanate from the lateral canthus and cross the malar prominence. The skin closer to the eye — skin that actually becomes the eyelid skin — is thin and stromatous, with a lot of ground substance and not a thick, well-defined dermis. Hence, when ZCI I is injected, the beading effect is more prominent. Patients report that it is two to three weeks before the implant smooths out. In this thin skin the implant beads look whitish and creamy, which also draws attention to them. These problems are more accentuated on the eyelid tissue, and less so laterally where the skin thickens. We often recommend that only the crow's feet lateral to the orbital rim be treated. However, a few patients want the whole line treated and are willing to put up with the beading during the first few weeks.

Only tiny droplets of material should be injected at each puncture site. Watch the skin closely; stop injecting after the first poof of Zyderm reaches the skin. Injecting more will produce a bead. With experience, a series of poofs along the axis of the line will produce the best results. Massage is usually necessary to blend and minimize the beading.

Another consideration is the cosmetic value of treating the crow's feet. On many faces they are beneficial, giving the face a soft, happy appearance. Because smiling is the etiology of most crow's feet — with squinting a distant second — marking the face when it is at rest with traces of smiles is not usually unsightly. The lines are curved and gentle and thus attractive, as opposed to the straight hack marks of the vertical glabellar lines or the sleep creases on the lateral forehead. There are definitely patients whose crow's feet should be treated: young people with persistent lines when there are no other lines on the face, or people with unusually deep lines, with straight lines, or lines crossed by straight sleep creases.

In this discussion of crow's feet we will include comments on two other cosmetic liabilities near the eye. Some people develop a sharp fold or crease that runs across the lower lid obliquely upward, beginning at the zygomatic junction of the orbital rim and ending near the medial canthus. This is a cosmetic liability that like crow's feet responds to ZCI.

Another problem is a depression at the midline on the lower eyelid-cheek groove (Fig 7–12). This depression is a significant cosmetic liability. It makes the face look sad. Clowns, when putting on a sad face, will paint a vertical line at this location to make the face look sad. We are unsure of the etiology of this feature; it is not related to facial movement and is not a skin change. Instead, it is a defect below the skin (hereditary or constitutional) indicated by loss of subcutaneous fat or depression in the subcutaneous musculature. ZCI or Zp will correct this defect in some patients, but in others filling the dermis at that depression produces a lump but does not correct the problem. Microlipoinjection has helped some, but it is too complicated a procedure for only one small depression. We hesitate to use silicone because it can create a palpable lump near the thin eyelid skin, but some doctors use it quite successfully.

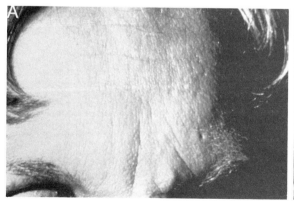 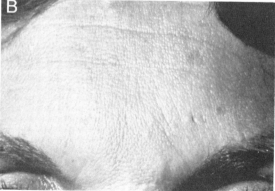

FIG 7–11.
Woman, 40 years old, with vertical creases in the glabella. **A**, before treatment. **B**, 4 weeks post-treatment with ZCI I, 1 ml.

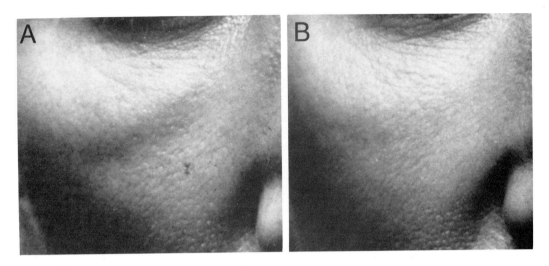

FIG 7–12.
Woman, 26 years old, with depression on the cheek just below the eyelid. **A**, before treatment. **B**, 4 weeks after treatment with 0.5 ml Zyderm I on each side.

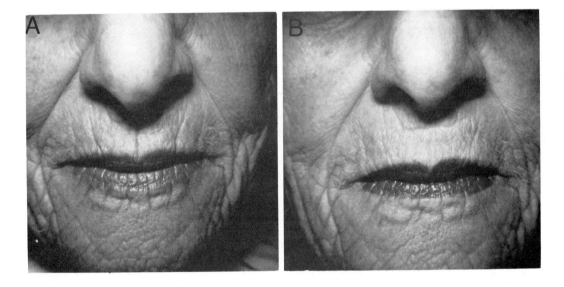

FIG 7–13.
A, woman, 73 years old, with sun-damaged skin and radiating perioral creases. Note the lipstick running. **B**, 6 weeks after treatment with ZCI I, 1.5 ml.

Treating the Perioral Area

The lines around the mouth are the second most common condition for which treatment is requested (Fig 7–13). They are mostly creases secondary to pursing both the upper and lower lips. Contrary to the most common assumption, smoking is not the cause. Most people do not really pucker when smoking. The most common cause is the way people purse their mouths during speaking and how they pronounce certain consonants such as "P" and "W." Only the most motivated individuals can retrain themselves not to pucker during speaking, but if they can, it is effective in reducing the radial perioral lines.

Men have fewer problems here because the skin is thicker and because the whisker follicles are so thick and numerous that the upper lip does not accordion-pleat as does the thin-skinned, vellous-haired female lip.

Before treating with ZCI, be sure the problem is movement-related creases and not massive sun-damage changes. From a distance, the actinically damaged upper lip will appear to have radiating lines — creases and minimal folds. But it will also have the color and texture changes of sun damage. These should be treated with dermabrasion, peel, or Retin-A. Movement-related creases, however, will be discrete in normal skin and can be correctly treated with a filler. The physician and the patient can be fooled by using a lot of a filler and blowing up the whole lip; the creases will be stretched out. But over-filling the whole upper lip area looks artificial and is not long-lasting. This mustache area should not be confused with the lips themselves (see below), and is called the cutaneous upper lip.

Treating the radiating lines of the lips is painful and perhaps should be treated last or blocked, as mentioned before. The best technique is to start at the vermilion and inject vertically for upper-lip lines. Start at the distal end of the line and inject toward the vermilion for the lower lines. Stabilization of the skin is achieved by pinching the lip with the nondominate hand or by pressing it against the patient's teeth. Massage helps to even out the implant.

Another perioral problem is the "drool groove" or the commissure grooves at the inferior edge of both commissures. These are a function of heredity, with the upper lip being longer than the lower (the most difficult to treat), or a function of aging where the cheek becomes more lax and a fold develops with its superior pole just below the commissure. This groove can cause trouble by collecting secretions, leading to perleche, and cosmetically by accentuating the lower corners of the mouth, producing marionette-mouth. Zp and ZCI II work well in these grooves.

The technique is simply to fill the space with ZCI. Because this skin is so stromatous, true intradermal placement is not possible in the amounts needed to fill the groove. Zp is probably the preferred agent because so much must be placed below the skin. The physician's gloved finger inside the patient's mouth and behind the treatment area not only detects the implant flowing in place but also creates a dam to keep the implant from shooting off in other than the desired directions.

Lips

At the time of this writing, it is a minor fad to have protruding, pouty lips. Just how long this fad will last is completely unpredictable, but for now Zyderm collagen is the filling agent of choice. We have used ZCI in lips since we first obtained it and discovered early on that the red-white line at the vermilion line could be enhanced by placing the needle into the skin at the lateral edge of the upper lip and injecting. The material snakes along the line, filling it better than can be done by trying to inject with the linear puncture technique. There must be anatomic space there because the Zyderm flows so regularly and predictably.

The fullness of the lips can be enhanced with ZCI. Either inject along the vermilion only, or fill in the entire body of the upper lip, enhancing the Cupid's bow. Sometimes just enlarging the central third of both upper and lower lips is adequate. With ZCI, the longevity of the correction is not great, but it certainly works well. Micro-lipoinjection may work as well here if the graft survival can be standardized.

For patients who want pouty lips, we inject ZCI II in the vermilion line space and ZCI I into the body of the lips. The lower lip is filled more than the upper. It is better to overfill because the lip swells quickly and it is so soft and spongy. The lips are swollen for a day or two, then settle down to what is hoped to be the desired fullness. The implant lasts only about three to four months in the lips.

Zyderm collagen is the best agent to use for the lips because it is temporary. It is not wise to use a permanent agent to encourage a fad. Fat implants or microlipoinjection also build spongy, full lips, but the results and longevity are quite

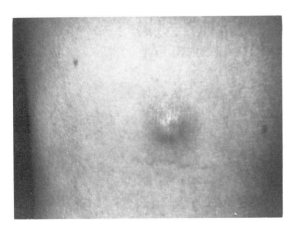

FIG 7–14.
A marked allergic reaction to ZCI at the skin test site on the volar forearm. The reaction was first noticed at 96 hours postimplantation and gradually resolved spontaneously within 4 weeks.

irregular (see below). Silicone works for this, but is permanent and takes several treatments to show.

Other Uses

Appropriate creases, soft shallow depressions, and soft scars anywhere on the body are correctable with filling agents. We have discussed only those areas where ZCI is used most often. It is also used for horizontal forehead creases and furrows (although sometimes the lines will be accentuated for several weeks), for horizontal creases at the bridge of the nose, for long, shallow, neck creases, and for some of the lines on the backs of the hands. There is a large podiatric experience with Zp (Keragen) implanted under corns on the feet.[15] ZCI has also helped chondrodermatitis nodularis chronica helices if surgery cannot be performed.

Complications

The complications from the use of Zyderm collagen implants (ZCI) and Zyplast implants (Zp) can be separated into three major categories: (1) true allergic reactions; (2) intermittent swelling; and (3) mechanical complications. This chapter will discuss each of these groups.

Allergic Reactions

For allergic and intermittent swelling, the clinical, immunologic, and histologic aspects will be presented. First, a brief discussion of the normal response to ZCI will provide helpful background.

At most test or treatment sites, a transient erythema develops which usually resolves within 48 to 96 hours.[16–19] Under light microscopy, periappendageal and perivascular lymphohistiocytic infiltrates develop around 7 days after implantation and can last as long as 90 days. The infiltrate does not appear to surround the implant, and a few quiescent fibroblasts which can be found within the clefts and crevices of the implant do not show any signs of depositing new collagen.

Allergic reactions are clinically similar at both test (Fig 7–14) and treatment sites (Fig 7–15). Within two or three days nearly 70% of the positive test-site reactions will become manifest. Many of the treatment-site reactions will also appear early, although a few test-site and many

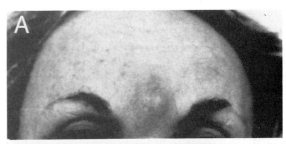
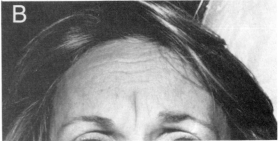

FIG 7–15.
A, an allergic reaction to ZCI at the treatment site on the glabella. It developed after multiple treatments, resolved spontaneously, and the patient developed a positive antibody titer to bovine collagen. **B,** the same patient 4 months later after complete resolution of the allergic reaction. No treatment was given for this reaction.

treatment-site reactions are delayed in onset. Sometimes the reaction will not show up until weeks or months after the implant has been placed.

The reactions are always located only at the injection sites and are indurated, elevated, erythematous, and occasionally pruritic. During the first few weeks, the reaction is more severe and gradually fades or becomes evanescent. Thus, short-lasting "reactions" are not true allergic reactions. If the reactions develop during the first six months after the test implant, the test site may also react. Most of the time, several or all of the treatment sites will react simultaneously. Rarely, only one site will react. In soft tissues the reaction may be only palpable, but over bony prominences it can be quite obvious and elevated. For example, the reactions in the nasolabial folds do not show as much as those on the glabella and forehead.

Rarely, the reaction will be extremely severe, with massive swelling and dusky erythema. The site feels almost cystic but usually is not (see cystic reactions below). These severe reactions can leave scarring.

The reactions fade out gradually after four to six months.[20] Some reactions will last a year and a few have persisted at 22 to 24 months. No treatments seem to shorten the reaction time. However, it may be necessary to offer treatment to some patients, mostly to alleviate anxiety. Temporary symptomatic relief and some reduction in edema are achieved with the nonsteroidal anti-inflammatory drugs, but antihistamines seem to be of little help. Systemic or intralesional steroids will provide temporary relief from both edema and erythema. However, treatment with steroids may depress the body's natural mechanisms for clearing the implant and thereby prolong the symptoms.

The best treatment for an allergic reaction is to warn the patient that it can happen. Reassurance that responses are self-limiting and that natural recovery takes place in an average of six months is the best therapy. Patient education about the possibility of an adverse reaction before testing should begin at the initial office visit and continue with reminders at subsequent treatment sessions.

Histologic examination of biopsies taken from test and treatment reaction sites are similar, and show that the epidermis is essentially normal. About one-third of the reactions show only a mild, almost normal perivascular, periappendageal infiltrate. The other two-thirds show granulomatous reactions of two types: diffuse granulomas (Fig 7–16), and palisading foreign body granulomas (Fig 7–17). In studies that have reported on allergic reaction histology, two types seem to be found with equal frequency.[16, 20–22] The diffuse granulomas develop earlier and the foreign-body-type later. It may be only a function of the elapsed time after the reaction began that these two types of histologic patterns are seen. The first stage of a reaction of Zyderm collagen may always be a diffuse granuloma and sometime later mature into a foreign-body type of granuloma.

Another explanation for the two types may be the location of the implant in the skin. In cases of the diffuse type, the implant is generally present in the deep dermis or subcutis. The palisading foreign-body type of granuloma is associated with deposits of ZCI in the mid to deep dermis. In work previously published by the author, it was demonstrated that the implant gradually sinks into and through the dermis with time.[23] It eventually is eliminated into the subcutis. The type of reaction that develops may be a result of where the implant is located, which is also a function of time elapsed after implantation.

Diffuse granulomatous nodules are composed of eosinophiles, lymphocytes, histiocytes, plasma cells, and occasionally polymorphonuclear leukocytes. A prominent eosinophilia dominates this type of lesion. The palisading foreign-body type of granuloma is overlaid with a mixture of lymphocytes, histiocytes, and plasma cells. The ZCI implant remains acellular and contains numerous foreign-body cells at the periphery.

Earlier studies confirmed that the bovine collagen implant could be identified within the granuloma with polarized light (Fig 7–18).[16, 17] These findings have been confirmed with more specific immunoperoxidase staining (Fig 7–19). Scattered foci of the host collagen entrapped within the implant can be identified by using the same techniques, because native collagen polarizes and ZCI does not.

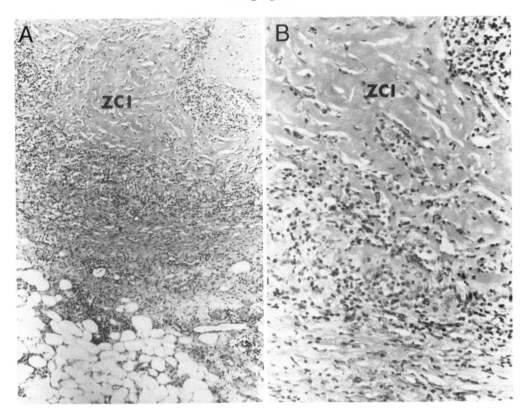

FIG 7–16.
A, biopsy of a diffuse granulomatous reaction in the deep dermis at a ZCI test site three weeks after injection. The cellular infiltrate is an admixture of eosinophiles, lymphocytes, histiocytes, and polymorphonuclear neutrophils, with a predominance of eosinophiles (hematoxylin-eosin, ×20). **B**, higher magnification of the same biopsy showing the diffuse distribution of the mixed inflammatory cell infiltrate permeating the ZCI (hematoxylin-eosin, ×40).

Immunologic studies on patients with reactions to Zyderm collagen reveal that 100% of the patients having hypersensitivity reactions have antibodies to ZCI.[24–27] These antibodies do not cross-react with human collagen or other mammalian collagen, nor do they form antigen-antibody precipitates. All of the patients have IgG antibodies and about one-third also have IgA antibodies.[10] The antibody titers persist longer than the clinical reactions.

Other studies for anti-ZCI antibodies by the ELISA assay have revealed that about 8.4% of the U.S. population have antibodies before exposure to ZCI and about 10% develop antibodies after exposure. However, the percentage of patients who develop clinical manifestations of allergy is much lower: approximately 3% react to the skin test and an additional 0.5% to 1.0% react on subsequent exposure.[22] It is assumed that

most people with pre-existing antibodies have become sensitized though dietary exposures.

There is a difference in the biological response to Zyderm and Zyplast, the gluteraldehyde cross-linked collagen.[23] Histologic studies comparing the two products showed that the Zyderm collagen is dispersed in the dermis as many small islands or droplets, whereas the Zyplast remains as relatively large accumulations. There is almost no fibroblastic invasion into the Zyderm collagen, while some Zyplast implants have many fibroblasts growing through the implant, and those fibroblasts appear to be in an active, secretory state. The larger implant, the preinjection cross-linking, and other unknown factors may contribute to the lower incidence of clinical reactions to Zyplast. Not enough antibody or histologic studies are available to provide any conclusions, but clinically there have been fewer reactions with Zyplast than the 3% on initial exposure and the 0.5% to 1.0% on subsequent exposures that has been the history of Zyderm.[31] Clinically, there have been examples of patients who had both Zyderm collagen and Zyplast implant in the same session. They later developed allergic reactions only at the Zyderm collagen sites.[32]

The Collagen Corporation has recently identified an unusual reaction that is characterized by draining vesicles or cysts.[28] More of these reactions have occurred in patients who were treated with Zyplast, but a few developed in patients treated with Zyderm collagen. At the time of this writing, fewer than 100 cases have been reported during the years 1983 to 1988. The incidence is rare, occurring in 1 of every 2,000 patients who received Zyplast implant or Zy-

derm collagen and Zyplast implant, and 1 of every 50,000 patients treated with Zyderm collagen alone.

The etiology of this reaction remains obscure. An atypical allergic hypersensitivity must be considered because approximately one-half of the patients had serology tests for antibovine collagen antibodies and of these, 80% were positive.

It is difficult to recommend therapy at this time because so little is known about cystic reaction. If the lesion is fluctuant, needle aspiration is recommended. If it is more like a ripe epidermal cyst, incision and drainage are necessary. Mechanical intervention must be predicated on whether or not such action will leave a better or worse scar. If the lesion is mostly indurated with little fluctuance, it might heal

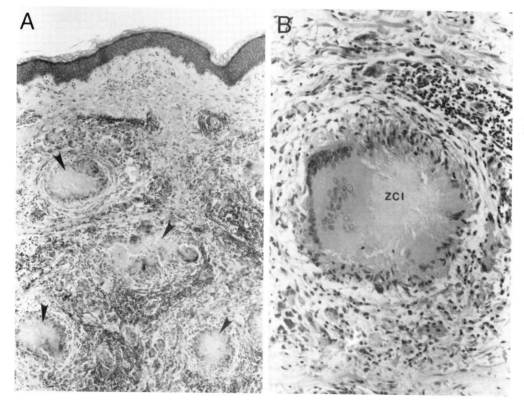

FIG 7–17.
A, biopsy of a foreign-body granuloma at a ZCI test site approximately two months after injection. Islands of ZCI (*arrows*) are surrounded by numerous giant foreign body cells (hematoxylin-eosin, ×20). **B.** higher magnification of one of the granulomatous nodules in **A,** showing the acellular, centrally located ZCI surrounded by giant foreign body cells and an outer covering of mixed inflammatory cells (hematoxylin-eosin ×40).

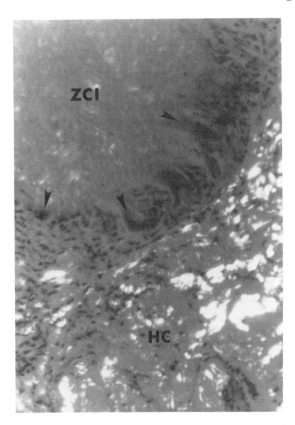

FIG 7–18.
Section from a biopsy of a palisading foreign body granuloma at approximately 6 weeks after test injection, stained by an indirect immunoperoxidase method using an anti-bovine type I collagen antibody. The bovine collagen implant is stained brown, while the host collagen in the right field is unstained. *Arrowheads* indicate giant cells (×100).

current intermittent swelling at treatment sites. This reaction can last up to three years. About 45% of these patients also experience erythema and induration during episodes of swelling. The reactions can be triggered by exercise, exposure to sun, menstruation, or ingestion of alcohol, cocaine, or beef. The implant sites appear perfectly normal between flareups. Not all of the implant sites react, and not always do the same sites react. Data from a retrospective study performed by the manufacturer indicate that many patients with intermittent swelling did have antibodies to bovine collagen. As soon as the swelling reactions clears, the patients can be treated

without drainage and the patient can be spared a scar. If the lesion has caused considerable skin necrosis, appropriate drainage may actually lessen the size of the scar. Any aspirated material should be cultured, and the patient started on broad-spectrum antibiotics. Intralesional steroids usually reduce the inflammation and may need to be repeated several times during the life of the reaction.

Intermittent Swelling

Another type of adverse reaction seen in approximately 1% of treated patients involves re-

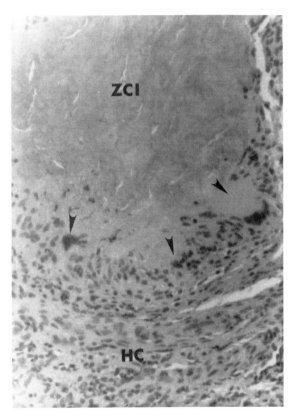

FIG 7–19.
Section from the same biopsy in Fig 7–17, viewed with polarized light, shows ZCI to be only weakly birefringent when compared with normal host collagen (HC) in the right field. *Arrowheads* indicate giant cells (polarized light, ×100).

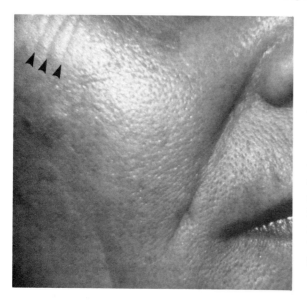

FIG 7–20.
Linear ridges (*arrows*) resulting from overcorrection with ZCI of a patient's crow's feet, shown three weeks after treatment. This condition resolves spontaneously without physical discomfort.

again with ZCI, without problems. After an intermittent swelling reaction, it is important to re-test the skin before treating again.

Mechanical Complications

The act of inserting a needle into the skin, even if it is only a 30-gauge needle, plus the injection of 1 to 2 ml of a moderately viscous material, will induce a small number of physical problems. Overcorrection is a complication with Zyderm collagen that fortunately will always be temporary (Fig 7–20). If the physician completely misplaces the implant and injects too much too high in the skin, it will migrate deeper within a few months. The problem of overcorrection becomes less frequent as the physician becomes more skilled. If the problem is discovered immediately, massage will help to smooth and reduce the size of the lump. Massage must be judicious so that the implant is not rubbed completely out of the skin, but only molded down to the proper level. Some doctors always mas-

sage a little to make the implant less visible from the beginning.

A small number of cases of localized tissue necrosis have been reported.[29] These happen more frequently with Zyplast implant than Zyderm collagen and most commonly on the glabella. Sometimes they heal without scarring and other times a flat, atrophic scar will result (Fig 7–21). It is theorized that in these cases too much collagen was pushed into too small an area of skin. Because the Zyplast is more robust and sets up as a relatively large bolus, a pressure necrosis develops. Another theory is that a dermal arteriole is occluded by direct placement of the implant on or in that arteriole. This leads to segment ischemia and necrosis.

True vascular occlusion has occurred. The

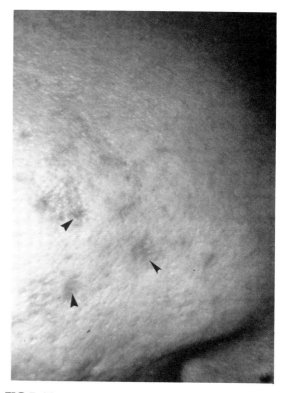

FIG 7–21.
Healing of areas of localized tissue necrosis following treatment with ZCI can result in hypopigmented, flat, atrophic scars (*arrowheads*). Test sites did not flare, and this patient was negative for antibodies to bovine collagen implants.

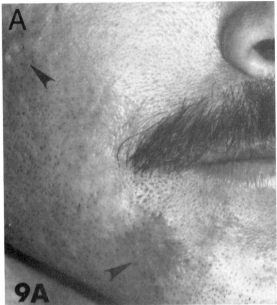

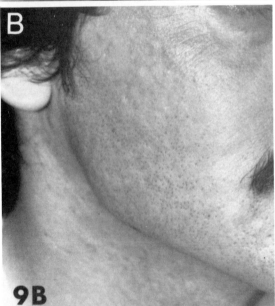

FIG 7–22.
A, patient with ischemia (*arrowhead*) associated with severe pain immediately following injection of ZCI. This is a suspected case of vessel laceration because the pain was transient and distributed over the labial artery. **B,** the same patient after a return to normal coloration that occurred within minutes of the initial injection. The patient did not show any adverse reactions after this treatment with ZCI or following any subsequent treatments with ZCI.

most serious is the one case reported of permanent, partial vision loss that occurred while Zyderm collagen was being injected into the glabellar region.[30] The author had one incident during the early clinical trials with Zyderm collagen in which an arteriole on the lower cheek was either entered or traumatized by the needle or implant (Fig 7–22). The cheek distal to the artery and the ipsalateral nasal ala immediately became ischemic and painful. After about two to three minutes, the involved areas became hyperemic and bluish. Within another three minutes, it all faded, with no short or long sequelae.

Bruising can almost be expected when intradermal injections of any kind are performed and is hardly a complication. However, the first time it happens it is upsetting to some patients. We are not aware of any way to predict which patients will bruise, except for those on anticoagulants. Bruising is unpredictable because it will happen only on some patients on certain days and not at all sites and not at all treatment sessions. There is no treatment for bruising but it may happen less often if only tiny amounts of collagen are injected slowly.

As with other mechanical complications, superficial infections have been reported at implantation sites. These infections resolve spontaneously or usually with antibiotic therapy, and without significant sequelae.[26]

Systemic reactions to ZCI have been considered but never proven. Flulike episodes have been reported following ZCI administration. Usually, if it happened once or twice, the patient was given no more of the product. These reactions never proved to be related to ZCI.

There have been attempts to link dermatomyositis to ZCI injections. There are only random temporal relationships of collagen-vascular episodes to exposure to Zyderm. However, intensive review by a panel of recognized experts in immunology, rheumatology, collagen vascular disease, and epidemology concluded that there are no theoretical or practical data to indicate that bovine dermal collagen, when prepared as Zyderm collagen or in other forms (e.g., sutures and hemostatic agents), can induce dermatomyositis or any of the other so-called collagen-vascular diseases. The panel also concluded that there is no evidence of cross-reactivity between antibodies to bovine collagen and human collagen; that antihuman collagen antibodies are found in untreated patients as a result of other disease processes and are not associated with the development of rheumatic disease; and that the incidence of rheumatic disease in patients treated with injectable collagen is the same or lower than that in the general untreated population. They closed with the following statement, "There are not current data to suggest that immunity to xenogeneic dermal collagen can precipitate autoimmune disease in man or in other species."[31]

Microdroplet Silicone

We purposely titled this section "Microdroplet Silicone" because we want to dissociate it from the other literature, controversy, and invective attached to the many silicone products and injection techniques. Microdroplet silicone refers to the injection technique in which amounts of silicone ranging from 0.005 to 0.01 ml are implanted at a single location per treatment, with a maximum total dose of 1 ml per patient visit.

For the purposes of this chapter and where referenced in this chapter, unless otherwise noted, silicone is a polydimethylsiloxane fluid with a viscosity of 350 centistokes (cS) which has been filtered and sterilized to remove heavy metals, low-chain-length polymers, and other impurities. This is most likely what is generally referred to as "injectable-grade silicone," which is different from "medical-grade silicone," Dow Corning's term for the product they manufacture which is used for lubricating disposable needles and syringes, coating containers for medicines and blood products, and as an emollient in lotions. Dow's medical-grade silicone has a viscosity of 360 cS.

The one new drug application (NDA) that was ever submitted to the FDA by Dow Corning was for a product they called MDX 4-4011, which was a purified, sterilized, 350-cS product. Some of the studies we cite were based on the use of

MDX 4-4011, and we are sure other references are not. It is our intention to discuss and recommend sterilized, purified polydimethylsiloxane fluid with a 350 cS viscosity injected by the microdroplet technique.

It is critical to divorce microdroplet silicone from all other products and techniques because of pseudoscientific or adverse reports in the scientific medical literature that relate the results of treatments with a multitude of products and mixtures labeled "silicone." While we have the luxury of making this important distinction in this chapter, the FDA, the public, and the media cannot be counted on to do the same.

Normal Histologic Response

In animal studies the early local response to both single and multiple injections of silicone was a mild round cell infiltrate that subsided in six months.[32, 33] In time, the silicone became encapsulated by the animal's own collagen. Sections showed thin-walled spaces widely separated in some cases but closely approximated in others, producing a honeycomb appearance. There was increased deposition of collagen around these spaces, with occasional giant cells and evidence of phagocytosis.[34] Similar reactions have been noted in humans.[35]

The above-stated normal tissue response to silicone in animals is probably similar to what happens in humans, although the evidence is circumstantial and some experienced users of the product do not believe it happens. Clinically, a postinjection erythema is not uncommon which fades over a few months; this would correlate with the nonspecific infiltrate. Capsule formation (or laying down of the animal's own collagen) is common with silicone breast implants, although these are bags of silicone that "bleed" a certain amount of higher-viscosity silicone. In addition, isolated biopsies have been taken of silicone which purport to show "collagen enhancement" around the implant.[36]

Microcapsule formation around each silicone droplet is an important theory for the users of this product because it is the rationale that explains why the correction appears to improve in four weeks and why the microdroplets will not migrate or, with native collagen encapsulation, are unlikely to be phagocytized. The theory does not fit the recommended treatment schedule of four weeks between visits. If the encapsulization were under way at four weeks, a much longer interval would be necessary to allow complete "collagen enhancement" to develop. Also, in cases of breast implants, only 40% develop a significant capsule, which leaves the silicone unencapsulated in 60% of cases. Painfully needed is a longitudinal histologic study in humans that chronicles what really happens to the microdroplets. We have approval from the Human Experimentation Committee of the University of California, San Francisco, to do just such a study, but the FDA-approved protocol was withdrawn when the sponsoring company decided not to pursue approval for their silicone.

Indications and Techniques

Silicone is a *permanent* implant that often "grows" a little after implantation — the encapsulation process. Never overcorrect. Always undercorrect. Experienced users may correct to nearly surface level, but for others it is best to stay safe and undercorrect.

Much of the literature describes using a glass tuberculin syringe never larger than 1 ml, with smaller ones recommended. Most physicians have settled on a 30-gauge needle either 1/2 inch or 1 inch long. A three-ring attachment helps the physician deliver the implant easily, smoothly, and without any uncomfortable pressure on the finger. However, we have happily used disposable 1-ml tuberculin syringes with a disposable 30-gauge, 1-inch needle. Medical lore maintains that because silicone is an effective lubricant, the needle will not stay on unless it is used with a Luer-lok. This is not so. We draw up the agent into the syringe with a 19-gauge needle, put on a 30-gauge needle, and inject (Fig 7–23, A and B).

As with other filling agents, magnification is strongly recommended.

The patient's skin needs to be clean but not sterilized. In most cases, alcohol wiping is adequate if the skin is clean.

There are no known allergies to this agent, and therefore no prior testing is needed.[36, 37]

As with other filling agents, anesthesia is not usually necessary. With silicone, the only significant discomfort is the needle stick (see the discussion on topical anesthetics above, in the discussion of ZCI).

Three injection techniques are generally used: multiple puncture, fanning, and tattooing. Multiple puncture is used primarily on creases and furrows, and places tiny droplets under the line, with repeated insertions starting at one end of the line and progressing toward the other. Physicians will develop individual habits about which end of the line to start on; it is a personal preference only. The fanning technique is for larger depressions such as poststeroid atrophy, hemiatrophy, or contour augmentations. The needle is inserted to the proper depth — just subcutaneously or deep dermis — and the needle

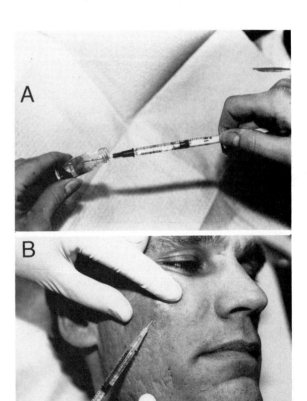

FIG 7–23.
A, silicone is drawn up through a 19-gauge needle into a disposable 1 cc tuberculin syringe. **B,** silicone is injected through a 30-gauge needle into a postacne scar.

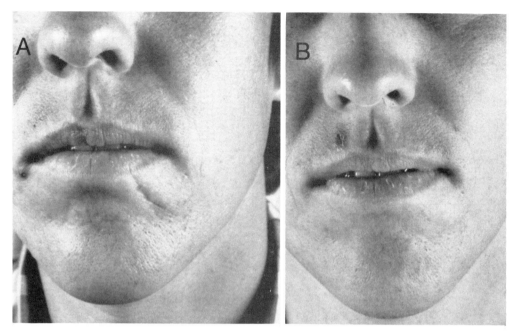

FIG 7–24.
A, post-traumatic, soft linear depressed scar on the lower lip area shown before silicone injections. **B**, the same chin 9 months after three treatments. (Courtesy of David Duffy, M.D.)

tip continuously moved. The agent is injected as the needle is both advanced and withdrawn. If there is some problem in placing the needle tip properly, injection might be made only upon withdrawal. By moving the needle rapidly, the amount at any one spot is minimal and intravascular injection problems are minimized. The tattooing technique includes rapid, shallow, sticks about 1 to 2 mm apart in a given area while pushing on the plunger. This deposits tiny droplets of silicone in the mid to high dermis. It is useful for very superficial lines around the crow's feet or area of the upper lip.

Scars

Postacne, (Fig 7–24) trauma, surgery, (Fig 7–25), or infection scars can be elevated to the surface of the skin, providing they are broad and distensible. Silicone is appropriate for atrophic scars where ZCI is not, because silicone can be placed just under the skin in the high subcutis (Fig 7–26). If the scar is distensible enough, it will be corrected by the implant. ZCI needs to be placed in dermis lacking in atrophic scars. As is particularly true with atrophic scars but also with any scars, the color and texture of the skin

at the base of the lesion should be normal or recontouring may not improve the appearance.

The scar depth and shape determine where the silicone is placed. A shallow defect that extends only into the dermis is recontoured by placing the silicone droplets in the mid to deep dermis. If the defect is a full-thickness skin depression, the implant goes into the high subcutis.

At each visit, spaced at least four weeks apart, inject about 0.005 to 0.01 ml through several entry sites at the proper depth. Try to place the material evenly under the entire defect to be elevated. Do not use more than 0.5 ml at any one scar site. The angle of the needle also depends on the required depth of placement. To lay it into the mid dermis, the needle angle to the skin will be between 30 to 60 degrees. For subcutaneous placement, the angle may be greater than 60 degrees. Different from the injection of ZCI for scars, *the needle should be moving slightly* while the plunger is depressed in order to implant many microdroplets, as opposed to one large drop.

Some silicone users recommend massage after injection (although some do not) to break up the implant into many droplets. Massage is certainly recommended if too much silicone is injected, and may help spread the material laterally and deeper. However, it is better to simply inject silicone in multiple microdroplets.

Creases and Furrows

Forehead lines, both verticle and horizontal, the horizontal lines on the radix of the nose, the smile lines (Fig 7–27, A and B), the perioral lines, earlobe lines, neck creases, and lines on the backs of hands have all been treated with silicone and reported.[36–38] The linear multiple puncture technique is most often used for lines. With time, the physician can learn to inject it without creating a "string of beads." Unlike ZCI, the object of each visit is not to erase the line (although shallow lines often disappear with one treatment) but to begin or continue to erase the line. After a few visits, when the line is minimized, the next or maintenance visit may be 4, 6, or 12 months hence. Deeper furrows in the smile line may require four to six visits to achieve correction and like all movement-related lines, will require maintenance. The tendency to fully correct furrows over bony prominences should be judged carefully. Silicone is permanent, and full correction may obliterate the furrow but create a fullness that looks strange forever. This is not a problem with temporary implants. Silicone treats an area, whereas Zyderm treats a specific line.

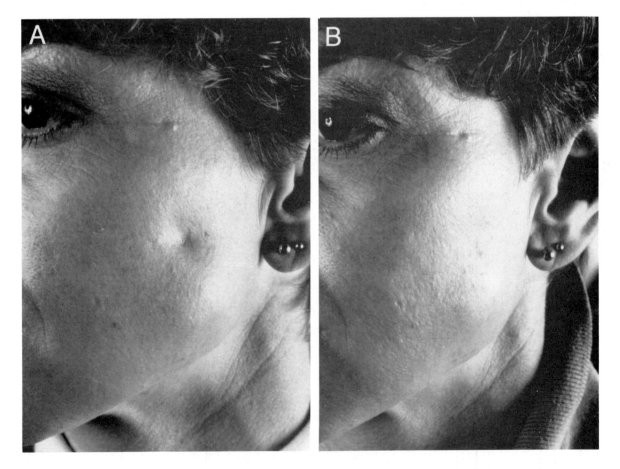

FIG 7–25.
A, steroid atrophy of longer than 6 months duration on the cheek. **B,** after treatment with silicone twice. (Courtesy of David Duffy, M.D.)

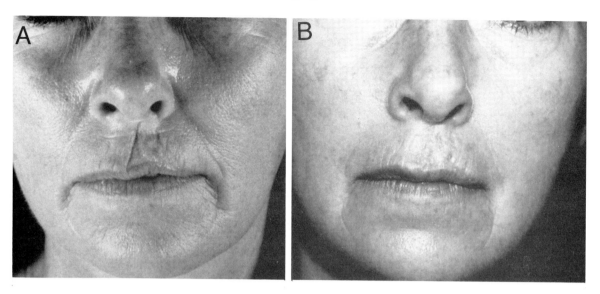

FIG 7–26.
A, medial side of the smile fold and the smile crease before silicone injection. **B,** 4 months after three treatments. (Photo courtesy of David Duffy, M.D.)

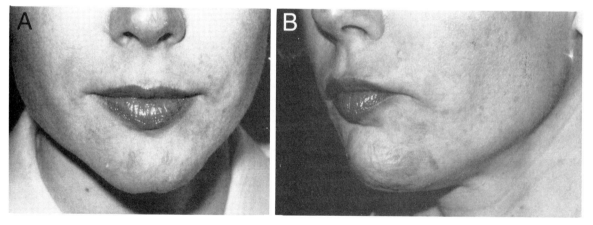

FIG 7–27.
A and **B,** persistent dusky erythema in the chin of 44-year-old woman treated elsewhere with silicone injections.

Postsurgical Refinements

After cosmetic surgery, especially surgery that reshapes firm structures, such as a rhinoplasty, irregularities sometimes develop. These small depressions or divots detract from the patient's total satisfaction with the procedure.[39] A few injections of silicone are wondrous in alleviating these nuisance irregularities.

Lips

The lips can be made more full with a few injections. The agent is placed along the vermilion in several visits. Unlike ZCI, which is injected just superior to the vermilion, silicone is injected within the red side of the line. Injecting anywhere around the lips is painful, and although topical anesthetics work on the mucosa, the epithelium is so much more keratinized at the vermilion that topicals do little. A field block is necessary for some patients; the infraorbitals are infiltrated for the upper lip and the mentals for the lower.

The labial creases — the perleche — can be filled with silicone. If the crease is in the thick skin of men and just lateral to the commissure, silicone works well. If, however, the crease is in soft, stromatous skin, as it is in women, and immediately inferior to the commissure, ZCI seems to do better even though it is temporary.

Podiatric Uses

There is a long experience of silicone use for foot problems, with clavi (corns) the most common. Relief of pressure spots and some neurotrophic ulcers has been accomplished with silicone.[36–40] A repeated microdose technique is required. Some reportedly poor outcomes may have been the result of trying to inject too much agent in one session. The locations where these problems usually occur are the weight-bearing surfaces of the metatarsal heads, the heels, and the interdigital web spaces (soft corns).

Except for the original investigations, a podiatric protocol was the only FDA-approved use of silicone injected freely into the skin since Dow Corning withdrew its application.

Complications

A reminder to the reader: We are discussing only techniques to inject microdroplet silicone. Happily, the incidence of adverse reaction is extremely limited. In a number of cases, probably fewer than 20%, a transient erythema will develop at the injection site only. It lasts from hours to three days and resolves spontaneously without sequelae. A few patients developed long-lasting dusky erythema which slowly responded to systemic or intralesional steroids (Fig 7–28). It has been argued that this reaction was from adulterated "silicone" or from massive overdosing. Those who are scrupulous in using the microdroplet technique do not report this adverse reaction.

In even a smaller percentage of cases a hyperpigmentation (blue-brown discoloration) will develop over the treatment site. This has been most commonly reported when postrhinoplasty defects were filled in.[37–41]

Itching, bruising, and infection have all been reported.[42, 43] These have been infrequent, self-limiting, and can be expected from any treatment that injects substances into the skin.

Overcorrection becomes a complication when a permanent agent is used. Overcorrection is easier to obtain with silicone than with the other injectables because with time silicone grows and the others shrink. We suspect there is a larger number of permanent overcorrections than reported because the reports have been by the "experts" with the agent and because it is

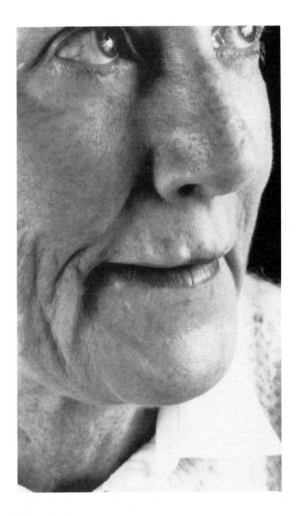

FIG 7–28.
Overcorrection of the upper lip with silicone shown 8 months after the last injection. (Courtesy of David Duffy, M.D.)

not FDA-approved. Nevertheless, the possibility of overcorrection underscores the need to administer only tiny amounts at each visit, and to wait the four-week minimum between treatments. The permanency factor, among others, has contributed greatly to the hesitation that legitimate medical manufacturing companies have about this product.

Human Adjuvant Disease

There are several reports in the literature of a polyarthritis condition that develops after silicone breast implantation.[44-45] We have not found any references to this problem as a result of use of the microdroplet technique. It is known that the older breast implants would "bleed" silicone and that patients developed the arthritis reported. The new bags are laminated with a material much less permeable to silicone and are called "low-bleed" prostheses. Whether the problem is related to a certain dose of silicone, the location of the bleed (i.e., breast tissue), or continuous exposure is not known. If reporting has been accurate, the microdroplet technique does not cause this problem.[47]

FDA Approval

There are many reasons why FDA approval is desirable: a constant, guaranteed source of pure material, acceptance and coverage from medical malpractice carriers, complete reporting of adverse reaction, more widely shared results — good and bad — and eventually a better understanding by the public and noncosmetic physicians of the safety of the microdroplet technique. At the time this book is written, it seems unlikely that there will be approval by the FDA in the foreseeable future.

Two well-capitalized, FDA-experienced, sophisticated medical companies initiated FDA new drug applications (NDAs) for injectable microdroplet-technique silicone. The FDA was receptive to these applications but on review of the initial submission of clinical protocols, required proof, based on animal data, of lack of immunogenicity, carcinogenicity, and teratogenicity. In addition, the FDA wanted proof that human adjuvant disease was not related to silicone and would not accept any of the past clinical studies as proof of clinical efficacy. These FDA requirements make it nearly impossible financially to prepare the necessary data and thus request approval. This product probably could not be patented — in any protective way — and thus the company investing the money to obtain approval would not be granted a use patent comprehensive enough to allow recovery of the initial investment.

Other serious problems with manufacturing and marketing silicone concern potential misuse, an issue that has bothered Dow Corning and all other potential manufacturers. The possibility of great amounts of silicone being injected into breasts, penises, hips, or cheeks scares any potential manufacturer. The legal ramifications are based on a misinformed public, as well as manufacturers' deep pockets and a legal profession that includes some members who might continuously "extort" defendants with cases that must be settled to protect the company's reputation. Therefore, this product must produce a very high profit to be worthwhile for any potential manufacturer. We do not expect to see this product widely available soon.

Microlipoinjection

Pierre Fournier, M.D., of Paris, who pioneered modern techniques of liposuction surgery and developed the system we rely upon for our lipoinjection technique has said that in liposuction we are concerned with the *remaining* tissues and thus we pay attention to hemostasis, even contour, and natural feel. With lipoinjection, however, we are concerned with the *viability of the lipocytes*. Therefore, our concerns turn to protection of the tissues during harvesting and reimplantation into the proper milieu. We completely agree, but how to protect and properly implant is still unknown. Generally, tissue transplantation is fairly successful if certain exacting criteria are met. For example, hair transplants can be kept out of the body for hours and vigorously washed; most of us have had an accident where the plugs were dropped or slightly crushed. These plugs seem to grow as well as nontraumatized plugs. Conversely, the upper limits of size are absolutely critical. Plugs 4.5 mm in diameter grow well, while plugs 5.0 mm in diameter usually do not grow hair or only grow hair at the periphery. A diameter difference of 0.5 mm makes a huge difference in growth.

The critical factors for successful "take" for fat injections have not yet been identified. In the meantime, the theories about why fat transplants do or do not take must all be given equal consideration — until the facts are known. We would like to propose the best or most successful technique, but we can only describe what we and others do, and follow the literature for proof about what really happens in fat-grafting.

History

In the historical search for soft-tissue augmentation techniques, fat has seemed a natural choice. Attempts at fat transplantation are not new.[48–50] At several points in the surgical literature, rudimentary experiments in autologous fat grafting are noted, beginning in the 19th century and proceeding to the present day.[51–53] Most of the early attempts at grafting fat involved the sharp dissection of bulk fat in pieces that were then placed into prepared pockets of subcutaneous tissue. The fate of these packets of fat was almost invariably, but not uniformly, ischemic necrosis, liquification, and absorption. In Peer's[53] oft-cited studies done in the late 1950s, it was observed that small pieces of fat, properly placed, lost at least 50% of their volume. At the time, surgeons looking for a higher volume survival rate were dazzled by the initial promise of silicone, and Peer's work slipped into medical obscurity.

In was not until the dramatic appearance of liposuction surgery in the 1980s that the possibility of fat grafting appeared once more.[54–57] Along with Georgio Fisher, Illouz, who developed the first successful liposuction procedures, was also seeing many referrals for lateral thigh depressions that were the result of overly vigorous fat removal by other surgeons. He began reinjecting viable fat harvested during liposuction to correct some of the depression.[56–58] In 1986, at the annual meeting of the American Society for Dermatologic Surgery, Pierre Fournier introduced to the U.S. his fat-grafting technique which he called "microlipoinjection."

Since then interest has exploded. With the laudably open American society, new instruments, new techniques, and clinical studies about microlipoinjection have filled meetings of cosmetic and dermatologic surgeons. Autologous fat-grafting is an outpatient surgical procedure for correction of minor defects and early changes of aging which meshes perfectly with the work and experience of many surgical dermatologists.

Histology

If this section of the chapter could be longer, the rest may be shorter because we could discuss the best method only. As it is, we will list the scanty data available and mention the various methods being tried. There are clear-cut differences in gross appearance and degree of associated fibrous tissue when comparing fat harvested from different sites. For example, the fat of the medial knee and inner thigh of women is quite soft and easily harvested, whereas the fat of the lateral waist "love handles" or upper outer buttock in men is much more fibrous and difficult to harvest. These differences have unknown impact on survival but make a significant difference in the ease of harvesting through a needle, how bloody the aspirant is, and how soft the implant becomes.[59]

We have information that proves that the size of the cannula used for harvesting fat affects viability. Campbell, et al. have shown that cannulas or needles smaller than 19-gauge damage lipocytes irreparably through mechanical shear forces.[60] Vacuum pressures generated by liposuction aspirators generally approach −1 atm (760 mm Hg), which "boils" the water from the fat cells. Interestingly, the pressures generated from the hand-syringe method advocated by Fournier rarely exceed 500 mm Hg, avoiding the desiccation caused by a stronger vacuum.

Reasonable theories about the impact of blood, insulin, and normal saline should be considered. The presence of free red blood cells in the graft, long known to be detrimental to full-thickness skin grafts, may adversely affect the survival of fat grafts. Hence, the inclusion of steps to "wash" the fat prior to reinjection. Ringer's lactate solution causes less stimulation of glucose metabolism in harvested lipocytes than

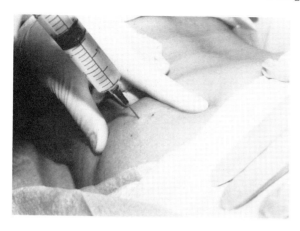

FIG 7–29.
Lidocaine "cocktail" being injected into donor site on the buttock.

does normal saline, implying that the microenvironment of the graft may be critical to its long-term survival.[60] Biochemical receptors on lipocytes may affect survival after transplantation.[60, 62] Therefore, a rinse in dilute heparin is part of some physicians' protocol.

Technique

The controversies about variations in technique begin at step one. The Fournier method harvests the fat gently into a disposable syringe of from 3 to 20 ml using only the negative pressure that can be generated by the syringe. Others trap the fat in specially designed containers during regular liposuction procedures, and transfer it to syringes for injection. We are theoretically opposed to the machine-harvested open methods because they have the potential of exposing the graft to bacteria, and unduly traumatize the graft by the machine suction and the extra handling.

Both donor and recipient areas are clensed with chlorhexidine (Hibiclens) and wiped with alcohol. A full surgical scrub is unnecessary. Betadine painting is also satisfactory. The patient is appropriately draped for a local procedure only. Also, the patient should be positioned so that gravity does not obliterate the depression being treated.

Heavy local anesthesia for the donor site may theoretically disrupt the cells or rupture cell membranes. It may eventually be proven that

injection of local anesthetics does no harm, but for now we have been using only dilute lidocaine (0.25% to 0.5%) with epinephrine (Fig 7–29). We try not to fill the space with anesthetic fluid as we do for the wet technique liposuction (see Chapter 13), but we do infiltrate the area. Fournier recommends the application of cold packs — cryoanesthesia — for 20 to 30 minutes. We and others[64] find this method too cumbersome and unpredictable, but we have seen it work well in Fournier's.

The anesthesia of the recipient area should be accomplished with as little distortion to the skin as possible. For the face, both regional and ring blocks meet this criteria. Again, cryoanesthesia may be effective. We use it more for the recipient area than the donor area because the injection is much quicker and less painful than the harvesting. For both donor and recipient areas a small drop of 1% lidocaine is placed at the needle entry site, because we use a 13- or 16-gauge needle. The procedure is so painless and quick that analgesics and tranquilizers are not necessary.

We have used the lateral thighs, the abdomen (preferably lower), the buttocks, and the knees, in that order, for donor fat for facial reinjection. We have heard physicians say they prefer fat from one area over another. Each area has been proclaimed "the best," but we have never heard exactly why. Certainly, fat color, fibrous content, and consistency varies with each area, but for a procedure that may have to be repeated several times, it is easiest to choose an area with plenty of fat to donate and an area that is easily accessible but where the bruises can be hidden by the clothing. The lateral thigh, the upper outer buttock, or the abdomen best meet these needs.

If the fat is to be harvested by machine as part of a liposuction procedure, the sterile preparation for that surgery will be included or take preference. Our bias now is that the machine suction is too traumatic and that the fat is exposed to too much manipulation. The following discussion details how we currently perform lipoinjection.

Several sites in the donor area are identified as entry sites and injected with 1% lidocaine. (Actually, the dilute lidocaine solution used in the donor site also works, but it is better to distort the recipient areas as little as possible.) Through these sites, a small incision is made with a #11 Bard-Parker blade (Fig 7–30). This entry is probed and dilated by the 13-gauge needle itself, or can be opened with any blunt instrument of appropriate size. Asken uses specially designed probes (available through Robbins Instrument Company of Catham, New Jersey),[64] and Fournier uses a graduated series of skin awls.[54] The entry-site scar is smaller to nonexistent if a tiny nick is made with the blade and the opening dilated than it is if the blade is used to cut open the skin. When we use the 16-gauge needle, the scalpel nick is unnecessary.

Needles with gauges of 13 to 19 work for syringe harvesting. We prefer a straight, 13-gauge steel needle with a 45-degree blunt bevel. Small cannulas, designed by Asken, which fit onto a Luer-Lok or onto suction tubing, work as well.[63] There is a wide array of suction tips for liposuction in all areas, but remember Dr. Fournier's admonition, "For fat transplants, be respectful of the lipocytes." The fat harvested through the 13-gauge needle appears macroscopically as small, clean microplugs of fat.

The needle is inserted into the subcutaneous area. Some physicians make several probing strokes before pulling any negative pressure on the syringe; others start right out with a suction. A few cc of normal saline in the syringe and needle help fill the dead space, making it pos-

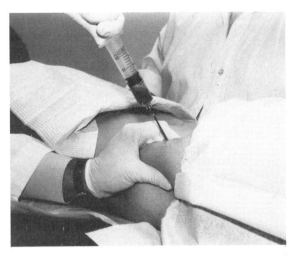

FIG 7–31.
Fat being harvested by pulling suction on the plunger and moving the entire syringe and needle in and out.

sible to obtain stronger negative pressure with the syringe. Once the tip is below the skin, the plunger is pulled out and held with the little finger or by a needle shoved through the plastic plunger. Other devices have been designed that clip onto the syringe to hold the plunger out. When we use a 10- or 20-ml syringe, we like to have an assistant hold the negative pressure, but for the 3-ml syringe, which we use the most, the little finger is adequate.

The syringe is moved in and out of the fat with a piston-like movement (Fig 7–31). Eight to ten strokes are made at each placement of the needle. The needle is then redirected and eight to ten more strokes are made until the area is fully harvested. The donor skin can be pinched up in the opposite hand or held in place by the flat of the opposite hand. As with any blind procedure, the amount of blood drawn up is unpredictable. If too much comes up, change locations; if only a little is collected, continue pumping and plan to wash the fat later. Each syringe can be filled only to two-thirds full because further withdrawal makes the plunger unstable.

Harvest as much fat (or more) as is estimated to be needed. The checks will require 10 to 15 cc each, the smile furrows about 5 to 10 cc each, the backs of the hands about 10 to 15 cc each. Morrow[17] has refrigerated excess harvested fat for three to four months and reports the viability

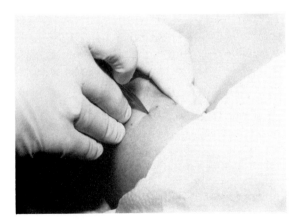

FIG 7–30.
Small nick made with no. 11 blade for entry site.

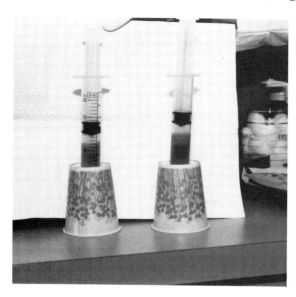

FIG 7–32.
Syringes filled with harvested fat standing to allow the fat to float up above blood and serum.

to be unchanged. If saving fat proves reproducible for all physicians, it would be prudent to harvest enough fat for several treatments.

The syringes are placed needle-end down in a container. The fat floats to the top, leaving an infranatant of saline, blood, and yellow fluid (presumed to be fatty acids from ruptured lipocytes) (Fig 7–32). This mixture is pushed out of the needle by depressing the plunger, leaving only the fat. If the fat is bloody, Ringer's lactate is drawn into the syringe, agitated gently, and discarded after allowing the fat to float to the top. Sometimes several washings are necessary to adequately clean the fat.

For implantation, the needle is changed to whatever size is desired; we sometimes use the same 13-gauge needle, or will change to a 16- or 18-gauge. The patient is positioned so that the areas to be treated are best presented. This maneuver is lost on patients who are heavily sedated or anesthetized — a serious drawback to the success of a procedure performed under general or IV sedation. The tip of the needle is inserted through a dilated nick, as in the donor area, if a 13-gauge is used, or simply pushed in if smaller needles are used. The needle is advanced to the distal point of the recipient area (Fig 7–33). The syringe is twisted off the needle

and the opening observed for a moment to be sure the needle is not in a vessel. Or, pull back on the plunger to see if any blood will aspirate. The fat is injected as the needle is withdrawn. It need be withdrawn only back to the entry site but not out of the skin. It can be advanced again to a new location from the same entry site. However, the syringe should be removed after each advancement to check for safe placement. Each area treated should be overcorrected by at least 100%. Within a few days, the swelling will resolve. What is resolved is unknown: edema, fat, or local anesthesia?

When the fat is all in, it can be molded by finger pressure (Fig 7–34). Often the operator places a finger in the patient's mouth to provide support for molding with the other hand.

Upon completion, a dressing may help stabilize the graft until the fibrin clots take over. An elastic tape works well for us. We trim it to fit over the entire graft with a rent cut in the center to allow the tape to fit snugly over the implant. However, we do not always use a dressing and the results do not seem that much different.

Postoperative cold to the sites, systemic antibiotics, and no facial movement are all individual physician preferences. There are no data to support such decisions. They require the art of medicine and are an advance defense for medical malpractice.

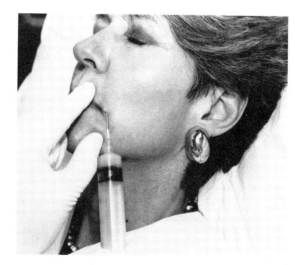

FIG 7–33.
Fat being injected into nasolabial furrow.

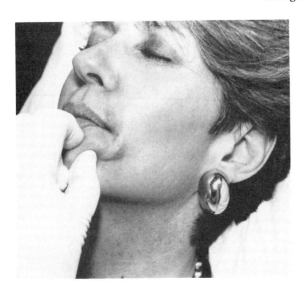

FIG 7–34.
Injected fat being molded.

Longevity

At this writing, the answer for questions about permanence of correction is "sometimes." While some aesthetic corrections are long-term, permanent correction is seen in less than one-half of those we have treated. The result is frequently about 30% to 40% retention of correction or none at all. The evidence for permanency and the acid test for fat-grafting is that the graft will enlarge when the patient gains weight. We have seen this happen, but it is not common. In some patients there is partial correction, and repeated grafts gradually fill in and seem to last. In others, each graft fails and then a subsequent one takes completely.

Indications

The reasons for fat grafting are threefold: (1) to correct contour defects secondary to subcutaneous atrophy from common cystic acne (see Chapter 8), permanent steroid atrophy, and the more exotic lipodystrophies (Fig 7–35); (2) to correct defects from traumatic fat atrophy following blunt trauma and overzealous liposuction; and (3) to treat the aesthetic changes in the aging face. The advent of fat-grafting has brought attention to the role of fat in the aging face, as discussed in Chapter 2.

Senile fat atrophy gives the appearance of the entire perioral cosmetic unit receding into the face. The smile lines deepen (Fig 7–36), the skin above the lip puckers, and the vermilion border loses its sharpness (Fig 7–37). The chin appears to recede, the cheeks hollow, and the skin above the brow and at the temple begins to sink. These are all areas where fat grafting and no other cosmetic surgical procedure will correct the true changes of aging. We are all familiar with the failure of face-lifting to restore the subcutaneous volume needed to restore the gentle and subtle contours seen in the three-dimensional face. In fact, the subtle three-dimensional changes affected by fat grafting are often lost in two-dimensional pre- and postoperative photographs.

Fat injections are not for wrinkles. Wrinkled areas can be blown up to where the wrinkles temporarily do not show, but this is the wrong treatment. Instead, a peel or dermabrasion should be used. Neither are fat injections for dermal-defect creases, which are treated so well with dermal fillers. It is elementary: fat injections should replace fat. We have experienced good results when we fill in hollow cheeks and temples (Fig 7–38). Rebuilding the perioral area and the furrows of the inferior portion of the smile line has also seen success. We have also had success with glabellar furrows, atrophic acne scars, atrophic traumatic scars, hemiatrophy and with puffing up lips.

Complications

To date, complications have been gratifyingly few. Bruising at the donor and recipient areas, some transient swelling and some asymmetry which evens out with time are the only problems we have encountered. We are not aware of other more serious problems from other physicians' patients or from what we have read in the literature.

Fibrel

This is an awkward time to write about Fibrel. The controlled clinical studies that were submitted as the application to the FDA have been shared at professional meetings and sub-

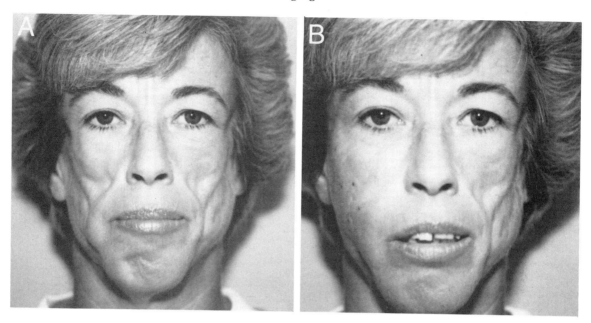

FIG 7–35.
A, woman, 41 years old, with lipodystrophy. **B**, after two treatments to one side only to more clearly define percentage of graft survival over time. (From Glogau RG: Perspectives: Microlipoinjection. *Arch Dermatol* 1988; 124:1340–1343 Used with permission.)

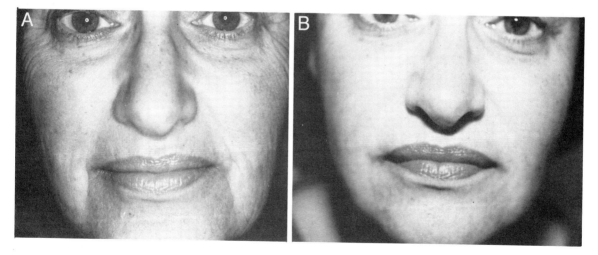

FIG 7–36.
A, woman, 47 years old, with deep meilolabial and perioral folds and furrows before fat grafting. **B**, 10 months after third session of fat grafting. (From Glogau RG: Perspectives: Microlipoinjection. *Arch Dermatol* 1988; 124:1340–1343. Used with permission.)

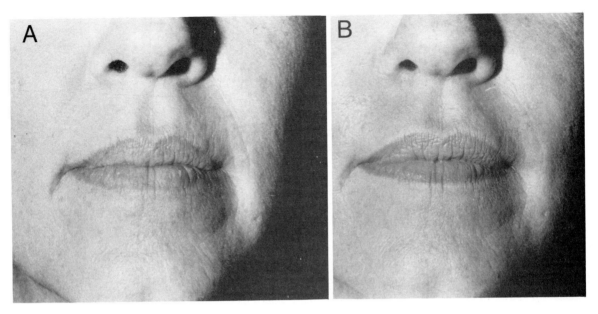

FIG 7–37.
A, woman, 52 years old, with rather flat upper lip. **B,** 12 months after treatment with one session of fat grafting. (From Glogau RG: Perspectives: Microlipoinjection. *Arch Dermatol* 1988; 124:1340–1343. Used with permission.)

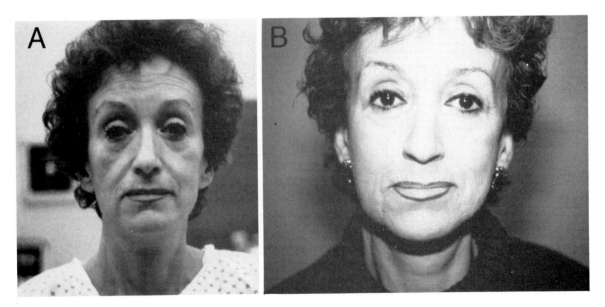

FIG 7–38.
A, woman, 47 years old, who has lost fat from the cheeks. **B,** 1 month after microlipoinjection.

sequently reported in the trade newsletters and cited in one multicenter study.[65] Careful attention to patient selection and protocol, plus the enthusiasm generated by participation in a formal study, often will bias both physician and patient. Often, the phase IV or open clinical use of a drug or device is the time when the "real" information is generated. Fibrel was approved by the FDA in 1988. Several months passed as Serono Laboratories, Inc., moved into production and began providing initial information to physicians. Consequently, in early 1989, our experience with the product is limited and there has not been adequate time for the trends of success and the scope of problems to be elucidated.

History

In 1944, Bailey and Ingraham published the results of their use of fibrin from pooled plasma as a hemostatic agent in surgery.[66] Spangler originated using fibrin to treat depressed scars.[67] He first published his early results in 1957 and by 1975 had accumulated more than 7,000 cases which, he reported, had good results 80% of the time.[68] Spangler's work imprinted the term "fibrin foam" in the literature. He would pull the foam that accumulated at the top of a tube in which blood was drawn and separate it into serum and cells. This foam is high in fibrin products. His complete technique was never published nor available commercially.

One of Dr. Spangler's residents, Sheldon Gottlieb, furthered the technique by formalizing it.[69] He called it the GAP repair technique because its recipe was a mixture of *g*elatin powder, *a*minocaproic acid, and *p*lasma from the patient; this was injected under scars. In a poster exhibit he reported 50% improvement in 75% of the 44 depressed scars he treated.

Serono Laboratories, Inc, lyophilized the gelatin and aminocaproic acid which was then mixed with the fibrin moiety from the patient's serum. This is the product approved by the FDA and now marketed by the Mentor Corporation in Santa Barbara, California, which bought the rights from Serono in 1989.

Implant Dynamics

When Fibrel is injected, a certain amount of tissue injury takes place. The recommended technique is to induce injury with a special cutting needle, a 20-gauge needle, and a zigzag pattern of needle placement. There is a release of clotting factors into the wound, which stimulates the clot. With time, the clot is organized and fibroblasts enter the area, eventually laying down new collagen. When Fibrel is injected, the physical injury plus the injected patient's own fibrin in the serum set up a clot around the gelatin matrix. The aminocaproic acid has antifibrinolytic action which stabilizes the clot. The ingrowth of fibroblasts is theoretically enhanced by the stabilized clot. Thus, the clinical improvement for depressed scars is theoretically twofold, resulting from the bulk of the implant and the localized fibroblast-rich clot. Studies with animals report that the implant becomes a sponge-like mass in the dermis and subcutaneous spaces. There is invasion of granulocytes and macrophages as well as fibroblasts. Eventually the gelatin sponge is replaced with new collagen and neovascularization.

The Product

Fibrel is sold in a sterile kit that has a long shelf-life at room temperature and contains everything needed for the treatment. A syringe in the kit contains the lyophilized mixture of 100 mg absorbable gelatin powder and 125 mg of epsilon-aminocaproic acid; these are reconstituted with 0.5 ml of the patient's serum and 0.5 ml of 0.9% normal saline. The syringe with the gelatin mixture is connected by a special adapter to the saline/serum syringe and the two are slowly mixed by making 10 to 12 passes of the solution from one syringe to the other. The Fibrel is then ready for injection. Once made up, it cannot be stored.

Many physicians experienced with the product do not use the needle or the syringe provided in the kit. A 27-gauge needle seems to be the most popular — a 30-gauge is too small — and a 3-ml disposable syringe will fit onto the adapter provided.

A skin test is made by diluting 0.05 ml of the Fibrel suspension 1:1000 with saline. The skin test is mandated by the FDA.

The gelatin in Fibrel is porcine. It will be interesting to follow the incidence of allergy to this product after it is used in several hundred thousand patients. All mammalian collagen is similar, and allergy to bovine collagen may occur in as much as 3% of the population, as learned from the Zyderm collagen experience. Several patients who are allergic to Zyderm collagen, however, have been treated with Fibrel without any untoward effects.

Treatment Technique

Four weeks before treatment, the skin test must be placed on the volar forearm. A positive reaction would be induration and erythema that persists longer than 24 to 48 hours. Late-onset findings are more suspicious of a positive test than immediate redness and swelling. The data presented to the FDA contained a positive skin test rate of 1.8% for a study population of 337 patients.

The technique is markedly different from that used for Zyderm collagen or silicone. Tissue wounding is helpful, and significant tissue reaction is part of the process. Consequently, a specially designed 20-gauge needle and cutting instrument is part of the kit. A pocket is created in the deep dermis or subcutaneous area under the depressed scar or furrow. The pocket is filled with the implant, and overcorrection of 50% to 100% is recommended. When treating shallower lines or soft, distensible scars, the pocket is less necessary, although the tissue-generated clotting factors enhance the implant reaction. Some physicians do not always create a pocket or make the wound, but rather inject Fibrel under the scar as they do with Zyderm collagen.

There are several different needle techniques. Multiple puncture, as used with Zyderm collagen, is the least used here because Fibrel is a less frequent treatment for shallow lines or creases. Creating a pocket and filling it is the most common technique because Fibrel is best for depressed scars. In the zigzag technique, the needle is threaded in an S track just under a linear scar. Once the mixture is injected, considerable molding to place it just below the scar or furrow is accomplished with finger pressure and massage from the surface. One or two treat-ment sessions are all that are necessary for most scars.

Fibrel injections are painful. Few patients can tolerate them without local anesthesia. The area is infiltrated circumferentially to the scar so as not to distort the scar, although this is not too critical because a large pocket is created below the scar and enough implant is injected to greatly overcorrect. A marked red/blue/violaceous area develops around the implant and the edema and discolorations last for 24 to 48 hours and even up to two weeks. This swelling is significant and one of the largest drawbacks to using this product.

Results

Clearly, the early experience with Fibrel suggests that its best use is for depressed scars. The clinical data submitted to the FDA was for scarring, and the initial investigators at 22 centers treated scars almost exclusively.[65] The number of scars that responded is similar to the data from Spangler's original work with fibrin foam. Approximately 50% of the scars were 65% improved.[70] What is important, however, is the longevity of correction: 85% of the reported patients maintained correction for one year, and new data released by the FDA since the product was approved show that 79% retained some correction for up to two years.[71] The experience with lines and furrows is so limited that longevity statistics are not available, but the impression is that the correction longevity will be shorter than for scars.[70] A small study of 264 rhytids on 100 patients has been submitted to the FDA.

Adverse Responses

Erythema, swelling, and nodules at the treatment site are the most common reactions. Only the nodules persist for more than one month and may be related to too high placement of the implant. The nodules are dusky red and in a few cases have left hyperpigmentation. They are unsightly and present a problem cosmetically. For treating scars, most patients consider this an acceptable trade-off, but for lines and creases, several weeks of red lumps diminish the value of the treatment.

Several cases of slough have been reported when Fibrel was used in the glabella area. This is probably the same phenomenon induced by Zyderm collagen. Too much agent leads to an ischemia and necrosis in that area.

The only systemic reactions reported were nausea, fainting, and headache, which probably represent usual responses to any study that must record *every* complaint from patients in the study.[72] True allergy develops in slightly less than 2% of the population. Whether the population that is allergic to Fibrel will be entirely different from the population that is allergic to Zyderm collagen remains to be seen. It would be helpful if the two populations did not cross, but both products use mammalian collagen.

At this time, it is fair to say that treatment morbidity from Fibrel is considerable. Patients and physicians need to be aware that postinjection swelling and discolorations are significant and not at all comparable to Zyderm collagen injections, which are quick and inconspicuous, although shorter-lasting in the treatment of scars.

References

1. Mcpherson JM, Wallace DG, Piez KA: Development and biochemical characterization of injectable collagen. *J Dermatol Surg Oncol* 1988; 14(suppl 1):7:13–20.
2. Mcpherson JM, Sawamura S, Armstrong R: An examination of the biological response to injectable, glutaraldehyde cross-linked collagen implants. *J Biomed Material Res* 1986; 20:93–107.
3. Mcpherson JM, Sawamura SJ, Conti A: Preparation of {³H} collagen for studies of the biological fate of xenogenic collagen implants *in vivo. J Invest Dermatol* 1985; 86:673–677.
4. Bailin PL, Bailin MD: Collagen implantation: Clinical applications and lesion selection. *J Dermatol Surg Oncol* 1988; 14(suppl 1):7:21–26.
5. Stegman SJ, Chu S, Bensch K, et al: A light and electron microscopic evaluation of Zyderm collagen and Zyplast implants in aging human facial skin. *Arch Dermatol* 1987; 123:1644–1649.
6. Stegman SJ: Zyderm, in Roenigk RK, Roenigk HH (eds): *Dermatologic Surgery*. New York, Marcel Dekker, 1988.
7. McCoy JP, Schade WJ, Seigle RJ, et al: Characterization of the humoral immune response to bovine collagen implants. *Arch Dermatol* 1985; 121:990.
8. Delustro F, Mackinnon V, Swanson NA: Immunology of injectable collagen in human subjects. *J Dermatol Surg Oncol* 1988; (suppl 1):7:49–55.
9. Cooperman LS, Michaeli D: The immunogenicity of injectable collagen II: A retrospective review of 72 tested and treated patients. *J Am Acad Dermatol* 1984; 10:647.
10. Cooperman LS, Mackinnon V, Bechler G, et al: Injectable collagen: A 6-year clinical investigation. *Aesth Plast Surg* 1985; 9:145–152.
11. Elson ML: Clinical assessment of Zyplast implant: A year of experience for soft tissue contour corection. *J Am Acad Dermatol* 1988; 18:707–713.
12. Bailin PL, Bailin MD: Correction of depressed scars following Mohs' surgery: The role of collagen implantation. *J Dermatol Surg Oncol* 1982; 8:845–849.
13. Millard RD, et al: A challenge to the undefeated nasolabial folds. *Plast Reconstr Surg* 1987; 37–46.
14. Cucin RL, Barek D: Complications of injectable collagen implants. *Plast Reconstr Surg* 1983; 71:731.
15. Croften BE, Delustro FA, Koretz MM, et al: Report on the clinical evaluation of glutaraldehyde cross-linked collagen (Keragen®) implant treatment of heloma. Durum and heloma molle. *J Foot Surg* 1985; 25:427–435.
16. Stegman SJ, Chu S, Armstrong RC: Adverse reactions to bovine collagen implant: Clinical and histologic features. *J Dermatol Surg Oncol* 1988; 14(suppl 1): 39–49.
17. Barr RJ, Stegman SJ: Delayed skin test reaction to injectable collagen implant (Zyderm). *J Am Acad Dermatol* 1984; 10:652–658.
18. Kligman AM, Armstrong RC: Histologic response to intradermal Zyderm and Zyplast (gluteraldehyde cross-linked) collagen in humans. *J Dermatol Surg Oncol* 1986; 12:351–357.
19. Kligman AM: Histologic responses to collagen implants in human volunteers: Comparison to Zyderm collagen with Zyplast implant. *J Dermatol Surg Oncol* 1988; 14(suppl 1):35–38.
20. Swanson NA, Stoner JG, Siegle RJ, et al: Treatment site reactions to Zyderm collagen implantation. *J Dermatol Surg Oncol* 1983; 9:377–380.
21. Brooks N: A foreign body granuloma produced by an injectable collagen implant at a test site. *J Dermatol Surg Oncol* 1982; 8:111–114.
22. Barr RJ, Long FD, McDonald RM: Necrobiotic granulomas associated with bovine collagen test site injections. *J Am Acad Dermatol* 1982; 6:867–869.
23. Stegman SJ, Chu S, Bensch K, et al: A light and electron microscopic evaluation of Zyderm collagen and Zyplast implants in aging human facial skin. *Arch Dermatol* 1987; 123:1644–1649.
24. Ellingsworth LR, DeLustro F, Brennan JE, et al: The human immune response to reconstituted bovine collagen. *J Immunol* 1986; 136:877–882.
25. McCoy JP, Schade WJ, Siegle RJ, et al: Characterization of the human immune response to bovine collagen implants. *Arch Dermatol* 1985; 121:990–994.
26. Cooperman LS, Mackinnon V, Bechler G, et al: Injectable collagen: A six-year clinical investigation. *Aesth Plast Surg* 1985; 9:145–153.
27. McCoy JP Jr, Schade W, Siegle RJ, et al: Immune responses to bovine collagen implants. *J Am Acad Dermatol* 1987; 16:955–960.
28. Shpall S: Zyplast collagen implant: Safety update (letter). 1988.
29. Menander KB: Zyplast collagen: Treatment suggestions (letter). 1987.
30. Cucin RL, Barek D: Complications of injectable

collagen implants. *Plast Reconstr Surg* 1983; 71:731.

31. DeLustro F, Fries J, Kang A, et al: Immunity to injectable collagen and autoimmune disease: A summary of current understanding. *J Dermatol Surg Oncol* 1988; 14:(suppl 1):57–65.

32. Rees TD, Ballantyne DL, Hawthorns GA: Silicone fluid research. *Plast Reconst Surg* 1970; 46:50–56.

33. Ashley FL, Braley S, Rees TD, et al: The present status of silicone fluid in soft tissue augmentation. *Plast Reconst Surg* 1967; 39:411–419.

34. Ballantyne DL, Rees TD, Seidman I: Silicone fluid: Response to massive subcutaneous injections of dimethylpolysiloxane fluid in animals. *Plast Reconstr Surg* 1965; 36:330–338.

35. Goulian D: Current status of liquid injectable silicone. *Aesth Plast Surg* 1978; 2:247–250.

36. Orentreich D, Orentreich N: Injectable fluid silicone, Roenigk RK, Roenigk HH (eds): in *Dermatologic Surgery*. New York, Marcel Dekker, Inc, 1988.

37. Webster RC, Fuleihan NS, Hamdan US, et al: Injectable silicone: report of 17,000 facial treatments since 1962. *Am J Cosmetic Surg* 1986; 3:41–44.

38. Duffy D: Silicone: A critical review, in Callen JK (ed): *Advances in Dermatology*, vol 5. Chicago, Year Book Medical Publishers, 1989.

39. Aronsohn RB: Reconstruction observation on the use of silicone in the face. *Arch Otolaryngol* 1966; 82:191–194.

40. Balkin SW: Plantar keratoses: Treatment by injectable silicone. Report of an eight-year experience. *Clin Orthop* 1972; 87:235–247.

41. Webster RC, Hamdan US, Gaunt JM, et al: Rhinoplastic revisions with injectable silicone. *Arch Otolaryngol Head Neck Surg* 1986; 112:269–276.

42. Selmanowitz VJ, Orentreich N: Medical grade fluid silicone. *J Dermatol Surg Oncol* 1977; 3:597–611.

43. Rees TD, Platt J, Ballantyne DL: An investigation of cutaneous response to dimethylsiloxane (silicone liquid) in animals and humans — a preliminary report. *Plast Reconst Surg* 1965; 35:131–139.

44. Piera H: Scleroderma after silicone augmentation mammoplasty. *JAMA* 1988; 260:236–238.

45. Brozena SJ, Fenske NA, Cruse W, et al: Human adjuvant disease following augmentation mammoplasty. *Arch Dermatol* 1988; 124:1383–1386.

46. Nightingale SL: Safety considerations with silicone breast prostheses. From the food and drug administration. *JAMA* 1989; 261:350.

47. Sergott TJ, Limoli JP, Baldwin CM Jr, et al: Human adjuvant disease, possible autoimmune disease after silicone implantation: A review of the literature, case studies, and speculation for the future. *Plast Reconst Surg* 1986; 78:104–114.

48. Newman J, Ftaiha Z: The biographical history of fat transplant surgery. *Am J Cosmetic Surg* 1987; 4:85–88.

49. Neuber F: Fettransplantation. *Chir Kongr Verhandl Deutsch Gesellsch Chir* 1893; 22:66.

50. Stevenson TW: Free fat grafts to the face. *Plast Reconstr Surg* 1949; 4:458.

51. Peer LA: *Transplantation of Tissues, Transplantation of fat.* Baltimore, Williams & Wilkins, 1959.

52. Saunders MC: Survival of autologous fat grafts in humans and mice. *Connect Tissue Res* 1981; 8:85.

53. Ellenbrogen R: Free autogenous pearl fat grafts in face — a preliminary report of a rediscovered technique. *Ann Plast Surg* 1986; 16:179.

54. Fournier PF: Microlipoextraction et microlipoinjection. *Rev Chir Est Lang Franc* 1985, no. 41, tome X.

55. Agris J: Autologous fat transplantation: A 3-year study. *Am J Cosmetic Surg* 1987; 4:2.

56. Illouz YG: De l'utilization de la graisse aspiree pour combler les defects cutans. *Rev Chir Esth Lang Franc* 1984; no. 40, tome X.

57. Newman J: Preliminary report on "fat recycling:" Liposuction fat transfer implants for facial defects. *Amer J Cosmet Surg* 1986; 3:2.

58. Illouz YG: The fat cell "graft": A new technique to fill depressions. *Plast Reconstr Surg* 1986; 78:122–123.

59. Glogau RG: Microlipoinjection: Autologous fat grafting. Perspectives. *Arch Dermatol* 1988; 124:1340–1343.

60. Campbell GL, Laudenslager N, Newman J: The effect of mechanical stress on adipocyte morphology and metabolism. *Am J Cosmetic Surg* 1987; 4:89–94.

61. Smith U: Human adipose tissue in culture studies — on the metabolic effects of insulin. *Diabetologia* 1976; 12:137.

62. Solomon SS: Comparative studies of antilipolytic effect of insulin and adenosine in the perfused isolated fat cell. *Horm Metab Res* 1980; 12:601.

63. Asken S: Autologous fat transplantation, Roenigk RK, Roenigk HH (eds): in *Dermatologic Surgery*. New York, Marcel Dekker, 1988.

64. Morrow D: Personal communication with S.I.S. 1988.

65. Treatment of depressed cutaneous scars with gelatin matrix implant: A Multicenter study. *J Am Acad Dermatol* 1987; 16:1155–1162.

66. Bailey OT, Ingraham FD: Chemical, clinical and immunological studies on the products of human plasma fractionation. XXI. The use of fibrin foam as a hemostatic agent in neurosurgery. *J. Clin Invest* 1944; 23:591–596.

67. Spangler AS: New treatment for pitted scars. *Arch Dermatol* 1957; 76:708–711.

68. Spangler AS: Treatment of depressed scars with fibrin foam — seventeen years of experience. *J Dermatol Surg Oncol* 1975; 1:65–69.

69. Gottlieb S: GAP repair technique. Poster exhibit. Annual meeting of the Am Acad Dermatology, Dallas, TX, December 1977.

70. Cohen IS: Fibrel, in Roenigk RK, Roenigk HH (eds), *Dermatologic Surgery: Principles and Practice.* New York, Marcel Dekker, Inc. 1988.

71. McGee E: Fibrel: A new gelatin matrix implant. *Cosmetic Dermatology.* Nov/Dec 1988.

72. Rosen T: Fibrel, a new implant material. *J Am Acad Dermatol* 1987; 16:155–162.

Eight

Surgical Management of Acne Scarring

The two primary methods for treating acne scars are discussed in Chapter 5, on dermabrasion, and in Chapter 7, on filling agents. This discussion elaborates on "cold steel" techniques used for some types of acne scars. When approaching the acne-scarred patient, inspect the scars both from a distance and close up. From a distance, two aspects should be discerned: the predominant type of scar present, and the scars that are the worst cosmetic liabilities. If the scars are mostly shallow craters, dermabrasion is indicated; if there are two or three deep tunnels with epithelialized bridges, some surgical revision is necessary first.

Close-up examination reveals the exact characteristic of each scar so the best method of treatment can be selected. Soft and depressed scars call for a filling agent; fibrotic and deep scars require excision of some type; deep, ice-pick lesions are best managed by punch replacement. Quite often, acne-scarred patients require more than one type of treatment. Develop a whole program and first discuss it with the patient. Working through that program may require numerous visits over several months.

Excision and Unroofing

Cutting out acne scars is something most of us have tried because it seems so obvious, but most of us have been disappointed with the results. The most meticulous technique and most

diligent postoperative care still do not render satisfactory improvement. Before cutting out a scar, remember that not all patients develop scars after acne lesions, and not all lesions scar. There was something that originally induced the scar formation at that site. Perhaps that factor(s) is still present. A large majority of patients who scar the worst from acne have thick, sebaceous skin and the glands remain active. Incisions in this type of skin invariably heal with ugly scars. Scars from the attempted repair or removal of acne scars are so often themselves unsightly that the technique should be undertaken only when the scars are very bad.

We excise lesions when there are cutaneous bridges, when there are draining cysts or tunnels that do not respond to medical management, or when there are protruding fibrotic masses (Fig 8–1). We have stopped almost entirely trying to excise small defects less than 3 mm in diameter. For years, we tried to do tiny ellipses with #11 blades and 6/0 suture, only to be rewarded with months of healing time and worse scars.

Some of the patients with the worst scars benefit simply from the removal of cutaneous bridges. Sebum and debris collect in the tunnels and become odoriferous and unsightly. A flat scar is preferable. Large, fibrotic scars have not been replaced by really acceptable scars no matter which method we have tried. Geometric broken-line excisions, simple fusiform excisions, or multiple Zs all end up with thick, or spread, but

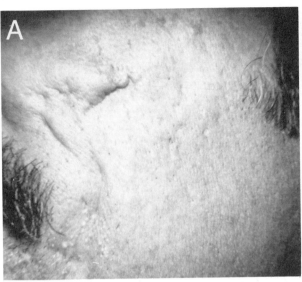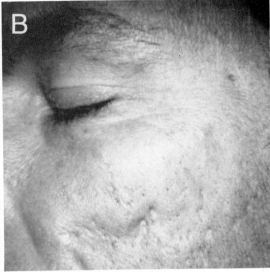

FIG 8–1.

A, man, 32 years old, with thick, sebaceous skin and an active acne cyst that has a skin bridge on the medial upper cheek. **B,** 3 months after the cyst was excised and closed primarily and some of the skin bridge was shaved off; the results are typical, with improvement but residual scars and bridges.

clearly visible scars. These new scars are worth the effort only if the original scar was large enough and protuberant.

Despite a lack of scientific basis for our preference, we have developed an opinion about the best time to perform these excisions. We used to excise or plane a lesion and wait 3 months before doing a dermabrasion. Now we do both procedures at the same time, and believe the healing and final scar are much more favorable (Fig 8–2). First, the tunnels are unroofed with a #15 blade, small cysts are ellipsed, and fibrotic scars shaved. The dermabrasion is undertaken in the usual manner. Then the incisions are sutured. Healing seems faster and the scars seem better when they are accomplished simultaneously.

Punch-Excision, Elevation, and Transplantation

Ice-pick scars that are moderate to deep in depth are problematic whether they are isolated, few, or many. Dermabrasion does not remove the deeper ones and filling agents do not work because of the narrow, fibrotic walls. The only good treatment is to punch them out. The size and appearance of the base of the scar determine whether to punch-excise, elevate, or transplant.

Punch-Excision

Punch-excision, followed by healing by second intention, is useful if the scars are very small — less than 2 mm in diameter. A few isolated or multiple lesions can be punched out and simply allowed to heal. The resulting small white scar is preferable to the light and makeup-catching ice-pick depression. This practice is even more satisfying when a dermabrasion follows immediately. Healing is faster, the patient has only one operation to contend with, and our opinion is that the final appearance is better. This is useful when there is a myriad of these small scars on heavy skin or on skin with a thick beard. We tend to use punch transplants when the skin is thin or smooth and when there are fewer lesions.

Punch Elevation

The punch-elevation procedure requires the visible base of the scar to be of good quality; smooth, normal-colored, and not fibrotic. Also, the scar must be straight-walled. If the diameter of the base is smaller than the diameter of the ostium, the base will not be large enough to fill the opening.[1] The punches must be the thin-walled, straight type. The technique is simple: choose a punch that has the same diameter as the scar, including the base; punch or cut out the skin at the base of the scar and extend the cut deeply enough into the subcutaneous tissues to allow the plug to float free; then gently squeeze and manipulate the plug upward until it is flush with the surface. Several processes anchor it in place: use of tapes, such as Steri-Strips, pressure until the fibrin clot forms, or sutures across the plug in a figure-of-eight pattern.

We do not commonly use this procedure. Only a few scars meet the criteria, and this procedure is more cumbersome than either of the other two methods. It is adaptable to treating scars larger than 3 mm in diameter if a round, circumferential scar is preferable to the original acne scar itself. If the skin at the base is of good quality, flat-based, depressed scars four to six mm wide can be punched and elevated and sutured in place. We do this if the fillers will not work and if the patient understands that the scar will be even with the surface but that there will be a round, circumferential scar.

Punch Transplantation

This is the mainstay of treatment for deep, ice-pick scars. It is most satisfactory for scars smaller than 3 mm in diameter. Although large scars — up to 5 mm — can be punched out and the grafts will take, there is a visible scar which needs to be a worthy trade-off.[2, 3]

If the patient has only a few ice-pick scars to treat, the scheme is used without other treatment. If there are many ice-pick scars and other types of scars which could benefit from a dermabrasion, the two procedures are scheduled sequentially with a minimum of 6 weeks between. Actually 3 to 6 months is ideal, but often patients do not want to wait that long between operations. It is challenging to try to decide whether the punches should be done followed by a dermabrasion, or if a dermabrasion should be undertaken followed by punch transplants for those ice-pick scars that did not abrade away. We do it both ways, trying to assess how many

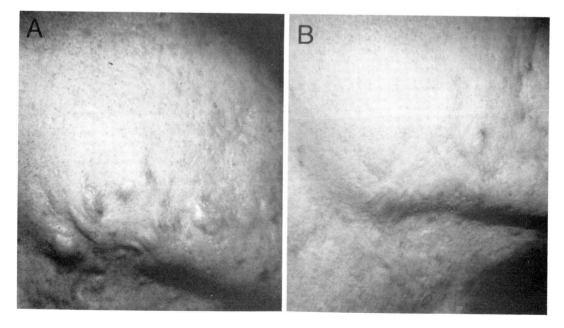

FIG 8–2.
A, man, 22 years old, with fibrotic, elevated acne scars and some skin bridges. B, 1 year after treatment that included unroofing the bridges, scalpel shaving of the fibrotic scars, and dermabrasion, all performed at the same time.

Surgical Management of Acne Scarring

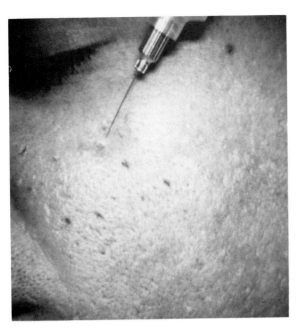

FIG 8–3.
Ice-pick scars, marked with gentian violet, being anesthetized before treatment.

scars will come out with the sanding. If our judgment is that most scars will, we do the dermabrasion first, advising the patient that a few punches may be necessary later. If we believe that not many ice-pick scars will come out with the abrasion, we do one or two sets of punch transplants first, and follow with abrasion. There is no reason why transplants cannot be inserted before and after an abrasion. It is interesting how the viewing eye works: when the deepest and most noticeable scars are eliminated, the lesser scars become more obvious. We always warn patients of this possibility.

After cleansing the face and the postauricular areas, mark the lesions to be treated. As with so many cosmetic procedures, we mark with the patient seated and watching in the mirror. Ask the patient which scars are the most bothersome and mark those first. Remember, success is on two levels: the real, total, aesthetic improvement, and the patient's perception of improvement. Also, patients only see their faces from the front. You need to remind them of other scarring that can be treated.

Local anesthesia with epinephrine is injected under each scar and behind the ear(s) (Fig

8–3). It is wise to wait 15 to 20 minutes after injection to allow the anesthetic to absorb so the scar is not distorted and to permit the epinephrine effect to engage. We mark each scar by pushing the tip of a gentian violet pen into it and twirling it. Just before we punch out a scar, we wipe it with alcohol, which reduces the amount of ink and cleanses the area again. If the scars are not well marked, bleeding, sponging gauzes, and developing interstitial edema all make it difficult to determine which scars were scheduled for treatment.

Donor sites are the postauricular sulcus, the posterior pinna—superior or inferior—the postauricular mastoid area, and the posterior lobe. Look at the skin on each of those areas for match in thickness, color, and texture, and lack of scars or active acne. The chosen skin should be a little thick, with some subcutaneous fat. Several areas may be needed for large numbers of grafts, and both ears can be used. Most often we harvest a row or two of plants from the sulcus. When these sites heal, they contract into a single-line scar right in the sulcus, which is minimally apparent.

The punches range from 1.0 to 3.5 mm in 0.5 mm increments, and are of thin-walled, internal-bevel, straight-cylinder design. They should be sharp. Each scar is punched out with a punch large enough to encompass the whole base and lateral walls of the scar. Leaving part of a scar wall or part of the base not only does not lead to the best cosmetic result, but also predisposes for inclusion cyst formation and wider scar formation at the periphery of the graft.

The punch is held over the scar perfectly perpendicular to the skin surface and pushed and twisted in without any lateral stretching of the skin (Fig 8–4). If while holding the skin taut lateral pressure is exerted, the round punch will cut an elliptical opening that will be impossible to duplicate on the donor site behind the ear. These plugs are lifted out with Bishop-Harmon or Graefe fixation forceps and discarded (Fig 8–5). Hold pressure for a few minutes while a clot forms. If many scars are being treated and they are of various sizes, record how many of each size have been taken.

The transplants are harvested. They are cut with a punch 0.5 mm larger in diameter using

Surgical Management of Acne Scarring

the same perpendicular motion and without any lateral pressure on the skin so the plants will be round and not elliptical. The plants are picked up with a small forceps and transferred to a petri dish that contains cool saline and a gauze square. Again, if there are several different-sized plants, some method of segregating them is necessary (Fig 8–6). We pick up the plug and stretch the tail of fat, holding it in place. We try to keep the fat on the plant and transplant it as well. The fat tail stuffs into the recipient site, acting as an anchor for the plug, and also fills in some of the space created by the scar removal. Because it is such a small graft, the take rate, even of the composite of fat and skin, is exceedingly high. The donor sites are treated with a chemical cauterant such as Monsel's solution. Or, just hold pressure.

Because some patients' donors contract or the recipient holes gape, it is a good idea to check a donor or two before cutting the entire crop. The plants are worked into the recipient openings. It is tedious, but experience speeds the process. After they are planted, a moistened cotton-tipped applicator helps tease them into the best position (Fig 8–7). Strange as it sounds, there is a best position for each plant. Push, twist, tease, hold until it pops into the right axis.

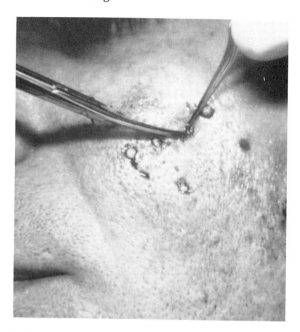

FIG 8–5.
The punched scars are lifted out and the fat tail is trimmed.

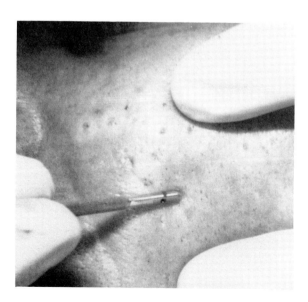

FIG 8–4.
Scars being punched out; the skin is held steady but not stretched so the excision will be perfectly round.

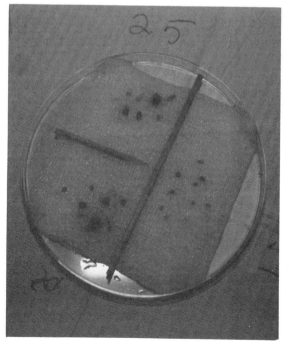

FIG 8–6.
The donor plugs are segregated by size, placed on gauze in a petri dish, and soaked with cool normal saline.

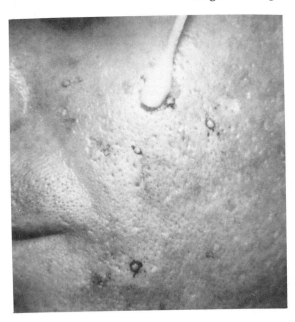

FIG 8–7.
A moist cotton-tipped applicator is used to tease the plugs into place.

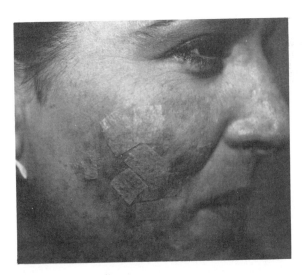

FIG 8–8.
The plugs are taped in place with paper tape; the tape is secured with medical skin glue.

Pressure with the patient's or assistant's hand for 3 to 5 minutes seats the plugs well. A stitch is seldom needed. After policing the area, the plugs are taped with Steri-Strips after first applying benzoin or a glue such as Dow Hypoallergenic Skin Adhesive (Dow Chemical, Chi-

cago, Illinois) or Mastisol (Ferndale Laboratories, Ferndale, Michigan) (Fig 8–8). Patients are advised not to eat food requiring heavy chewing, to laugh, or to engage in excessive facial movement for the first 24 hours. We ask patients to keep their faces dry, not because the moisture makes any difference, but so they will not manipulate the plants.

Patients are seen again after 5 to 7 days for tape removal. Acetone, hydrogen peroxide, or an adhesive remover such as Detachol (Ferndale Laboratories) on a cotton-tipped applicator are maneuvered to carefully lift off the tapes. The grafts look like red papules and go on through the healing phase of crust, edema, induration, contracture, and maturity. It takes three to six months for a graft to fully mature. During the contraction phase, grafts often mound up and become dome-shaped (Fig 8–9). There is no reason the tops cannot be burned off with an electrodesiccator or planed off with a dermabrader. A scar forms at the periphery of the graft, but when the whole transplant is smaller than 3 mm it is much less visible than the dark hole of an ice-pick scar.

The best areas for punch transplants are on the cheeks (Fig 8–10, A and B). The chin is a far

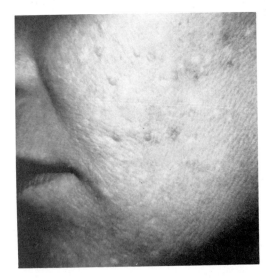

FIG 8–9.
The punch transplants 6 weeks postimplantation. Some have begun to develop a dome shape, which may settle with time, or may be burned off with the electrodesiccator.

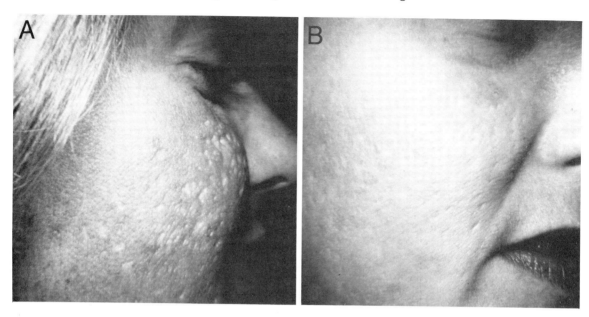

FIG 8–10.
A, woman, 28 years old, with severe ice-pick acne scarring on the cheeks. B, 6 months after two sessions of punch transplants and a full-face dermabrasion.

second and the cutaneous upper lip a distant third for punch survival and improved cosmesis. Tiny punches — 1 to 1.5 mm — are workable on the nose, but if the skin is very sebaceous, the poor tissue match diminishes the value of the effort.

This discussion has been limited to ice-pick scars smaller than 3 mm in diameter. The punch transplant procedure can also be used to fill in larger and more irregular depressed scars (Fig 8–11). The results are variable but in combination with a dermabrasion or as part of multiple procedures to improve the overall appearance, the fill-ins, although not perfect, can help.

Complications

There are few problems, and when the size of the graft is less than 3 mm, those problems are relatively minimal.

Fall-Out

Grafts fall out about 5% of the time; they are a composite graft which is not sutured in place. Facial movement is probably the most common reason for fall-out, and the areas around the mouth are, understandably, where it happens most. If the patient returns in a day or two, we just put in a fresh plant. If the recipient hole has been open for several days, we freshen the hole and replant.

Scarring

Occasionally the scar around the edge of the graft becomes widened and is more apparent than desired. Time helps — 6 to 12 months — and if a dermabrasion is scheduled, it will soften the demarcation line.

Hyperpigmentation

The grafts may hyperpigment or hypopigment. There is not much to do to prevent or treat either event. Because the graft is small, both changes are unnoticeable, and for such a small area, makeup is quite sufficient.

Depressed Graft

Actual sinking of the graft or scar contraction may cause this. If the graft sinks enough to again be a cosmetic problem, it can be replanted with a slightly larger plant.

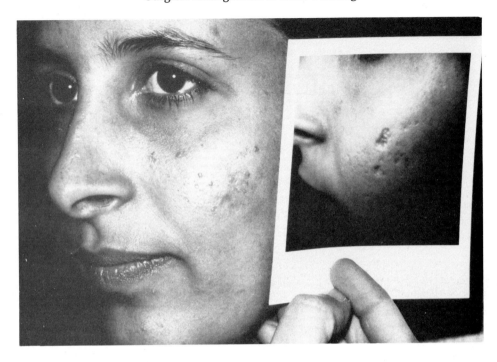

FIG 8–11.
Woman with deep scars larger than 3 mm in diameter on the cheek, shown in the photograph *(right)* held by the patient. Her cheek is shown 3 months after excision and primary closure of the larger pits and punch transplantation of the smaller ones.

References

1. Orentreich N, Durr NP: Rehabilitation of acne scarring. *Dermatol Clin* 1983; 1:405–413.
2. Johnson WC, Baker GK: Use of steel pins in hair transplantation. *J Dermatol Surg Oncol* 1977; 3:220–221.
3. Johnson WC: Treatment of pitted scars: Punch transplant technique. *J Dermatol Surg Oncol* 1986; 12:260–265.

Nine

Tattoo Removal

The disclosure by George Schultz, U.S. secretary of state 1981–1988, that he has a tattoo on his derriere did not elevate tattooing to social acceptability. It is still a juvenile means of self-adornment for most, and a cult marking or indication of a distorted self-image for a few. The problem is when the bearer wants the tattoo removed. In addition to whatever pressures induced the patient to come in to talk about removal, there is always some nagging embarrassment. Consequently, the tattoo-removal patient may be difficult to communicate with. Then by the time he or she is informed about the prolonged procedure and healing time, the scar potential, and finally the cost, which is at least 10 times greater than the initial fee, an unhappy person sits before you.

Experience has taught us that we need to collect the fee before we schedule the patient for tattoo removal. Almost more than for most cosmetic procedures, photographs, signed informed consents, and exacting communication about procedure and risks are necessary.

Excision

Excision and primary closure is the single best method for tattoo removal because it consistently removes all of the pigment and exchanges the tattoo for a surgical scar which the patient can ascribe to any chosen cause. It is a one-stage process for all small and medium-sized tattoos, with minimal surgical morbidity. Excision is designed to encompass all or as much of the tattoo as possible and still close primarily. S- and T-shaped designs are perfectly acceptable. The incisions are carried to the subcutaneous plane, with dissection under the tattoo at the same level. Use peripheral undermining as necessary, and standard closure.

If the tattoo is so large that the closure is tight, it may be acceptable to close under tension and accept the spread scar that will ensue (Fig 9–1). The advantage of performing only a single-stage procedure that leaves a "traumatic" scar is paramount. On the extremities, nonabsorbable sutures can be left in for weeks to prevent dehiscence while the scar tissue bridges the gaps and gains strength.

When the tattoo is large or irregularly shaped, staged excisions are indicated. One side, or one-half, or a segment out of the middle is removed and closed primarily. Some 6 to 12 months later, the rest is excised. Flap coverage is certainly acceptable if the final appearance is good enough to have been worth the trade-off. Usually the tattoo is not worth trading for a graft, especially on the trunk or extremities where grafts often are not cosmetically wonderful.

Tissue Expansion

This relatively new area of surgery has application for tattoo removal.[1, 2] Expanders placed on one or several sides of a tattoo on the extremities or trunk might provide enough extra

Tattoo Removal

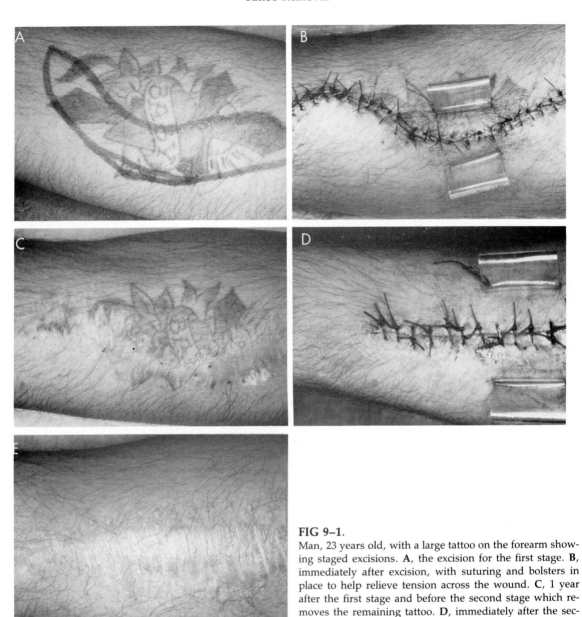

FIG 9–1.
Man, 23 years old, with a large tattoo on the forearm showing staged excisions. **A**, the excision for the first stage. **B**, immediately after excision, with suturing and bolsters in place to help relieve tension across the wound. **C**, 1 year after the first stage and before the second stage which removes the remaining tattoo. **D**, immediately after the second-stage removal. **E**, 1 year after the second and complete removal.

tissue within 6 to 8 weeks to remove the tattoo and close primarily.[3] Although the incidence of complications such as infection, skin necrosis, and bag extrusion is fairly high with expansion, placing an expander under the healthy and normal skin around a tattoo of an otherwise well patient should be accompanied with a low rate of trouble. Also, the inconvenience and unsightliness of the expanders is minimized on the ex-

tremities, where they can be covered with clothes.

Good results have been reported on the trunk and upper extremities with expansion, but the leg has an almost unacceptably high rate of serious problems.[4] The results of many research studies are just now appearing in the literature. It appears that the result of expansion is to slightly thin the dermis and slightly thicken the epidermis, which are not contraindications for tattoo removal.[5]

The problems with expansion and the time and equipment required lead to high cost. As mentioned above, so many tattoo-removal patients are miffed at the cost of a simple excision that the added $300 to $500 for the expander, the additional six to ten office visits, and the cost of the initial instillation will certainly limit the number of patients who choose this procedure.

Intraoperative Expansion

Even newer and possibly more in tune with the needs of the dermatologic surgeon is intraoperative expansion. We have experimented with this technique and our very preliminary results are exciting. While the wound is open during removal of the tattoo, expanders are slipped under the skin on one or several sides. We have been using Foley catheters with 30 ml and 75 ml bags after cutting off the distal tip of the catheter. The bags are inflated until the skin is tight but not white for ten minutes; then the fluid is let out for five minutes. Inflating to blanching means that the pressure against the skin is greater than the arterial pressure.

The inflation/deflation is repeated three or four times. This varies with the anatomic area. The back and shoulders expand easily and quickly, the forearm more slowly. We gain about 15% to 30% more skin from all sides for our closure. This extra skin is often enough to remove all of the tattoo in one step and to effect closures that are under less tension and thus cause less scar spreading (Fig 9–2).

Dermabrasion

All of the methods other than excision involve partial removal of the pigment, followed by some manipulation to induce further or complete pigment extrusion. If a tattoo was professionally applied, the pigments are placed consistently in the dermis. Nonprofessional, self-administered, prison, or traumatic tattoos have pigment from the high dermis to the subcutaneous fat. Clearly the latter type are harder to remove without inducing serious scarring, and excision might be best.

The tattoo is cleansed and anesthetized with lidocaine. One of the spray refrigerants is also adequate anesthesia, but the frost, blood, and tissue debris make visualization of the abrasion depth more difficult. If the hair is thick, it should be shaved carefully. Use the instrument you are most comfortable with. We use the diamond fraise, but those facile with the wire brush may prefer it. The critical factor is not speed of abrasion but controlled *superficial* wounding.[6] As the epidermis comes off, the tattoo will actually brighten. Abrade to the level of pinpoint bleeding, or the upper dermis. Hemostasis is accomplished with a chemical cauterant such as 30% aluminum chloride in alcohol.

It is tempting to "sand that whole tattoo out of there." This is just the thing not to do. Dermabrasion is most commonly performed on the face, where the wounds to the level of the reticular dermis seem to heal without scarring. On the trunk and extremities, the whole dermis is much thicker or composed mostly of compacted collagen fibers. Wounding into this collagen leaves scars.

Wire-brush abrasion is more practical on the face for nonprofessional and traumatic tattoos. Both have pigment irregularly spread through the skin and the experienced wire-brush derm-

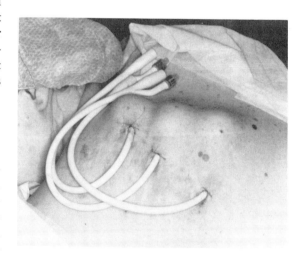

FIG 9–2.
Intraoperative tissue expansion. Three Foley catheters are pictured, inserted over the scapula with bags inflated. Expanded tissue will permit primary closure of large lesion in that area.

abrader can go after little bits and pieces of pigment on the face without inducing scarring.

Several recipes have been developed to induce additional pigment spitting without deeper wounding. The first is to simply paint gentian violet over the abrasion and cover it with a light dressing such as Telfa. Then have the patient scrub the wound vigorously daily with soap and water, which delays healing and seems to cause more of the pigments to "spit" onto the dressing. We have seen Telfa dressings come off with an impregnated mirror image of the entire tattoo.

Another plan is to lightly dermabrade and cover the wound with a tannic acid mixture (two parts tannic acid, one part glycerin, one part distilled water). The area is lightly dermabraded a second time, making a slurry of the tannic acid mixture and the debris of the abrasion. Silver nitrate sticks are rubbed over the area until a thick, rubbery crust is formed. When this separates some weeks later, a great deal of the pigment is included with the crust.

An additional technique to combine with superficial dermabrasion is to scissor-excise small but deep collections of pigment.[7] Particularly when the tattoo is nonprofessional, traumatic, or small, pick up small pockets of tissue containing pigment with small-toothed forceps and cut them out with Gradle or iris scissors. These tiny wounds may or may not scar — there is a much less chance of scarring when the procedure is done in conjunction with dermabrasion.

Laser

A wound of controlled depth is just what lasers can deliver. They are tried on tattoos and produced acceptable results.[8, 9] The argon and carbon dioxide lasers were compared and found to give similar results for tattoos.[10] Originally, the laser operators traced around the tattoo and removed the pigment but ended up with a wound, then a scar, that looked like the bird or snake they were removing. With experience, the laser wound included surrounding skin and was made into a patch that camouflaged the shape of the tattoo (Figs 9–3 and 9–4).

The same problems that accompanied the superficial wounding techniques followed treatment with the laser: ghosting, scarring, irregular results, pigmentary problems, and of course a few spectacular complete removals without scarring. As was true of all physicians treating tattoos, the laser doctors soon found themselves treating the developing hypertrophic scars with intralesional and topical steroids. The laser approach also required several sessions to treat the whole tattoo.

In the early 1980s combined techniques were developed for use with the laser.[6] After 3.0 to 4.0 W argon laser exposure of 0.5 seconds, the area is cleansed with 100% acetone. It is then covered with 40% to 50% urea in petrolatum base and tightly covered with Elastoplast tape. The assumption is that the urea slows healing and causes more pigment to be expelled. This dressing is left in place for a week. Ruiz-Esparze and colleagues published a variation of this procedure; they used 50% urea in petrolatum after treatment with a defocused CO_2 laser with a continuous output of 10 to 15 W.[11, 12] The wound was lightly covered with gauze. The dressing was changed daily with reapplication of the urea ointment until the wound was completely healed, as early as five days or as long as two weeks.

Salabrasion

This technique may have begun in antiquity with a Greek physician named Aëtius in 50 A.D.[13] Or it may have been learned from the natives of the South Pacific islands. There was a paper in the German medical literature in 1935 about salabrasion.[14] In the 1970s in the U.S. there was a resurgence of interest in the technique and papers with histologic evidence demonstrated good results with the technique.[15–17]

The tattoo can be anesthetized with lidocaine but the hypertonic salt solution of the abrasion will numb the skin adequately. Ordinary table salt works well; some physicians prefer rock salt. Some sort of firm handle is needed — wooden door knobs have been used — to wrap gauze squares around. The apparatus is dipped into tap water and then into the salt. The tattoo is held taut and abraded with the salt. The rubbing must continue through the various layers of skin from glistening to light pink, to bright

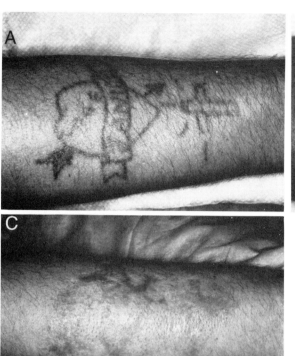

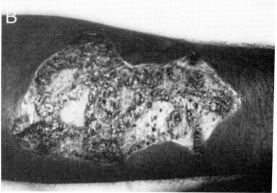

FIG 9–3.
A, professional tattoo on forearm. **B**, immediately after argon laser treatment. **C**, 3 months later, with still more fading expected. (Courtesy of Roy Grekin, M.D.)

red. It is necessary for the whole tattoo to have the bright red appearance. It takes a long time to achieve this goal, which is the limiting step for most practitioners. This method was more popular in the military, where corpsmen took up the rubbing, or in training institutions, where the residents did the job. The salt is rinsed off and the area dressed. Again, wound stimulation with gentian violet and Telfa is a required part of the procedure.

The results have been spectacular in some hands[18] but there have also been the expected complications of scarring, pigmentary irregularities, and irregular results, with ghosts of the tattoo still present.

Scarification

The folklore of the American Indians tells of some tribes that made multiple small, linear, superficial incisions in the skin over a tattoo. Goat's milk was applied and the area bandaged with a cloth. The pigment would be drawn into the eschar. Prisoners have made multiple scars over tattoos to remove them with some success. In 1888, Variot described a similar method of using linear skin incisions, scratches, or punctures over tattoos for removal.[19]

In recent times, David Duffy, M.D., tried concentrations of TCA 50% to 90% with poor results. He scarred the patient but only partially removed the tattoo. He also tried to remove tattoos with multiple punch-excisions made with 1- or 2-mm punches traced along the tattoo lines. This too resulted in unacceptable scarring and incomplete removal of the pigment.[20]

Miscellaneous

The infrared coagulator has been tried on many different cutaneous lesions. Its two basic components are a power transformer and a handpiece. An electronic timer in the transformer monitors the exposure time within a range

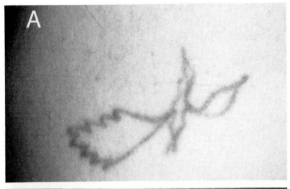

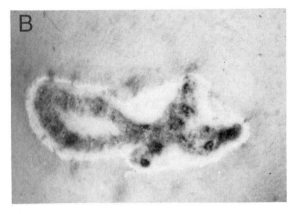

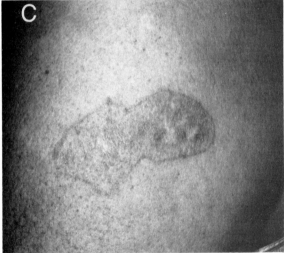

FIG 9–4.
A, nonprofessional tattoo on the shoulder. **B**, immediately after treatment with argon laser. **C**, 6 months posttreatment with good resolution and healing. (Courtesy of Roy Grekin, M.D.)

of 0.25 to 3.0 seconds. A tungsten halogen lamp centered in a gold-coated reflector delivers the infrared light through a quartz tip. Essentially, the light is so focused and strong that it destroys the skin lesions by heat.

Results of using the infrared coagulator for destroying tattoos were compared with those of a carbon dioxide laser.[21] The infrared coagulator had the advantage of more rapid healing time while giving similar cosmetic results, but the CO_2 laser removed all the pigment in a single treatment.

References

1. Radovan C: Tissue expansion in soft-tissue reconstruction. *Plast Reconstr Surg* 1984; 74:482–486.
2. Argenta LC, Marks MW, Pasyk KA: Advances in tissue expansion. *Clin Plast Surg* 1985; 12:159.
3. Hallock GG: Refinement of the radial forearm flap donor site using skin expansion. *Plast Reconstr Surg* 1988; 81:21–25.
4. Manders EK, Oaks TE, Au VK, et al: Soft-tissue expansion in the lower extremities. *Plast Reconstr Surg* 1988; 81:208–217.
5. Johnson PE, Kernahan DA, Bauer BS: Dermal and epidermal response to soft-tissue expansion in the pig. *Plast Reconstr Surg* 1988; 81:390–395.
6. Clabaugh W: Removal of tattoos by superficial dermabrasion. *Arch Dermatol* 1968; 98:515–521.
7. Robinson JK: Tattoo removal. *J Dermatol Surg Oncol* 1985; 11:14–16.
8. Goldman L, et al: Laser treatment of tattoos: A preliminary survey of three years' clinical experience. *JAMA* 1967; 201:841–844.

9. Goldman L: Effects of new laser systems on the skin. *Arch Dermatol* 1973; 108:385–390.

10. Apfelberg DB, Maser MR, Lash H: Argon laser treatment of cutaneous vascular abnormalities: progress report. *Ann Plast Surg* 1978; 1:14–18.

11. Dismukes DE: The "chemo-laser" technique for the treatment of decorative tattoos: A more complete dye-removal procedure. *Lasers Surg Med* 1986; 6:59–61.

12. Ruiz-Esparze J, Goldman MP, Fitzpatrick RE: Tattoo removal with minimal scarring: The chemo-laser technique. *J Dermatol Surg Oncol* 1988; 14:1372–1376.

13. Berchon E: *Historie Medicale du Tatouage.* J B Bailliere et Fils, Paris, 1869.

14. Klöekorn GH: Eine einfache methode der entfernung von tätowierunger. *Dermatol Wochenschr* 1978; 101:1271–1275.

15. Manchester GH: Tattoo removal: A new simple technique. *Calif Med* 1973; 118:10–12.

16. Crittenden FM Jr: Salabrasion — removal of tattoos by superficial abrasion with table salt. *Cutis* 1971; 7:295–300.

17. Koerber WA Jr, Price NM: Salabrasion of tattoos. A correlation of the clinical and histological results. *Arch Dermatol* 1978; 114:884–888.

18. Price N: Salabrasion. *J Dermatol Surg Oncol* 1979; 5:905.

19. Variot G: Nouveau procede de destruction des tatouages *C. R. Soc Biol* 1888; 8:836–838.

20. Duffy D: Personal communication, 1987.

21. Groot DW, Arlette JP, Johnston PA: Comparison of the infrared coagulator and the carbon dioxide laser in the removal of decorative tattoos. *J Am Acad Dermatol* 1986; 15:518–522.

Ten

Treatment of Keloids

It is crucial to differentiate between a true keloid and hypertrophic scar. The prognosis for a hypertrophic scar, even without treatment, is fair to quite good. The prognosis for a keloid, however, even with treatment, is guarded. A hypertrophic scar indicates a physiologic response to injury and certain genetically determined events during healing; the keloid is a manifestation of inherited collagen metabolic variations. Keloids are rare and hypertrophic scars are common.

From a practical standpoint, patients must not be told they have a keloid when indeed they have a hypertrophic scar. A history of keloid formation puts all future doctors on guard and warns them that this patient does not heal normally. Most of the time it was *not* a true keloid and the patient does not form keloids. The physician must go ahead and take the risk that the past event was at most a hypertrophic scar. If the patient is told that he or she has a tendency to form keloids (when this is not the case) the doctor may escape blame for an unsightly scar, but all doctors in the future must either not operate on the patient or take the risk of having the patient say that any less than a perfect result is the doctor's fault because "I told you I formed keloids."

The best differentiation clinically is still the simplest: if the lesion grows beyond the peripheral boundaries of the original wound, it is a keloid. If it is hypertrophic or elevated but within the same boundaries as the initial wound, it is a hypertrophic scar. Keloids develop on the up-per back, chest, shoulders, jaw, and earlobes. Pain is more often associated with true keloids but itching is found with either. Keloids are more common on younger people, especially dark-skinned individuals, for example blacks and Hispanics. Keloids arise from trauma, but in teenagers who are undergoing a rapid growth phase, medical conditions like acne and virus scars also incite keloid growth.

Hypertrophic scars demonstrate a rapid growth phase in the first 3 to 5 months after the inciting trauma, then plateau, and become smaller over the next 6 to 12 months. They arise in people of all ages but less often in patients over 60 years old. They are predictable on the back and other areas where the skin is thick and frequently stretched. The incidence is higher when the wound closure is poorly designed and there is tension across the wound edges, or when an infection develops that interferes with regular healing. A salutory response to intralesional steroids does not differentiate the two lesions, but recurrence typically implies a keloidal process.

Composition

The development of a keloid, a hypertrophic scar, and a normal scar are somewhat similar.[1] One difference is in the growth potential of fibroplasia, both in the amount of tissue formed and in the time it takes to develop. Numerous enzymes have activity that is higher in keloids than in hypertrophic scars. One of these enzymes is proline hydroxylase.[2] Collagen synthesis is markedly elevated in keloids and only slightly elevated in hypertrophic scars, compared to normal scars.[3] Whether this is the function of overproduction or underdissolution is not clearly worked out in the literature.[4] It is clear that there is a great increase in fibroblastic activity,[5] and that activity correlates with the rapid growth of the lesion and the pain and itching that develop.[3]

The failure of normal collagen breakdown as a mechanism is further supported by the clinical dissolution of the lesion when treated with IL steroids. The steroids may remove collagenase and/or protease inhibitors, thereby allowing activation of the collagenase with subsequent breakdown and resorption of the excessive collagen.[6]

Treatment and Management

The management of keloids is an ongoing program. Some treatments with surgery or radiation combined with intralesional steroids may "cure" keloids, but usually do not. Once a keloid is flattened, the patient is painstakingly advised that it may regrow at any time. This may occur in a year or two, or in only a few months. In at least 50% of keloids, particularly on the chest or shoulders, pain and/or itching is problematic. Patients become accustomed to the appearance of the growth, but the discomfort will bring them in for treatment. Fortunately, the symptoms respond quickly to treatment.

Intralesional Corticosteroids

For those keloids that develop on the face, the trunk, and the extremities, and that are small to moderate in size, intralesional steroids are the best treatment. Patients are advised that there is a good chance the growth will become larger if surgery is attempted. For a new lesion which may be a hypertrophic scar, intralesional steroids are suggested because they are the best way to manage that as well.

Triamcinolone acetonide has become the mainstay for intralesional injections.[7–12] It has a longevity of 3 weeks and if there is systemic absorption, 40 to 60 mg given every 4 to 6 weeks is not dangerous. There is some systemic absorption, but it happens slowly over 4 to 6 weeks. Triamcinolone hexacetonide (Aristospan) has been tried in the past, but too many patients retained the crystals for months to years; some crystals had to be excised. The starting dose is a clinical judgment. It is prudent to begin with 10 mg/ml and to assess the response in 2 to 4 weeks. However, most true keloids are resistant to that low dose, so the starting dose may as well be 20 to 30 mg/ml. We do not start with 40 mg/ml, but have worked up to that full dose when the lesions did not respond to lower concentrations and the patient suffered no side effects.

The administration technique varies depending on the pain induced and the firmness of the lesion. Most keloids are firm, almost tense, before treatment (hypertrophic scars are more rubbery) and therefore the first few treatments are difficult and painful. We use a 30-gauge needle on a Luer-Lok syringe and force the medicine into the center of the lesion. If it is resistant, we may have the patient come back in a week, hoping the keloid is softer, and reinject. It has been recommended that the steroid suspension be blasted in with a Dermajet or Madajet.[13] These instruments make it possible to treat some of the tougher lesions and some patients prefer the gun to the needle.

It is probably best after a few treatments, however, when the keloid is softer and the patient's trust has built, to inject through a 30-gauge 1-inch needle. The medicine works more evenly if it is infiltrated throughout all parts of the growth. It is harder to accomplish that with the jet unless the tissue is soft and homogeneous. Also, with 30 or 40 mg/ml triamcinolone, deposits will crystalize out. If the medicine is placed too near the surface of the keloid, it may ulcerate; if the medicine is placed too near the normal skin at the edge, the skin may atrophy.[14]

Freezing the keloid and injecting one day later is another method that can be used to soften it. It is probably only the interstitial edema that separates the tough collagen fibers. This technique is a shorter freeze than using cryosurgery as a treatment modality (see below).

The pain of injection and prolonged postinjection pain are separate but material problems.

Injection pain is worse during the first few treatments, most likely because the lesion is so tough. If, after several treatments, treatment is still painful, anesthetize the entire lesion by putting in a ring block of lidocaine and some below the keloid. Do not try to actually numb the lesion itself. For posttreatment pain, the patient may have to come back the next day for reinjection of the local anesthetic. Seldom does the pain persist for more than two days. Encourage the patient to persevere because the pain lessens with subsequent treatments.

Surgical Excision

Many keloids look like they could just be cut out and done away with. A few can. Most will recur, however, and a substantial number will return larger, more unsightly, and symptomatic. The ones we choose to excise are well-delineated and were caused by a specific event such as a pierced ear or an accident rather than an ongoing or recurrent medical condition or trauma. The technique of excision is standard, with no special instruments or sutures used. The closure is designed to evert the wound edges without tension, and few or no buried sutures are used. We never try to excise keloids on the chest, shoulders, or upper back.

The recommendation for intralesional steroids is less commonly seen in the general and plastic surgery literature. It is actually stated that this treatment does not work, but we know it does and use it for the majority of the cases we see. In that last statement lies the answer to this apparent contradiction. There is a difference in the referral pattern between the specialities; surgeons see the large (>20 sq cm), multiple keloids; dermatologists see the smaller, localized ones. We do not advise trying to treat multiple or large keloids with intralesional steroids and have great empathy for the patients who have them and the doctors who try to treat them.

The unique keloids that form on the pinna are especially disposed to surgical excision (Fig 10–1, A to D). Whatever was the inciting nidus is long gone (e.g., the earring is out) and the keloid is usually too large and fibrous for intralesional steroids. Excision should be designed so the walls of the keloid become a flap for defect repair. If the lesion is excised and a flap or graft is necessary for closure, and if a recurrent or second keloid develops, the situation is worse. Therefore, try to utilize the keloid skin for repair. The large protuberant type of keloid typically shells out as one large, fibrous mass, leaving the skin intact. Design the pattern for excision and the closure to take advantage of the best skin on the lesion. Some areas are atrophic while others are perfectly normal.

Whether or not to make the incision extramarginal or intramarginal is still controversial.[15] For large keloids or linear lesions under stretch, the intramarginal incision has the merit of allowing the closure sutures to be placed in scar tissue. Pulling on scar tissue does not incite further scar spread or induce more keloids. When the keloid is small and isolated, particularly if the lesional skin is discolored or atrophic, extramarginal incisions are superior.

All excision surgery should be combined with further treatment. For the size and type of keloids we treat, that second treatment is intralesional steroids. Begin injections when the sutures are removed, or within the first four weeks postoperatively. Continue injections every six weeks for the first six months. If there is no sign of recurrence, slack off to every three months and then inject as needed. Alert the patient to come in for an injection at the first sign of regrowth or symptoms. Warn patients that they may go two to five years before a keloid appears again.

Depending on its availability, the size of the lesion, and the standard of care in a given country, radiation therapy is combined with surgical excision.[16–18] Using 1.7 mm of aluminum half-value layer, administer a one-time-only dose of 500 to 1,500 roentgens or give three alternate-day doses of 300 to 500 roentgens. Begin the radiation the day after the excision, or at least when the sutures come out. Obviously, appropriate shielding is important and radiation is not recommended on the neck.

Pressure

Pressure garments or dressings help reduce hypertrophic scars.[19] What they do for keloids

Treatment of Keloids

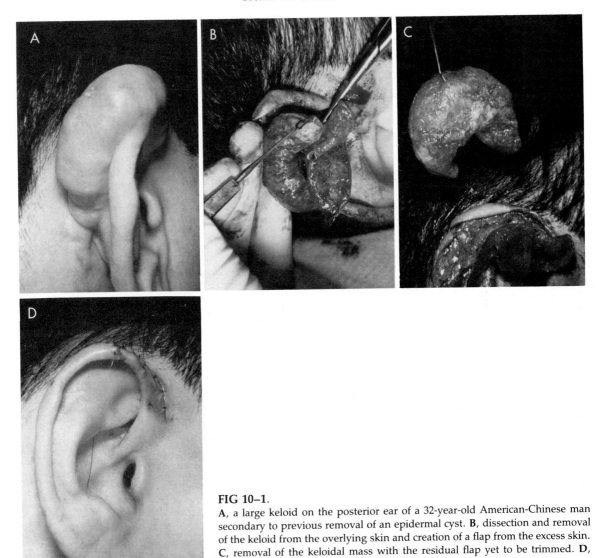

FIG 10–1.
A, a large keloid on the posterior ear of a 32-year-old American-Chinese man secondary to previous removal of an epidermal cyst. **B**, dissection and removal of the keloid from the overlying skin and creation of a flap from the excess skin. **C**, removal of the keloidal mass with the residual flap yet to be trimmed. **D**, final reshaping of the skin over the ear with suture closure.

is questionable.[20] For pressure to be effective, it must be applied firmly for 18 to 20 hours per day for 6 to 12 months. The special pressure garments for this purpose are uncomfortable and hot. Second and third sets are needed for a change and they are expensive, not to mention ugly. Only those patients with terrible scars — with keloids over large areas, such as burn victims — are motivated enough to wear such contraptions.

There are a few clip-on or sew-on devices that may be tenable on the earlobe.[21] They are disguised as clip-on earrings and hold pressure on both sides of the lobe. These are the only devices we recommend for applying pressure.

Cryotherapy

Small, discrete lesions will flatten with one or several moderate freezes.[22] The scar is still present, but flattened. The color may stay the same, or hyperpigment or hypopigment, which is a consideration in dark-skinned people. The patient may or may not need local anesthesia for the treatment. For reasons we do not know, cryotherapy is excellent for postacne scars on the trunk. Perhaps these are a special type of hypertrophic scar. In addition, special instruments have been designed.[23] The ordinary spray instruments or even cotton-tipped applicators all work.

Laser

The CO_2 laser has been used to excise keloids within the margins of the lesion; they are then allowed to heal by second intention.[24] The theory is that the laser reduces the fibroplasia which is thought to be the etiology of the keloid. The early success of the cases treated by laser were tempered when scientifically designed comparative studies showed no superiority of the laser over cold steel surgery.[25]

Miscellaneous

Physicians in Africa who encounter huge and debilitating keloids will excise the lesions and put the patients on methotrexate.[26] It is given intramuscularly 15 to 20 mg every 4 days for 2 weeks before the surgery and 12.5 to 15 mg orally or IM daily for 3 of every 4 weeks for 6 months postoperatively.

Injectable bacterial collagenase has shown promise in an experimental clinical setting.[26, 27] Tretinoin cream 0.05% may help with long-term use.[28] Early and limited studies have been reported with interferon alpha-2b used to prevent keloids in those prone to develop them.[29] In New Zealand, topical application of silicone gel was used to flatten hypertrophic scars and keloids secondary to thermal burns.[30]

References

1. Mancini RE, Quaife JV: Histogenesis of experimentally produced keloids. *J Invest Dermatol* 1962; 38:143–181.
2. Cohen IK, Diegelmann RF, Keiser HR: Collagen metabolism in keloids and hypertrophic scars, in Longacre AC (ed): *The Ultrastructure of Collagen.* Springfield; Charles C. Thomas Publishers, 1976.
3. James WD, Besanceney CD, Odom RB: The ultrastructure of a keloid. *J Am Acad Dermatol* 1980; 3:50–57.
4. Ala-Kokko L, Rintala A, Savolainen ER: Collagen gene expression in keloids: Analysis of collagen metabolism and type I, III, IV, and V procollagen mRNAs in keloid tissue and keloid fibroblast cultures. *J Invest Dermatol* 1987; 89:238–244.
5. Abergel RP, Pissurro D, Meeker CA, et al: Biochemical composition of the connective tissue in keloids and analysis of collagen metabolism in keloid fibroblast cultures. *J Invest Dermatol* 1985; 84:384–390.
6. Diegelmann RF, Bryant CP, Cohen IK: Tissue alpha-globulins in keloid formation. *Plast Reconstr Surg* 1977; 59:418–423.
7. Ketchum LD, Smith J, Robinson DW, et al: Treatment of hypertrophic scars, keloids, and scar contracture by triamcinolone acetonide. *Plast Reconstr Surg* 1966; 38:209–218.
8. Murray JC, Pollack SV, Pinnel SR: Keloids: A review. *J Am Acad Dermatol* 1981; 4:461–470.
9. Kiil JC: Keloids treated with topical injections of triamcinolone acetonide: Immediate and long-term results. *Scand J Plast Reconstr Surg* 1977; 11:169–172.
10. Maguire HC: Treatment of keloids with triamcinolone acetonide injected intralesionally. *JAMA* 1965; 192:325–327.
11. Griffith BH, Monroe CW, McKinney P: A follow-up study on the treatment of keloids with triamcinolone acetonide. *Plast Reconstr Surg* 1970; 46:145–150.
12. Griffith BH: Treatment of keloids with triamcinolone acetonide. *Plast Reconstr Surg* 1966; 38:202–207.
13. Vallis CP: Intralesional injection of keloids and hypertrophic scars with the Dermojet. *Plast Reconstr Surg* 1967; 40:255–262.
14. Jemec GBE: Linear atrophy following intralesional steroid injections. *J Dermatol Surg Oncol* 1988; 14:88–90.
15. Engrav LH, Gottlieb JR, Millar SP, et al: A comparison of intramarginal and extramarginal excision of hypertrophic burn scars. *Plast Reconstr Surg* 1987; 81:40–45.
16. Ollstein RN, Siegel HW, Gillooley JF, et al: Treatment of keloids by combined surgical excision and immediate postoperative X-ray therapy. *Ann Plast Surg* 1981; 7:281–285.
17. Levy DS, Salter MM, Roth RE: Postoperative irradiation in the prevention of keloids. *Am J Roentgenol* 1976; 127:509–510.
18. Malaker K, Ellis R, Paine CH: Keloid scars: A new method of treatment combining surgery with interstitial radiotherapy. *Clin Radiol* 1976; 27:179–183.
19. Kischer CW: Pressure treatment of hypertrophic scars. *J Trauma* 1975; 15:205–208.

20. Bremt B: The role of pressure therapy in management of ear lobe keloids: Preliminary report of a controlled study. *Ann Plast Surg* 1978; 1:579–581.

21. Kischer CW, Shetlar CL, Shetlar MR: Alteration of hypertrophic scars induced by mechanical pressure. *Arch Dermatol* 1975; 111:60–64.

22. Sheperd JP, Dawber RPR: The response of keloid scars to cryosurgery. *Plast Reconstr Surg* 1982; 70:677–681.

23. Meltzer L: A cryoprobe for the therapy of linear keloid. *J Dermatol Surg* 1983; 9:111–112.

24. Onwukwe MF: Treating keloids by surgery and methotrexate. *Arch Dermatol* 1980; 116:158.

25. Greenberg S, Krull EA, Watnick K: Comparison of CO_2 laser and electrosurgery in the treatment of rhinophyma. *J Am Acad Dermatol* 1988; 18:363–368.

26. Bailin PL, Ruiz-Esparza J: The CO_2 laser treatment of keloids. *J Dermatol Surg Oncol*

27. Pinnell SR: Injectable bacterial collagenase appears promising for keloids. Presented at American Academy of Dermatology annual meeting, San Antonio, Texas, 1987.

28. Panabiere-Castaings MH: Tretinoin seems effective drug for keloids. *J Dermatol Surg Oncol* 1988; 14:1275–1276.

29. Berman B: Interferon alpha-2b promising for keloid prevention, treatment. *Skin and Allergy News*, May 1989.

30. Mustoe T, Ahn ST, Monafo W: Silicone gel appears inexplicably to flatten, lighten hypertrophic scars from burns. *JAMA* 1989; 261:2600.

Eleven

Blepharoplasty and Brow-lift

Blepharoplasty

More and more dermatologists are being trained in blepharoplasty. It is a rewarding operation that is entirely appropriate for office surgery. There are many patients whose only cosmetic surgery need is for a blepharoplasty, and the rapport they have with the dermatologist may make them more comfortable having that person improve the appearance of their eyes.

Blepharoplasty is not an easy surgery, even for the experienced. All physician skills are called into play for this operation. A working knowledge of basic and specific anatomy of the eyelids and periocular structures is essential; regular practice of basic dermatologic surgical techniques and specific, detailed understanding of this operation and its variations are requisite. Blepharoplasty, more than any other procedure described in this text, requires careful attention to every detail, beginning with the consultation and continuing through the examination, preoperative planning, anesthesia, surgery, and follow-up.

Several medical specialists perform blepharoplasty: ophthalmologists, ophthalmoplastics, otolaryngologists, dermatologists, and general plastic surgeons. There is a great deal to learn from the viewpoint of each of these specialists. Try to read the relevant literature on this subject in each speciality. About twice a year a trip to the medical library to review each speciality's journals will expose you to what is up-to-date in blepharoplasty. For a review, attend a blepharoplasty course given by a speciality different from your own. It is exciting to see well-guarded icons in one discipline thoroughly trashed by another discipline. More important, cross-speciality exposure stimulates careful inspection of current surgical practices and often induces growth and better understanding.

Preoperative Evaluation

Preoperative evaluation (Table 11–1) is undertaken twice, first and most extensively during the initial consultation, and then again on the day of surgery. At first glance, obviously redundant skin and puffy eyelids are easily detected. But sometimes the pathology is subtle — something the patient has recognized and which prompted the visit. While you and the patient exchange pleasantries and rapport-building is under way, watch the patient for asymmetries, for differences in eye, eyelid, and brow movement, for tight squinting, for scleral show, and lid irregularities. Several anatomic structures contribute to the appearance of the upper third of the face. Just which ones need a correction must be discovered or you and everyone else will wonder what went wrong.

TABLE 11–1.
Preoperative Evaluation

Surgical need
History
Physical examination
   Symmetry
   Brow location
   Lid redundancy
   Fat herniation
   Tear adequacy
   Lower-lid extropion
   Skin quality
Ophthalmologic examination
Photographs
Instructions

History

Any medical history of thyroid malfunction is important. Swelling of the eyelids from allergies, hormonal variations, or occupational hazards affect the longevity of the outcome. Any problems with the eye, visual or traumatic, or dryness or irritation should be fully explored. The true or perceived hyperpigmentation of the lid skin must be noted, as discussed in the etiology of wrinkles. The dark coloring may be from pigment or from tissue overhang. Is the crepey skin from sun damage or are the creases from smiling? A blepharoplasty will change either condition little, if at all.

The history of this cosmetic procedure includes the chief complaint: what the patient perceives as his or her problem, and also precisely what the patient sees. It is time for that mirror to come out; all discussion must identify exactly what the patient is talking about by having the patient look into the mirror and point to the real or imagined defect. The patient's observations and your findings must be documented. Do not speak with euphemisms or jargon. Speak clearly about the complications. Use the terms "loss of vision" and "unequalness." Stress that a change in appearance will result.

Physical Examination

For the meticulous physician — and every physician performing blepharoplasty needs to be meticulous — an orderly approach helps keep the task manageable and reduces the chance of missing a finding. Start at the top and work down. Marked asymmetry of the forehead lines signifies uneven movement of the brows, which may be a nerve deficit or just an expression trait. Nevertheless, you and the patient must analyze why the unevenness occurs.

Next, examine the eyebrows for evenness and location, which should be just over the orbital rim. If the brows are low, move them back to the proper position just overlying the bony supraorbital rim and observe how that affects the appearance of the upper lids. If nearly all of the redundant skin disappears, the problem is with the eyebrow and not the eyelid. Much of the time, in our judgment, only a small portion of the problem is brow. However, we read and hear discussions by others about how often a brow-lift is needed in conjunction with a blepharoplasty. If the brow-lift did not have some major drawbacks (see below), we might agree. Also, if there is sagging elsewhere on the face,

repairing a ptotic eyebrow can produce a look that is more surprised than pleasant.

The skin immediately inferior to the brow may be eyelid skin or noneyelid skin. Usually there is noneyelid skin there which in only a few millimeters becomes eyelid skin. The noneyelid skin is thicker and wider over the lateral one-half of the upper lid area. This is a very critical observation because it is best to excise redundant skin only from the thin, soft, eyelid skin and not up into the thicker, noneyelid skin. The suturing together of eyelid skin to noneyelid skin creates a thick, noticeable line.

Examine the upper lid redundancy and try to estimate how much is skin, fat, or skin and fat. Picking up the skin with fingers or forceps will help. If there is a large protrusion laterally, is it a ptotic lacrimal gland? If it is a ptotic gland, repair and fixation should be part of the plan for surgery. If there is irregular attachment of the levator aponeurosis manifest by lid lag or uneven size of the palpebral fissure, note that and show it to the patient in the mirror. Many times it is impossible to modify, and is not a procedure most nonophthalmologists want to perform. Also notice the presence and location of the palpebral fold. It may be low or nonexistent, as in the Oriental eye, or very high in some women. In planning the operation, determine where the new fold will be placed.

Study the excursion of the upper lid. Does it close completely without lagophthalmos? Do both lids blink together? Is there protrusion of the globe? Is there edema around the eye or erythema of the lid skin? Any of these findings may alert the physician to other pathology which it is far better to know about before the surgery.

Try to evaluate the tear function. It used to be easier: do a Schirmer test and discover how well the tears are formed. Nowadays, it is understood that the "dry eye" is much more complex than just the production of the watery component of the tears as measured by the Schirmer. Tears have three layers: water, mucus, and oil. Each comes from a different gland and each affects the dry eye differently. Blepharoplasty probably does not influence these glands as much as it does the slope of the lower lid or the position of the puncta. Shifting the slope of the lower lid margin, which normally tilts downward toward the medial canthus, affects normal tear flow across the eye and into the puncta. Discovering a history of dry eye problems is almost more important than performing a Schirmer test. A relative dry eye does not preclude performing a blepharoplasty, but it means that skin removal from both upper and lower lids should be conservative. The lids must close after surgery. It does help prepare for the postoperative protection of the cornea.

Examination is more complex for lower than for upper lids. Skin redundancy should be assessed, and it should be kept in mind that true excess skin is usually a small part of the problem. Granted, there are some patients with massive skin redundancies — called festooning. For these patients, it is the skin that must be removed and it can be taken from the lid margin edge or in some cases from the cheek margin. Lower lids have two additional common but important features — fat protrusion and laxity of the lower lid margin.

Fat pad herniation is not usually a true herniation of fat through the orbital septum, but a combination of weakness or stretched orbital septum and fat protrusion. (New techniques specifically address this finding.) Note which pockets protrude when the patient is sitting. The pockets may show more if the patient tilts the head slightly forward and gazes upward. Also, gentle finger-pressure on the globe will cause the fat to bulge. The names of the fat pockets is in question. Whether or not there are three or two with multiple lobes becomes academic. Most surgeons talk about two pockets in the upper lid: the middle pocket, which may have a lateral extension, and the medial pocket, which is a white rather than yellow and is more posterior behind the orbital septum. The lower lids have three pockets: lateral, middle, and media, which are all well-defined (in some patients). Clinically, note where the bulges are and plan to remove them during the surgery.

Lower lid laxity is finally getting the attention it deserves. Partially, this is because of new and better operations, but also because of complications of pull-down and scleral show. Now that transconjunctival lower lid lipectomy is widely practiced, a more critical look at the percutaneous lower lid technique is revealing that increased scleral show lateral to the limbus has been far more common than we have wanted to admit.[1, 2] Additionally, a slight outward rotation of the lower lid produced a very subtle "look" stigmatic of having had the eyes "done." The lower-lid laxity is tested by picking it up between the fingers, pulling it out about 3 mm, and letting it snap back. The properly tense lid will snap back; the lax one will ooze back. Also, some older lids will have a slight outward rotation at the margin.

Planning for lower-lid blepharoplasty should incorporate corrections for these problems. The most simple is to do a skin-muscle technique and increase the tension on the lower orbicularis by a suspension stitch. Or, a lid wedge can be performed through skin and muscle or just muscle; the wedge can be at the lateral canthus or on the lateral one-half of the lid. Or, the lipectomy and septum tightening can be approached transconjunctivally, with no risk of further weakening the lid or of creating any downward pull of the lid.

Examine the quality and color of the skin of the lids and the periorbital area. Hyperpigmentation is not going to be corrected but certain shadows may be changed. Sun-damaged skin will not change, and combined or alternative procedures such as peeling can be recommended. The incorporation or removal of some benign lesions should be discussed and planned.

Ophthalmologic Examination

We recommend to nonophthalmologists that blepharoplasty candidates have a complete eye exam. We ask the patients to go to an ophthalmologist and say that they need a preblepharoplasty examination. Or, we write down specifically what information we want: examination of visual acuity, fields, pressure, tear function, slit-lamp of the cornea, and fundoscopy. If the patient is young and having only a minor "tuck," this examination may not be as necessary, but we are more comfortable having it on record. For older patients, it frequently uncovers problems that were not anticipated. For medical insurance to pay for the upper lid surgery, a visual field examination must be on record to prove loss or restriction of upper lateral gaze.

Instructions and Photographs

Many times the decision to proceed and schedule the surgery is not made at the first consultation. If it is, if the patient comes back for a second visit, or if the patient calls back and schedules by phone, a system should be in place with the office staff to insure that the patient has received complete instructions about what will happen on the day of surgery, and immediate and long-term follow-up. This information can be mailed or given directly to the patient.

Whether or not the patient should have had nothing to eat or drink for several hours before surgery is directly related to how much anesthesia is going to be used. We do the procedure under local anesthesia, and an occasional patient is given Demerol and Compazine intramuscularly just before surgery. Therefore, we want the patient to have eaten the appropriate and usual meal on the day of surgery. We advise no alcohol the night before, no aspirin or nonsteroidal anti-inflammatories the week before, and a shower the night before or the morning of surgery. Patients should wear no facial makeup, wear loose-fitting clothing, have arranged for transportation home, and have an adult with them the first night after surgery.

At one of the initial visits a good series of photographs should be taken: frontal, lateral, and oblique of each eye. Depending on each doctor's habits for filing photographs, the pictures may or may not be available on the day of surgery. If they are, a Polaroid copy can easily be made from the original photograph. Even better, a Polaroid snapshot can be taken of the patient sitting up just before any surgical preparations or drugs are given. The pictures can be put up on the wall or a light stand or wherever they can be visible throughout the surgery. The benefit of being able to consult the pictures after the patient is reclining, anesthetized, and halfway through the operation is invaluable.

Anesthesia

Local anesthesia is the principal anesthesia used for all of the techniques of blepharoplasty and brow-lifting. Lidocaine is infiltrated into the skin and fat and drops into the conjunctival space. The physician's choice and routine dictate how much additional medicine the patient receives. This may include preoperative sedatives and analgesics, surgeon-administered or anesthetist-administered, twilight sleep during the first injections of local, even light sleep with the patient able to respond to commands throughout, may be employed. Deep anesthesia is unnecessary.

We use lidocaine 1% with epinephrine 1:100,000 injected directly into the lid where the surgery will be performed. Others use 2% lidocaine, or Marcaine 0.25%. Some like to add hyaluronidase to the cocktail to permit easier spread of the local. For the uppers, we hold gentle pressure over the lid for a minute or two, which seems to reduce the ecchymoses from the needle and speed agent spread. All of the excess volume should be absorbed before starting so that the lid skin is again soft and pliable. Also, the wait should be long enough for the full epinephrine effect to occur, to minimize bleeding.

Once the skin is opened, a few milliliters of agent should be put into the fat pads because the cutaneous infiltration seldom achieves the deeper anesthesia needed for the lipectomy behind the septum. The same is true for the lowers. For reasons we can only surmise, the wound edge closer to the lid margin loses numbness rapidly and often requires a second injection before the closing sutures are made. Because we prefer that the patient not feel any pain after the initial needle sticks, we make it a habit to reinject the inferior wound edge after the lipectomy is completed on each eye. When we begin closure, the site is well numbed.

Techniques for Upper Lids

Marking

We mark the patient before any medications are given, with the patient sitting up and watching in the mirror. Or, the patient should at least look in the mirror when we have completed the marking. Once in a while patients question the marks, which gives us an opportunity to explain further what we plan to do before the operation — far better than *after*. Other doctors will mark patients after they are anesthesized and lying down. Obviously, it does not make a great difference.

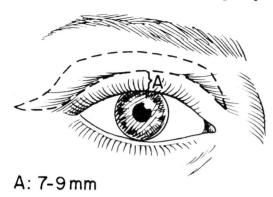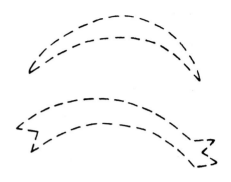

A: 7-9 mm

FIG 11–1.
Upper lid blepharoplasty design variations.

No matter which type of marking pen we use, the movement of the upper lid soon smears the mark. Gentian violet pens now come with a tiny point, which is the best so far. A broken wooden cotton-tipped applicator dipped into brilliant green also works well. Some physicians wait until the anesthesia has taken effect, and mark with shallow scalpel cuts.

Design

Several contingencies impact on the upper-lid design. If a brow-lift (discussed below) is to be included, that surgery should be completed first — before any marking or anesthesia to the lid. If the lower lids are also being operated on, the upper surgery is performed before the lower, although the technique planned for the lower lids affects the design of the uppers. If a skin or skin/muscle technique is planned, an absolute minimum of 8 mm must be left at the lateral canthus between the lateral poles of the incisions. How low the lateral extension of the lower incision is placed, and how far and at what angle it extends out onto the lateral orbital rim in the crow's feet, must take into account the required width of the isthmus of skin between the upper and lower lid surgeries. If a transconjunctival approach is to be used on the lowers, the placement of the upper lateral extension is not critical, nor is it important if there will be no lateral extension past the line of the lateral canthus.

Because many patients have more loose skin on the lateral one-third of the lid, and many have crow's feet they do not want, it is natural to extend the design out onto the lateral orbital rim.

This extension helps reduce lateral hooding, but is not necessary. Adequate tissue is removable within the confines of the lid by performing dog-ear repair techniques or Burow's triangles. Removing the redundant skin over the lateral orbit will temporarily pull out a few radial furrows and creases.

The trade-off is the scar. Incisions and excisions lateral to the lid itself fall in skin that is thicker and has many more adnexa. Consequently, healing is considerably different. The line remains red and thickened for months. The scar may be visible for years, although not always. Eyelid tissue heals with a fine white scar which is naturally hidden in the palpebral fold. The scar that heads across the orbital rim is noticed because it is straight, visible, and different from any of the regular lines in the area.

The placement of the lower edge of the incision is the next decision (Fig 11–1). Measuring it is one way to decide. At the midpupillary line, the distance from the lash line to the lower incision (and the location of the suture line which becomes the all-important palpebral fold) is often around 5 to 7 mm for men and 7 to 9 mm for women. This line may stay at the same distance for the lash line all across the lid, or it may dip closer to the lash line at either the medial or lateral end. The line can be higher on a woman if she desires a large-lidded look and wants to use colored eye makeup below the fold.

Another guide is to place the incision in the natural palpebral fold line if it is there, and in an even and pleasing location. Many times it is not, or only parts of it will be retained. Some surgeons recommend placing the incision at the upper pole of the tarsal plate. Again, that is all right if that line is even and appropriate, but there is no anatomic reason why it should go there. It is doubtful that the line should remain as high as the top of the tarsus in the lateral one-third of the lid, at the lateral canthus, or beyond.

The design at the medial pole of the incision is usually a simple 30-degree corner that begins just superior to the punctum. If there is excessive redundant skin, a small dog-ear or M-repair can be built into the corner. The same is true at the lateral pole if it is to end on the eyelid and not travel out onto the area of the crow's feet.

The upper incision line sweeps up from the medial canthus and is placed to remove just the right amount of skin — obviously a harder line to place. There are several suggestions. With the patient seated, use the nondominant hand to pull up on the eyebrows, thus pulling the excess skin away; mark the lower line; then let the skin fall down to its natural position, where it will bunch up and lie over the proposed inferior line. In your mind's eye, picture that line through the redundant skin and draw the second line right "over" the first. Then again raise the brow, pulling up the lids. The location of the upper line will illustrate the true amount of skin to remove. In most patients, there will be more skin to remove at the lateral half than the medial half.

Another aid is to have used hyaluronidase in the anesthesia so the skin is doughy. Green fixation forceps are designed to gently pick a length of skin so that an estimate of how much to remove can be grasped between the tips. Be careful to observe where the skin changes from eyelid skin. Keep the incisions well within the boundaries of that soft, thin skin, leaving enough superior to the upper line to suture eyelid skin to eyelid skin. We cut the lower line on the line and the upper line just inferior to the line, which builds in a few millimeters of safety. It is always better to go back and take more skin — although it is difficult to get it cut as evenly — than to take too much.

An alternate approach to the upper line is the Silver Segmental Technique.[3, 4] After the lower incision is made, gentle, blunt undermining of the entire upper lid frees the skin in a natural cleavage plane (Fig 11–2). Whatever else

had been planned for the operation, usually lipectomy, is completed. When all is completed and hemostasis has been obtained, the loose, redundant skin is pulled downward over the pretarsal incision. Three vertical marks are made across the lid, essentially dividing it into thirds. A gently curved line is drawn horizontally, just over the site of the pretarsal incision below. Cuts are made with scissors through the skin on the three vertical lines to the level of the horizontal line. These cuts permit a precise look to see if just the right amount of tissue is being removed. If too little, cut the vertical line farther superiorly. If too much, less skin will be sacrificed at that site. This technique avoids the chance of cutting off too much with the en bloc method.

Skin, Muscle, and Fat Removal

Whether the skin is taken out completely or in segments, as described by Silver, it is fairly easy to dissect it up from the underlying stroma and muscle. A slow but gradual surgical trend is toward removing more and more muscle. In the upper lid, an area of muscle 3 to 5 mm wide is removed from the preseptal portion of the orbicularis (Fig 11–3). We have not yet added large amounts of muscle removal to our technique, although those who have believe the removal deepens the palpebral sulcus and sharpens the newly created palpebral fold. We have felt our folds were adequate, and have not really seen a need to change our technique. In the lower lid, we trim any muscle overlying the tar-

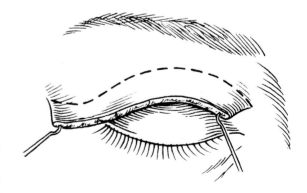

FIG 11–2.
Silver method for upper lid blepharoplasty. The lower incision is made and the redundant skin is pulled down and transected as needed.

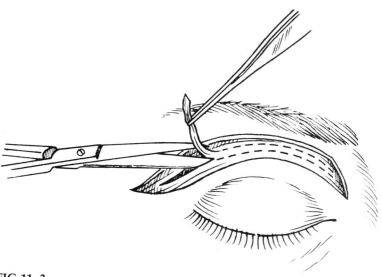

FIG 11–3.
Removal of a strip of preseptal orbicularis oculi muscle. The width of this strip varies.

sus. In some patients there is actual hypertrophy of the pretarsal muscle which produces the "Michelin Tire Man" look. We note this preoperatively and plan to trim. On others, if there is excess muscle when the skin muscle flap is draped over the lid, it is trimmed.[5] We probably trim muscle on at least one-half of our lower lid blepharoplasties.

Some surgeons like to mark and cut the incisions with a scalpel and then use a small blunt-nosed scissors such as a Gradle or Wescott to dissect off the skin. Habit makes it difficult not to use a #15 blade. The #15c is approximately half the size of a regular #15 and is a similar shape. It is supposedly comparable to the #67 Beaver blade but fits a standard scalpel handle.

In our version of the technique, the skin is dissected off and a 2-mm strand of preseptal orbicularis muscle is picked up with Bishop-Harmon or jeweler's forceps and the lateral edge of the wound. A strip 2 mm wide is cut all across the open wound. Through this second layer of exposure the orbital septum can be seen, and with a little manipulation or gentle pressure on the globe, the fat below can be seen as visible or bulging. In some patients with an incontinent septum, runny lobules of fat are found lying just under the muscle.

Before the septum is opened or probed is a good time to stop any bleeders and verify the anatomy. Check at the upper lateral edge of the wound for the lacrimal gland (the orbital lobe of the gland). It can be seen or palpated under the septum, and inferior to the orbital rim if it is ptotic or enlarged. It is firmer than the fat and has a more grayish color. Visually, it is possible to mistake the gland for fat, but if the gland is caught in forceps or desiccated, the feel and response is so different from fat that the error is quickly recognized. Minimal damage to the gland is of almost no consequence; tearing or damage to the ducts from the gland has potential harm because there are only six to eight openings. A markedly ptotic gland should be repaired when it is discovered. A fine, permanent suture is passed through the periosteum of the under surface of the orbital rim as far back as can be reached from the upper lid wound. The suture is then passed through the capsule of the lacrimal gland with one or two turns and tied, with the knot placed as far under the bony orbit as possible.

Another anatomic feature that should be located is the tendon of the superior oblique muscle, which passes from the trochlea on the medial orbital wall to its insertion in the sclera. For a short segment, it lies just above the white upper-lid medial fat pad and is at risk if that pad is not opened carefully or if clamps are not used judiciously. The tendon can be located by placing the little finger pulp just inside the upper medial orbital rim and palpating the trochlea. Then place the little finger horizontally so the lower border rests at the level of the medial canthal tendon. The medial fat pad will lie at the midpulp, and the superior oblique tendon and pulley will lie a few millimeters above the upper border of the finger. It is easy to avoid this tendon if the medial fat pad sac is opened carefully and the fat gently teased or squeezed out and if the instruments are not pushed into the space.

A small vessel is commonly found passing superiorly and medially just under the orbicularis. The vessel lies between the medial margin of the middle fat pocket and the medial pocket. Also, the medial pocket is on a different plane than the middle; it is more posterior. The lateral fat pocket as such is still controversial. Its existence is talked about but the anatomists stress that the middle pocket can extend laterally and that the fat laterally is simply submuscular and not in a pocket.[6]

When removing the strip of muscle, be sure

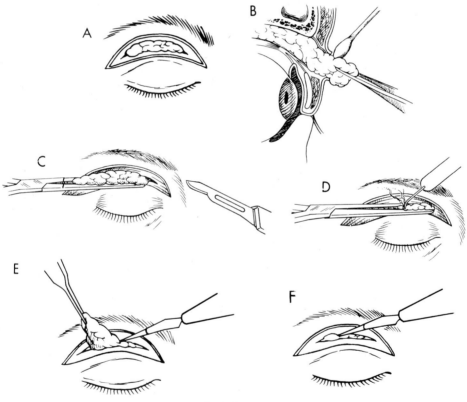

FIG 11–4.
A, the septum is opened; the underlying fat may protrude spontaneously or may need to be gently teased out and trimmed. **B,** teasing the fat out. **C,** the fat can be clamped and cut off. **D,** the fat can also be clamped and electrodesiccated. **E** and **F,** in some cases, the fat can be desiccated only. **G,** the lid is closed with running sutures; some surgeons leave one or both ends of the suture free so it does not bunch up with the lid movement.

it is removed from the upper preseptal section of the orbicularis. Pick up a bit of muscle in toothed forceps and with scissors carefully dissect up and trim off the desired width of muscle. Removal that is too low will expose the levator aponeurosis, a structure of immense importance. Should the levator be exposed near its insertion, it will be more difficult to locate the fat pocket, and the chance of injuring or getting the levator caught in a suture is greater. Injuring or suturing the levator may affect the even and symmetrical excursion of that lid, which produces a significant cosmetic and functional defect.

At this point of the operation, the offending, protuberant and/or herniated orbital fat is treated (Fig 11–4, A to G). Again, there is controversy so diametric that one cries for scientific data to answer the questions. First, should the septum be opened? For years it has been probed and the fat has been pushed out through one or several holes. Seldom has there been any recommendation to close the septum. Henry Baylis, M.D., a very experienced ophthalmoplastic surgeon, suggests that the septum be opened widely for good control over fat trimming and removal, but also to prevent any retrobulbar pressure build-up from hemorrhage or edema. Conversely, recent papers describe treatment of the fat without opening the septum.[7] A Davol electrical muscle stimulation (EMS) 2,000 bipolar diathermy system was used to probe through the septum and cause lipolysis. The advantages mostly relate to less surgical morbidity.

Open treatment of the fat with electrosurgery, however, is becoming much more popular.[8, 9] It was not too long ago that the absolute dogma for trimming the fat involved careful teasing out, clamping, cutting above the clamp, and electrodesiccation of the stump *before* release. It was even advised by some that the fat stump be sutured to completely eliminate any chance of bleeding. Many others must have had the same experience we did: a little lobule of fat would remain, and if we just hit it with a zap of the desiccator or cautery it would vaporize. There seemed to be no untoward effects. This principle has been expanded; the cautery instruments (of choice) work efficiently and safely for fat destruction.

At this time, we open the septum above the middle pocket, carefully pressure the globe to cause fat bulging (if it is not already opened), and with scissors, trim the top off the sac. Once in a while there seems to be more than one sac. When the fat rolls out, we insert scissors to open that space wider. Under direct visualization, the fat is trimmed by design — only what falls out or most of what can be safely cut out if we are trying to make a deep sulcus. This deep sulcus look is usually the wish of the patient. Large lobules of fat are clamped and removed with the desiccator. If vessels are visible, they are clamped and cauterized. Stray bits of fat and small, random lobes are simply hit with the cautery or desiccator. The end point is determined by consulting the preoperative photos, the patient's wishes, and the doctor's judgment. Regardless, gentleness and meticulousness are the keys.

(Throughout this discussion, cautery and desiccation have been used interchangeably. Historically there have been theoretical reasons why bipolar desiccation was considered safer than monopolar desiccation: battery operated cautery was less traumatic than desiccation; this company's product was better than another's, etc. Experience has proven that which electrosurgical unit is used makes little difference. It is the physician's choice.)

The operation is completed to this point on one eye. Anesthesia is touched up particularly along the lower edge of the wound. The eye is covered with a moist gauze and the other eye is operated on to this same point. Then we return to the first eye and inspect for bleeding, missed fat, symmetry — now that we have done the other eye, if there was a great anatomic difference not noticed before surgery, it is investigated with the wounds open.

Closure

The septum and muscle do not need to be closed. The skin seems to heal equally well with interrupted or running sutures — permanent or absorbable. The mild chromic gut sutures dissolve in five to seven days, avoiding the need for removal which may pinch. Not having a specific day when the patient must be rescheduled is a benefit for both patient and doctor. Sometimes the gut only partially dissolves and the patient may call describing "tiny worms" coming out of the suture line. For years we have enjoyed closing with 6/0 Prolene subcuticular running sutures. More recently we have switched to Novafil, which is less stiff. The closure is begun laterally, looped over the surface at the midpoint, brought out at the medial canthus, and taped to the glabella. The loose end allows the thread to move as the lids open and close. This give completely eliminates puckering which so often develops along the closure. The puckering probably does not affect the long-term result, but it looks much smoother during the first few days. Also, removal is simple: the center loop is snipped and each end is pulled out.

Another closure variation is determining whether or not to include levator aponeurosis fixation. Depending on the height and placement of the inferior wound edge incision, the inferior wound edge may not be directly overlying one of four structures: (1) the upper edge of the pretarsal orbicularis; (2) the cut edge of the preseptal orbicularis, depending on how much muscle was removed; (3) the orbital septum, if the placement of the new fold is to be high; or (4) the levator aponeurosis if the placement is just at or slightly superior to the superior edge of the tarsus. Fixation of the skin suture line to any, some, or all of these underlying structures helps deepen and define the new palpebral fold.

There are five situations where this stitch may be indicated:[10] (1) converting an Oriental eye to look more Caucasian; (2) when a patient with a ptotic brow does not want a brow-lift; (3) when there is a pre-existing, very low palpebral fold; (4) when a patient has two lid creases that are not very definite; and (5) when a patient preoperatively has a lid crease so far back and upward beneath the orbital rim that the patient looks gaunt or hollow-eyed.

Clear nylon or Prolene is often used to fix the skin suture line to the aponeurosis with a bite of muscle included. The first stitch is located at the midpupillary line, 2 to 3 mm above the upper edge of the tarsus. (The tarsal border is easily found by gently everting the lid.) The stitch passes through the aponeurosis carefully so as not to penetrate the underlying conjunctiva, then up through muscle and through the inferior edge

of the skin, and tied. Several of these interrupted stitches are evenly distributed along the length of the opening. Then the skin is closed side-to-side in the manner of choice.

No dressings are required. Reinforcing the suture line with Steri-Strips or even closing the entire line with Steri-Strips is acceptable. Cooling the lids with ice or specially designed bags filled with a gel helps reduce swelling and ecchymoses, and also the stinging that occurs as the anesthesia wears off. The ice is applied in the office while the patient recovers. Patients are advised to continue the cooling for 20 minutes of each hour until bedtime. The eyes should remain at rest throughout the remainder of the day, with no television, no reading, and no routine chores.

The lids have a special predilection for developing suture tracts, or epithelialization of the suture pathway through the skin. It is surmised that tract formation is related to the length of time the sutures are left in. Snipping the tops off or lightly desiccating the tiny pseudomilia helps them disappear faster.

Techniques for the Lower Lids

Three techniques will be discussed: skin only, skin and muscle, and transconjunctival. The indications are based on the pathology. Baggy skin by itself calls for skin-only removal, but this is the least common situation. Bulging fat only, the most common situation, is treated with a skin/muscle or a transconjunctival approach. A combination of excess skin and muscle with bulging fat is treated with a skin/muscle technique. Senile ectropion or lid laxity also require a skin/muscle design for simultaneous repair.

The preoperative visits, taking of photographs, and patient preparation discussed above are the same for surgery on the lower lids as they are for the uppers. Anesthesia is different only for the transconjunctival approach, where it is administered from the conjunctival surface. Trying to numb the conjunctiva from the skin side does not work well and is also awkward.

Skin Only

For those few patients with only redundant lower lid skin, an incision is made in the crease, present in half the population, about 2 mm below the lash line. This cut is made with a scalpel or started with a nick laterally and completed with scissors. A stitch with a 3/0 suture is sometimes placed through the midpoint of the lower tarsus, pulled over the forehead, and clamped with something like a hemostat for weight. This stitch pulls up and stabilizes the lower lid for the operation; it is removed when surgery has been completed.

The skin is dissected carefully from the underlying orbicularis under the entire lid, using small, blunt-nosed scissors. Staying in the plane just under the skin and above the muscle reduces hemorrhage. In patients with thin skin, buttonholing is possible. When the undermining is completed, secure the bleeders with cautery or electrodesiccation and proceed to the same place on the other eye.

To close, drape the skin upward and laterally pull out the redundancy. Holding the skin up gently with a moist cotton-tipped applicator, ask the patient to look upward and open the mouth. This maneuver puts the maximum tension on the lower lid skin at the inferior lateral canthus. Leave enough skin to cover the lid during this exercise. First trim the excess skin by cutting the wedge of skin that is pulled up and over the lateral portion of the incision line. A tacking suture at this point helps; it can be replaced later. Because the redundant skin has been pulled up and laterally, there may be quite a lot of excess skin in the wedge to be excised. The lateral extension of the incision may need to be lengthened to accommodate the dog-ear at this corner. Cut that extension laterally, not inferiorly or obliquely. Like the lateral extension of the incision on the uppers, that component of the scar shows the worst and longest, and patients complain about it.

When the corner is trimmed and sutured, the rest of the excess skin, now pulled up and lying over the rest of the incision line, is trimmed with scissors. The amount taken will be less as you move medially. Little will be sacrificed medial to the midpupillary line. The bulk of the skin is taken out at the lateral canthal wedge.

A few interrupted sutures at the lateral edge and a simple running subcuticular suture ade-

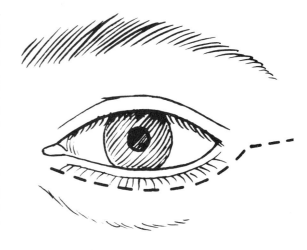

FIG 11–5.
The incision for lower-lid blepharoplasty. The lateral extension of the incision is horizontal and not pointing downward.

quately close the incision. Dressings are not needed.

Skin/Muscle

The initial cut is a stab wound at the lateral canthus made in the horizontal plane (Fig 11–5). Blunt-tipped scissors are used to probe the wound deeply to the bony orbit and then turned and tunneled under skin and muscle along the lower lid 3 to 4 mm below the lash line. The scissors are brought back to the stab wound and used to cut through the skin and muscle. The scissor blades are not held perpendicular to the skin surface but angled 45 degrees, with the outer blade cutting the skin more superiorly than the inner blade cuts the muscle. This incision is carried medially to about 2 mm from the punctum. The skin muscle flap is grasped with fine-toothed forceps, such as Adson or Brown-Adson forceps, and lifted away as the scissors spread the fine stroma between the muscle and the septum.

The septum is opened over each pocket, as needed. There is nothing wrong with one long incision. As with the upper lid, several methods of removing the fat are evolving.[11] The method of tease out, clamp, cut, desiccate, and remove clamp works well and safely. More electrocautery and less clamping is also in vogue. And for cases with minimal fat protrusion, particularly younger patients, cauterizing the fat through what is nothing more than a puncture hole, followed by cautery or desiccation of the septum itself, seems to produce adequate results. The theory is that if the problem is a weak or herniated septum, tightening or strengthening the septum by generating scar tissue is a valid approach.

In the 1950s Castañares[12] and more recently Rees[13] described the location of the "classic" lower lid incision as 1 to 2 mm below the free border of the lower lid. This has served well the hundreds of physicians who have done thousands of blepharoplasties. However, in the past year or so, critical examination of lower-lid blepharoplasty results reveals unhappiness with the shape of the lower lateral lid margin. The jargon for this look is "round eye," and it is a function of one or several factors: (1) increased scleral show between the limbus and the lower lash margin; (2) medial displacement of the lateral commissure; (3) increased slope of the lateral one-third of the lid; (4) a flattened, unanimated pretarsal component of the orbicularis; and (5) a healed, unnatural line from the incision scar. The lower lid is just a bit short of ectropion.[14]

Several diverse theories account for this constellation of findings. The most popular is that the scar that develops in the plane undermined to create the flap — just above the septum in the skin/muscle flap, or just above the muscle in the skin-only flap — undergoes contraction, tugging downward on the lower-lid margin and its support tissues. This pull ever so slightly displaces the lateral lower lid and the canthus. Another theory blames unphysiologic sacrifice of pretarsal and preseptal orbicularis which leaves inadequate but too tight support for the tarsus. Another conjecture is that an incision only 2 mm below the lid margin is not a natural line and that the vertical contraction of that scar twists the lower lid slightly outward.

One proposal, by McCollough and English,[14] is to make the skin incison inferior to the lower edge of the tarsal plate, or 4 to 6 mm below the lash line. The muscle is incised as a second incision with scissors under direct vision immediately below (posterior) to the skin incision, creating a skin/muscle flap inferior to the incisions and a skin flap only superiorly. The theory is that the pretarsal orbicularis is left intact to provide the smooth, hammock-like support for the lid margin.

Another solution, rapidly becoming the more customary, is the transconjunctival approach for lower-lid lipectomy (discussed below).

Lower Lid Technique

For several years we have performed a combined-technique lower lid blepharoplasty.[15] The skin incision is located 2 to 3 mm below the lid margin and starts with a horizontal cut at the lateral canthus (Fig 11–6). Only the skin is dissected down above the muscle for a few more millimeters. This step takes a little time because it is not unusual to encounter bleeders. Then the muscle is bluntly separated in a sweeping curve that begins just below the punctum and extends as far laterally as will be necessary to remove all of the fat. (Clinically, try to determine before the operation whether or not there is too much fat in the lateral pocket.) The septum is now visible and is opened as much as necessary for fat extrusion.

This design lowers the incision scar to just below the tarsus, preserves the muscle hammock of the pretarsal orbicularis, develops a skin/muscle flap that reduces the potential for scar contraction, decreases bleeding, and more easily exposes the septum. The closure includes trimming fat and skin separately so that each is tailored as needed (Fig 11–7). The muscle suspension and muscle debulking at the preseptal level are easily accomplished without too much worry of weakening the supporting hammock of the pretarsal muscles (Fig 11–8). The skin flap is still supported laterally, and the scar line is in a more favorable location (Fig 11–9).

Correction of a Lax Lower Lid

Moderate or severe lid laxity should be corrected as part of the lower-lid blepharoplasty. The lid-shortening procedure is used for very lax, senile lids, and the muscle suspension is for those with only slight or moderate looseness.

A lid-shortening is the same operation as the pentagonal or wedge removal procedure. Full-thickness lid is excised followed by a side-to-side closure. Most very lax lids need only about 5 to 7 mm removed. The easiest location to take out the tissue is at the junction of the lateral one-third and middle one-third of the lid. Skilled eyelid surgeons sometimes prefer to take it out at the lateral canthus, but the muscle approximation is more tricky there.[16, 17]

Plan the blepharoplasty in the ordinary manner. When the skin or skin/muscle flap has been elevated, do the shield-wedge resection. Cuts are made with Stevens tenotomy scissors, cutting exactly vertically through the tarsal plate but angling to a midpoint inferior to the tarsus — thus the title pentagonal. A careful technique is to cut only one side of the wedge through and through. Then test close, using hooks or small-toothed forceps, to see how much lid needs to be excised to develop a smooth but tight lower lid. The proper amount is removed and the closure is a three- or four-layered closure. Starting with tarsal suture(s) (the lower lid tarsus is not as well defined or as wide as the upper) and being careful not to put a loop of suture through the lid conjunctiva, follow with lid margin, muscle, and skin sutures: 6/0 or 7/0 Dexon for the

buried sutures, and suture of choice for the skin. Then continue and complete the rest of the blepharoplasty.

Skin and muscle or muscle suspension techniques improve the results of lower-lid blepharoplasty when there is mild laxity of the lid margin and when the skin is heavy.[18, 19] Webster et al. recommend a longer and higher lateral extension of the incision which includes the supero-lateral pull on the skin alone if it is thick, and on the skin and muscle if a skin/muscle flap has been developed.[20] The preseptal orbicularis muscle is imbricated to the lateral orbital periosteum, or a wedge is excised and the muscle edge is sutured to the periosteum. The skin is draped over the high lateral extension and closed with an M-plasty.

The muscle suspension methods are directed toward a real problem and help, but are not as easy to perform as they sound, nor are they trouble-free. Especially in the very patients who need a blepharoplasty, the orbicularis is not the well-defined, substantive structure it might

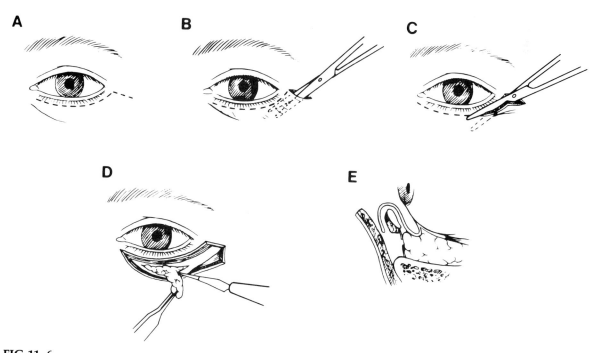

FIG 11–6.
Our technique for the lower lids. **A,** the incision is made about 2 to 3 mm below the lash line. **B,** the skin is dissected down with scissors, about 5 mm. **C,** the skin is cut with scissors. **D,** a strip of preseptal orbicularis oculi muscle is removed to expose the septum, and the fat protrudes when the septum is opened. **E,** a lateral view of the operation.

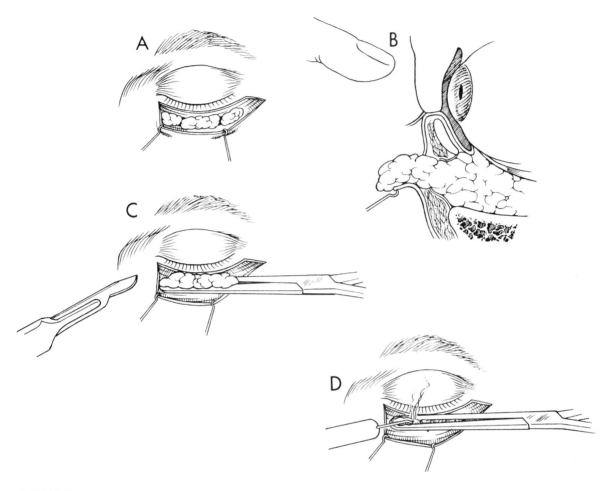

FIG 11–7.
A–D, as with the upper-lid fat, the skin may be clamped and cut, or clamped and electrodesiccated, or in some cases just desiccated.

be. Finding a strong band of muscle that will withstand the rigors of being sutured to the lateral orbital rim is not always possible in these patients, where the muscle is weak, thin, or spread out. The next problem is the bulge of imbricated muscle, or the bulge composed of muscle ends and enough suture to hold it together, that lies over the preorbital rim muscle and is fastened to the periosteum. These bulges and ridges cannot be completely trimmed away or the suspension itself will be lost. Unless thick skin is draped over the repair, the irregularity will show for many months.

Transconjunctival Lipectomy

For years, eyelid cosmetic surgeons have known that in a large majority of lower-lid op-erations, very little skin was removed. The lipectomy was all that was indicated in many patients, and was the most rewarding part of the operation for many others. But how to remove the fat without having to open the skin and muscle with all of the incumbent morbidity? Thus, the transconjunctival (TC) approach was developed.[2]

In all patients who have problems with bulging lower-lid fat and minimal problems with lid laxity or redundant skin, the TC lipectomy is the treatment of choice. It may be combined with upper-lid surgery, brow surgery, lower-lid margin tightening, rhytidectomy, and resurfacing procedures such as dermabrasion and chemical peel.

After numbing the conjunctival sac with

Blepharoplasty and Brow-lift

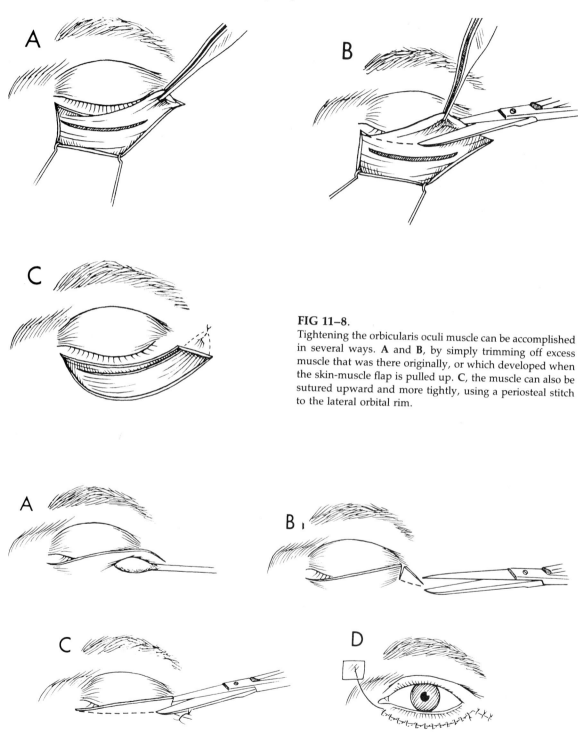

FIG 11–8.
Tightening the orbicularis oculi muscle can be accomplished in several ways. **A** and **B**, by simply trimming off excess muscle that was there originally, or which developed when the skin-muscle flap is pulled up. **C**, the muscle can also be sutured upward and more tightly, using a periosteal stitch to the lateral orbital rim.

FIG 11–9.
A, the skin is closed by first gently draping it up and over the lash line. **B**, a perpendicular cut is made at the lateral canthus to gauge how much redundant skin there really is. **C**, after the lateral edge is trimmed and sutured, the remaining redundant lid is excised. **D**, the lid is closed with running sutures.

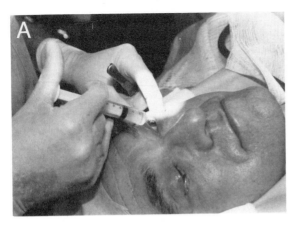

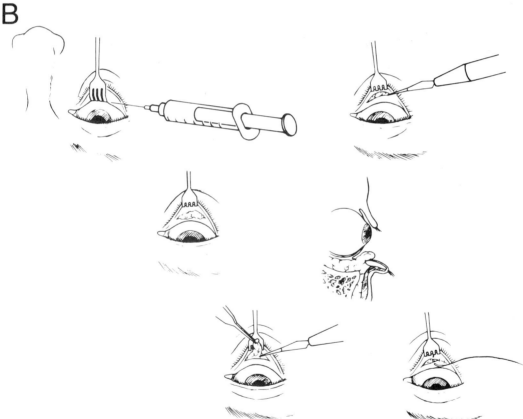

FIG 11–10.
A, in the transconjunctival technique, local anesthesia is injected through the conjunctival sack. **B,** first the fat pads are anesthetized through the conjunctiva. Next, the conjunctiva is incised and opened so the fat is visible. The fat flows easily through the opening and can be grasped and excised. Finally, a stitch or two closes the conjunctiva. (All views are from above patient's head.)

drops, the local anesthesia is injected through the conjunctival sac; it fills the same areas of the lower lid as when it is injected from the skin surface (Fig 11–10). Also inject behind the orbital rim to numb the fat pockets. Leave ample time for the full epinephrine effect. Sometimes the anesthetic agent will infiltrate the sympathetic nerves of the globe and the pupil will dilate. Do not be surprised if this happens on one eye only.

A Jaeger retractor is placed over the cornea and into the inferior fornix. A 3- or 4-mm pronged, blunt, heavy, rigid retractor holds the lower lid away. Electrocautery, electrodesiccation, laser, or scalpel all work to incise the conjunctiva and mucosa of the lower lid. Start laterally and cut toward the medial side (Fig 11–11). After 5 to 6 mm is opened, check the location of the incision to be sure it exposes the fat that lies in the pockets superior to the orbital rim. As the incision is carried medially and a little more laterally, be careful to follow the curve of the lid and not just make a straight incision which is seen by the surgeon above and behind the field. A straight incision will become more and more superior on the lid on both sides of the starting point; the curved line will stay the same distance from the lid margin, as it should.

The fat is immediately visible and often flows into the lower conjunctival sac (Fig 11–12). It is trimmed as before with clamping and cutting and desiccating, or clamping and cutting, or just desiccating. The laser is not the best tool for fat excision because the tissue being vaporized must be backed with moist cotton or gauze. Pulling the fat out and over a moist backing is an extra step that is also somewhat cumbersome. In addition, it interferes with the most difficult part of the TC lipectomy — judging how much fat to remove. When the standard anterior approach

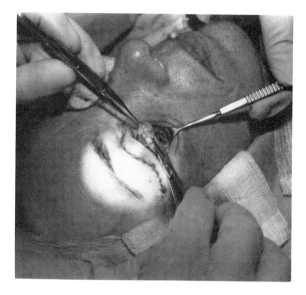

FIG 11–12.
The fat is grasped gently and trimmed appropriately. Electrocautery can also be used for the fat trimming.

to lower lids is used, the fat to be removed is either self-extruding and lying there, or is extruded by putting gentle pressure on the globe. However, it is considerably different with the TC approach.

From the conjunctival side, the opening looks down onto the suborbital fat spaces. The surgeon sees the excess or protuberant fat and its continuation back under the globe. Conceivably, too much fat from under the globe could be removed rather easily. One guideline is to trim the fat off at a level parallel to the anterior edge of the bony orbital rim.[6] It takes some experience to make this judgment.

The only other anatomic structure in this area is the inferior oblique muscle. It originates on the bony orbital floor of the maxilla, just lateral to the nasolacrimal duct, and courses backward and temporally in the infraorbital fat. It is this section of the muscle that could be injured during a lipectomy. The muscle is visible during the TC approach, but would not normally be injured unless the surgeon were not careful with clamps and electrocautery instruments. The injury would be difficult to detect because the resulting diplopia would be manifest on upward gaze only.

Several 5/0 or 6/0 absorbable interrupted su-

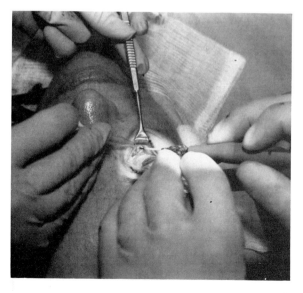

FIG 11–11.
A Jeager retractor pulls the lower lid away and down to expose the conjunctival side of the lid through which an incision is made with electrocautery in this example.

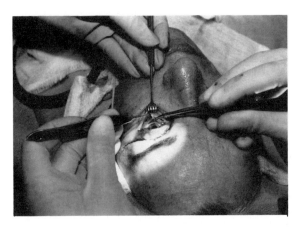

FIG 11–13.
Absorbable sutures are placed to close the posterior lid wall.

tures partially close the septum (Fig 11–13). The conjunctiva does not need closure. Conjunctival injection, redness, and irritation are common for a few weeks, but otherwise it is nearly trouble free (Figs 11–14 through 11–16).

Complications

Hematoma

Hematomas can occur from bleeding at any level of a blepharoplasty wound. Retrobulbar hematomas are the most severe and are potentially dangerous (see below). The hard decision is deciding whether to and when to drain the hematoma. If it is large and easily noticeable within the first 12 hours after surgery, it is probably best to open the wound, find the bleeder (if possible), irrigate well, and re-close. Some retromuscular hematomas do not become apparent until several days later when the swelling has dissipated. Either drain the hematoma in the first 2 to 3 days, or wait 7 to 8 for it to liquefy. A nick with a #11 blade will allow it to drain, and is adequate opening to irrigate through. Hematomas allowed to resolve on their own may leave a larger scar that may be visible or palpable through the thin eyelid tissue. Intralesional triamcinolone acetonide 5 mg/ml every three weeks will speed the resolution.

Retrobulbar hematoma fortunately is rare but is probably the most frequent cause of blindness.[21] It is probably caused by puncturing a vessel during the administration of the local anesthetic. It could also be caused by a bleeder in the fat pedicles, but this is less likely and would have been seen. The signs are obvious. The eye becomes stony hard and proptotic. The lids are forced back from the globe and the eye pro-

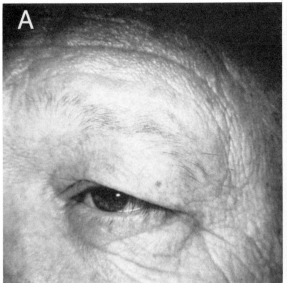

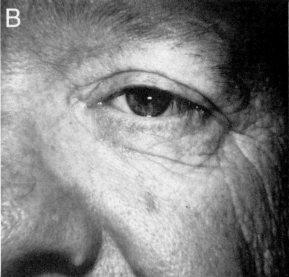

FIG 11–14.
A, man, 48 years old, before an upper lid blepharoplasty. **B**, 3 months after surgery.

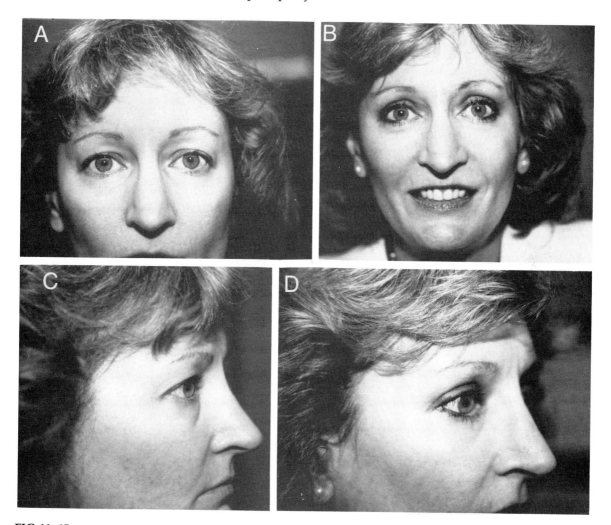

FIG 11–15.
A, woman, 41 years old, before and after upper and lower lid blepharoplasty. **B**, 2 months after surgery. **C**, same woman preoperatively, lateral view. **D**, lateral view postoperatively.

trudes. If there are any signs of deep hemorrhage, the wound, including the orbital septum, must be opened immediately. The operating surgeon can do this at once and should seek consultation with appropriate ophthalmologists. Diuretics such as mannitol or diazoxide, cold compresses, and medical reduction of blood pressure help reduce the pressure within the globe. Deep pain, wound-edge bleeding, changes in vision, orbital swelling or globe protrusion are all important findings. Blindness may also be caused by increased intraocular pressure.

Keratoconjunctivitis Sicca or "Dry Eye" Syndrome

It is hoped that any pre-existing predilection to dry eye would have been picked up in the history or physical examination. It may have arisen de novo from the surgery or have been subclinical before. Many factors can contribute to this one symptom, so do not wait too long to assume it is a temporary problem that will resolve spontaneously. Which component of tears is affected — the lacrimal production and drainage system, the angle and contact of the lids with the globe, medicinal or mechanical irritation are all possible culprits. A specific diagnosis is needed for proper treatment. Seek consultation with another physician who can do a complete dry eye work-up.[22]

The most common cause of dry eye post-blepharoplasty is a simple-exposure keratitis that results from the eyes not closing completely during sleep. If there is any sign of inadequate closure, we instruct the patients how to cover the eyelids and tape them closed for sleep. They are advised to insert an ophthalmic ointment at bedtime and shown how to use wetting drops during the day. As the edema settles out, the lids close better.

Formerly we tested patients for Bell's phenomenon, which was believed to be a protective reaction for the cornea. But it does not work consistently enough to protect during sleep, even in those patients who demonstrate it.

Asymmetry

Often the skin redundancy covered the asymmetry before surgery and the asymmetry becomes noticeable afterwards. Naturally, it is best to discover it before surgery and to talk with the patient about how to correct it, if possible. Certain cases are not correctable, but some are. The problem may not have been noticed before and then the patient thinks the operation went awry. We try to prepare patients for unexpected events and offer to correct any problems we can. It is part of building a reputation to correct even the smallest defects at a later date. Actually, offer the correction as soon as you think it can be done.

Lagophthalmos

Inability to close the eyes completely can be expected for the first 24 to 48 hours after an upper-lid procedure. The lids should not remain open more than 3 mm, however, or dry eye and corneal irritation will ensue. Treatment with methylcellulose drops will often prevent symptoms until the condition corrects itself.

The most common cause is excessive skin removal. If resolution of the edema does not correct the problem within a week or so, the lid incision should be opened and a full-thickness skin graft sewn in.

Blepharoptosis — Drooping of the Upper Lid

Injury to the levator aponeurosis is the cause of blepharoptosis (if it did not exist prior to surgery). This trauma happens more frequently when a lipectomy is performed in which the medial edge of the levator is exposed where it lies between the medial edge of the middle fat pocket and the medial fat pocket. The levator also could have been caught in the sutures that closed the skin. This finding does not always imply surgical misadventure. It can arise from

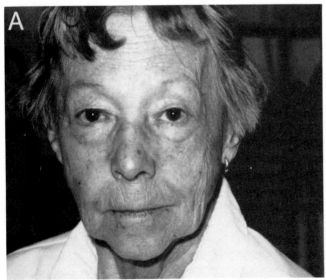
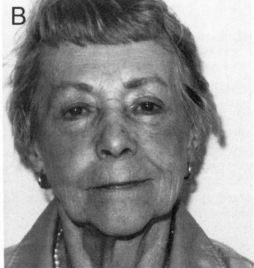

FIG 11–16.
A, woman, 67 years old, before upper and lower lid blepharoplasty. **B,** 14 days after surgery.

postoperative edema and bleeding that produces disinsertion of the levator. The droop often corrects itself within a few weeks. If it does persist, a second operation with levator repair may be necessary. It is not always possible to repair it completely.

Ectropion and Scleral Show

These findings are secondary to the same mechanism — too much skin removed from the lower lid, or scar contraction after lower-lid blepharoplasty. Every so often time will soften the look, but not always. Tiny drops of triamcinolone acetonide 5 mg/ml injected into any firm areas may help. If the downward pull is marked, the suture line should be opened and a full-thickness graft placed.

Miscellaneous

Infection is extremely rare and nearly always responds to appropriate antibiotics. There is one report of an orbital abscess.[23] Dysesthesias also are rare and thought to be the result of injury to the terminal branches of the ophthalmic division of the trigeminal nerve.[24] Some dysesthesias may persist for years; some respond to intralesional corticoids.

Brow-lift

Examination of the patient helps determine whether or not a brow-lift is needed. Ptosis medially makes the patient look angry or uncomfortable, while lateral ptosis produces a sad or tired look. The lateral hooding must be analyzed to determine which components are responsible: the brow ptosis or the lid redundancy. Obviously such analysis is critical to which operation is chosen.

The percentage of blepharoplasty patients who should also have a brow-lift varies with the desires of the patient and the experience of the surgeon. Some patients, particularly women who are into high fashion, want a lot of skin showing inferior to the lateral brow. Often these women look great when they are dressed up and wearing makeup. At other times, however, many look surprised rather than pretty. Try to assess how patients will look in all situations after having this surgery.

Some surgeons believe nearly every patient can benefit from a brow-lift in conjunction with upper lid blepharoplasty. We suspect that these doctors have a bit of a bias for a certain look. We find that there is a population of both men and women who truly need the brow-lift — and sometimes a brow-lift only — because of the low position of the brow and excessive hooding laterally. Another group of women want a brow-lift for that look. In our practice we do a brow-lift on about 10% to 12% of our upper lid blepharoplasty patients.

The brow-lift is not a permanent procedure. Like a face-lift, it falls within a few years. The heaviness and laxity of the skin determine which lifts will last and for how long. Raising a ptotic brow, even if necessary, when the whole face also needs lifting, creates beauty only if the face is looked at segmentally.

The brow-lift operation can be designed at several different levels: suprabrow, mid- or upper forehead, forehead-hairline junction, or within the hair, which is called a coronal lift (Fig 11–17). Each has its advantages and disadvantages. The following physical findings help determine where skin removal will be located.[25] An important factor is the height of the forehead and hairline. If the forehead is already high, skin removal should be from the forehead skin itself, either suprabrow or midforehead. The coronal approach will accentuate the problem of a high hairline and broad forehead. In men who are bald or balding frontally, the coronal scar will not be hidden and may actually bring attention to the receding hairline. In men or women with sharp and curved hairlines, the addition of a scar at that line may sharpen it even more, producing an artificial or batlike face. Deep forehead creases help decide in favor of a mid- or upper-forehead approach. The creases imply loose and movable skin on the forehead, and the scar line will be more camouflaged by the creases and other horizontal lines. Skin thickness and color affect how inconspicuous the scar may be. If the corrugator muscles are very active, they may need transection; this is only done well under direct vision, using a coronal approach of one type or another.

Suprabrow Position

This design is more appropriate for medical

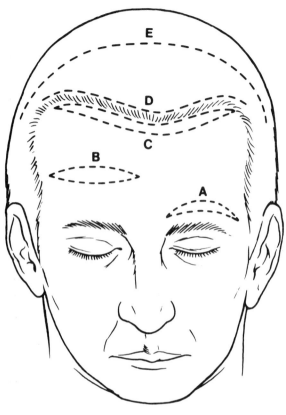

FIG 11–17.
Diagram of various incisions for a brow lift. **A**, suprabrow. **B**, midforehead. **C**, pretrichal. **D**, posttrichal or bat-wing. **E**, coronal.

that the brow should be lifted. There is significant stretch or return in the first few months after the operation, so extra elevation should be designed into the measurements.

One technique is to have the patient seated and relaxed, with the brows in their regular, ptotic position. With a marking pen, draw the line of the inferior edges of the supraorbital bony rim. With the fingers, elevate the brows to where you and the patient think they should be placed and again mark the skin just at the inferior edge of the supraorbital rim. The distances between the two lines indicates the amount and shape of the skin to be removed above — wherever on the forehead the ellipse of skin is to be taken. Another technique is to pinch up the forehead skin and estimate how much and in what design it should be removed. Again, take a bit more than will perfectly position the brows to allow for later stretch and fall-down.

The incision through the skin is made perpendicular to the surface, although a few doctors believe that oblique incisions and eventual over-eversion of the wound edges reduce scarring. This is difficult to prove, and we are unaware of any proof in the literature. However, some good physicians believe it helps. Following incision, the skin is removed. At which level to undermine and whether or not to plicate muscle are ongoing variables discussed frequently. For the suprabrow-lift, little undermining is done in either direction; only a skin removal is performed.

After hemostasis is achieved, the next decision concerns the suspension sutures. Again, there are diametrically opposed opinions about the necessity of a suspension suture. To put in one or several, select a permanent suture material such as Prolene or Supramid. Start deep behind the brow and place the stitch through the dermis under the brow; pull the brow up to its new location and push the needle through the periosteum at the proper location to anchor the brow; tie, with the knot buried. The periosteal loop is best achieved by first bluntly dissecting a small opening through the frontalis muscle in order to actually see the bone. Usually we place about three of these buried, permanent, periosteal horizontal mattress sutures per brow. The skin is closed with the repair of choice.

or functional brow-lifts than for cosmetic reasons. The scar is visible for many months, even in those people in whom the scar eventually fades. The scar line shows more because it is curved rather than linear like the other forehead lines, and because it highlights and demarcates the brow. Many people have a tapered brow edge with hairs that go in several directions and get smaller and smaller — just like the scalp hairline — rather than in an abrupt line. When a scar is placed just above the thicker hairs, it accentuates the natural "soft" brow margin and makes it look painted or artificial.

The suprabrow-lift is used only when the lateral brow is ptotic. Elevating the medial brow places a straight line scar across the glabella, which looks terrible. An ellipse or fusiform excision should be planned, with the maximum width the same distance and on the same plane

Midbrow Position

This ellipse of skin removal is located in the mid- or high forehead. So that there will be less tendency to produce a scar that looks like it runs across the whole forehead,[26] this ellipse is often located at a different height on each side of the forehead. The measurements are made in the same way as for the suprabrow lift: the lines are drawn in the skin, as for a suprabrow lift, and transferred to the midforehead with calipers. The midforehead lift works for raising the whole brow or either end selectively. The width of skin excised equals the distance the brow is to be elevated; the location of the excision is directly superior to the part of the brow that is to be elevated.

After the skin is removed, undermine inferiorly only. Dissecting above the frontalis is easy until the fibrous attachments are encountered just superior to the brow. The nerves and vessels are in or below the muscle. Do not undermine much below the brow laterally, because the ophthalmic branch of the trigeminal may be transected. Then place several permanent suspension sutures as described above. A variation of this procedure is to remove a small ellipse of muscle and close the muscle in one layer. Alternatively, it is possible to imbricate the muscle with an absorbable suture to tighten it in the vertical plane.

The skin is closed with the edges slightly everted. We do not recommend trying to dissect over the glabella or doing any cutting of the corrugator from this approach.

Hairline Approach

The entire forehead can be opened from a hairline incision, called the pretrichal incision (as opposed to a midcoronal incision), or the incision can be limited to both sides. Also, the incision could be extended into the sideburn hair to access a mini-face-lift laterally. This location is chosen if the patient needs a whole forehead incision and brow-lift but the hairline is already too high. In patients with thick frontal hair, some forehead skin and hair-bearing scalp are sacrificed to prevent raising the hairline too much.

The markings and incisions are made as described above. Undermining is done above the frontalis to the level of the brow. For this incision, the surgeon may only incise the upper edge of the ellipse, undermine, pull up and drape the skin flap over the incision, and then excise only the excess.

If the incision is made completely across the forehead, the corrugator is accessible. When the patient has deep, vertical furrows on the glabella and they are observed frequently making these lines, transection of the corrugator is indicated. The frontalis muscle must be cut from the back of the skin and the muscle body itself scissors-excised as well. The supratrochlear nerve runs from its foramen *through* the muscle, so carefully tease the muscle from the nerve. Transection of the nerve will result in an extended period of forehead numbness. The supraorbital nerve, however, is inferior to the muscle and located far enough laterally that it is seldom at risk.

Muscle removal needs to be fairly complete. The overlying skin never shows any depression from muscle loss, but if the muscle is not removed evenly, the glabella may look bumpy.

Coronal Brow-lift

When the patient needs a brow-lift, a forehead-lift, and corrugator muscle excision, this is the approach to use if the frontal hairline is naturally low enough to withstand some further elevation. The scar from this approach is completely hidden by the hair; in addition, this approach provides the best access to the corrugator.

The incision is often flying-bird-shaped in men and like a giant C in women. If the coronal lift is done in conjunction with a face-lift, the incision does not extend as far laterally. Otherwise, the incision extends down onto the sideburn area to effect a little lateral pull on the temples, which further reduces the upper lid hooding.

The entire forehead is undermined in the plane between the frontalis muscle and the periosteum of the frontal bone. All the periosteal muscle attachments are released over the forehead, including the lateral supraorbital ridges. As the skin and muscle flap are turned down, the supraorbital vessels and nerves are identified and preserved. The corrugator muscle is exposed and carefully dissected off the supra-trochlear nerve.

If marked forehead wrinkling is also a problem, some of the frontalis muscle can be incised or excised in a transverse direction. Take care not to extend any frontalis cuts lateral to a line vertically from the junction of the middle two-thirds and lateral one-third of the eyebrows. This preserves the eyebrow-elevating function. If some of the frontalis is excised, there will be an adhesion of the muscle to the periosteum, but this lasts only a few months and resolves spontaneously.

When the muscle work is completed, the skin is draped over the forehead and the proper amount excised. Closure of choice is completed. Flying-bird incisions help reduce the elevation of the midportion of the forehead. The same preservation is possible if the forehead is pulled up and *laterally*, rather than just upward.

Some controversy exists about whether this lift should be undermined under the muscles and galea, or subcutaneously.[27] There are several reports of prolonged, even permanent, numbness and itching of the scalp posterior to the incision when the undermining was done in the subgaleal plane.[28, 29] The subcutaneous approach is more tedious and there is some risk to the ophthalmic branch of the facial nerve when dissecting over the lateral orbital rim, but the achievable results can be good.

Complications

Only rarely is there numbness, and if it happens it is usually temporary, although we have seen it last up to a year. The scar is the most common and persistent problem. Dermabrasion on the forehead is helpful to blend out raised scars, but not helpful for white, atrophic scars, or in patients with dark or easily pigmented skin. Occasionally there is asymmetry which can and should be corrected by a repeat procedure. And, the results of a brow-lift are not permanent.

References

1. Mackinnon SE, Fielding JC, Dellon AL, et al: The incidence and degree of scleral show in the normal population. *Plast Reconstr Surg* 1987; 80:15–20.
2. Baylis HI: Blepharoplasty. *Oculoplastic Newsletter*, No. 1 Fall 1987.
3. Silver H: A new approach to the operation of blepharoplasty. *Br J Plast Surg* 1969; 22:253–256.
4. Field LM: Principles of Silver's segmental technique applied to upper and lower lid blepharoplasty with and without direct browpexy. *Am J Cosmetic Surg* 1988; 5:93–96.
5. Zide BM: Anatomy of the eyelids. *Clin Plast Surg* 1981; 8:623–634.
6. Baylis HI: Personal communcation, April 6, 1989.
7. Sachs ME, Bosniak SL: Nonsurgical fat removal in cosmetic blepharoplasty: A new technique. *Ann Plast Surg* 1986; 16:516–520.
8. Colton JJ, Beekhuis GJ: Use of electrosurgery in blepharoplasty. *Arch Otolaryngol* 1985; 111:441–442.
9. Wolfley DE: Blepharoplasty: The ophthalmologist's view. Symposium on the aging face. *Otolaryngol Clin North Am* 1980; 13:237–263.
10. Webster RC, Smith RC, Hall R: Blepharoplasty: Prevention of the "sad or round eye." Proceedings of the Fourth International Symposium on Plastic and Reconstructive Surgery of the Head and Neck 1983. St Louis, C.V. Mosby Co., 1984.
11. Cook TA, Derebery J, Harrah ER: Reconsideration of fat pad management in lower lid blepharoplasty surgery. *Arch Otolaryngol* 1984; 110:521–524.
12. Castañares S: Blepharoplasty for herniated intraorbital fat: Anatomical basis for a new approach. *Plast Reconstr Surg* 1951; 8:46–58.
13. Rees TD: Surgical procedures, in *Aesthetic Plastic Surgery*. Philadelphia, WB Saunders Co., 1980.
14. McCollough EG, English JL: Blepharoplasty. *Arch Otolaryngol Head Neck Surg* 1988; 114:645–648.
15. Klatsky SA, Manson PN: Separate skin and muscle flaps in lower-lid blepharoplasty. *Plast Reconstr Surg* 1981; 67:151–156.
16. Shagets FW, Shore JW: The management of eyelid laxity during lower eyelid blepharoplasty. *Arch Otolaryngol* 1986; 112:729–732.
17. Lisman RD, Rees T, Baker D, et al: Experience with tarsal suspension as a factor in lower lid blepharoplasty. *Plast Reconstr Surg* 1987; 79:897–905.
18. Mladick RA: Muscle suspension lower blepharoplasty. *Plast Reconstr Surg* 1979; 64:171–175.
19. Foerster DW: A new method for tightening the orbicularis oculi muscles in blepharoplasty. *Aesth Plast Surg* 1979; 3:265–269.
20. Webster RC, Davidson TM, Reardon EJ, et al: Suspending sutures in blepharoplasty. *Arch Otolaryngol* 1979; 105:601–604.

21. Mahaffey PJ, Wallace AF: Blindness following cosmetic blepharoplasty — a review. *Br J Plast Surg* 1986; 39:213–221.
22. Graham WP, Messner KH, Miller SH: Keratoconjunctivitis sicca symptoms appearing after blepharoplasty. *Plast Reconstr Surg* 1976; 57:57–61.
23. Rees TD, Craig SM, Fisher Y: Orbital abscess following blepharoplasty. Case Report. *Plast Reconstr Surg* 1983; 73:126–127.
24. Klatsky S, Manson PN: Numbness after blepharoplasty: The relation of the upper orbital fat to sensory nerves. *Plast Reconstr Surg* 1981; 67:20–22.
25. Connell BF: Eyebrow, face, and neck lifts for males. *Clinics in Plast Surg* 1978; 5:15–28.
26. Cook TE: Blepharoplasty and brow-lift. Presented at Facial Cutaneous Surgery Meeting. March 27, 1989, Copper Mountain, Colo.
27. Wolfe SA, Baird WL: The subcutaneous forehead lift. *Plast Reconstr Surg* 1989; 83:251–256.
28. Viñas JC, Caviglia C, Cortiñas JL: Forehead rhytidoplasty and brow lifting. *Plast Reconstr Surg* 1976; 57:445–449.
29. LeRoux P, Jones SH: Total permanent removal of wrinkles from the forehead. *Br J Plast Surg* 1974; 27:359–363.

Twelve

Basic Face-lift

Face-lifting has been performed and talked about in Europe since the beginning of this century. For some reason — perhaps because plastic surgeons in the U.S. only wrote about reconstruction — the operation was never really discussed openly here. The operative design started with skin removal only, and the amount of skin removed was increased until the incidence of spread scars and slough became too great. Then the trend evolved toward more undermining until the flaps were joined submentally. It was popular in the 1970s to talk about the surgeon and the assistant shaking hands under the flaps under the chin. Undermining helped, but was far from the whole answer to making rhytidectomy a lasting operation.

Cutting, plicating, or sewing the platysma was the next general improvement. Indeed, pulling the posterior edge of the platsyma back and suturing it to the sternocleidomastoid fascia with or without a cut in the muscle was helpful in reducing submental banding.[1,2] And, unbeknownst to the operators, in many cases the platysma plication produced a superficial musculo-aponeurotic system (SMAS) tuck because of the close proximity of the two structures.

In 1976, Mitz and Peyronie described the SMAS.[3] They showed that there is a continuous sheet of fascial tissues in the face and neck that envelops the frontalis muscle and the platsyma muscle, is separate from and overlies the parotid fascia, and is quite thick in the pretragal area. This sheet of tissues becomes attenuated anterior to the masseter muscle and parotid gland. Although many variations are used today, some form of SMAS tightening is incorporated into most rhytidectomies.

The most recent refinement has been the incorporation of liposuction. Not having to make a long, submental incision — or any incision there at all — and having the ability to defat the neck, the jowl, and the flaps has greatly improved both early and late results.

SMAS and Platysma

A modern-day lift would most likely be substandard if one or both of these structures were not manipulated as part of the procedure. For the purposes of this discussion, we define plication as a folding on itself and fixation. Imbrication is to cut, undermine, slide over, excise excess tissue, and suture. These terms describe the two primary ways the SMAS and the platysma are shortened and tightened. Because the SMAS envelops the platysma and because the platysma is often thin, sometimes comprising only a few muscle strands between the fascial layers, we and others speak of these structures almost as one unit. One surgeon includes the overlying fat as part of the same structure.[4]

The two categories of SMAS-platysma surgery are (1) opening the SMAS, dissecting under, and pulling it up, or up and back, and suturing it in place, and (2) plicating the SMAS

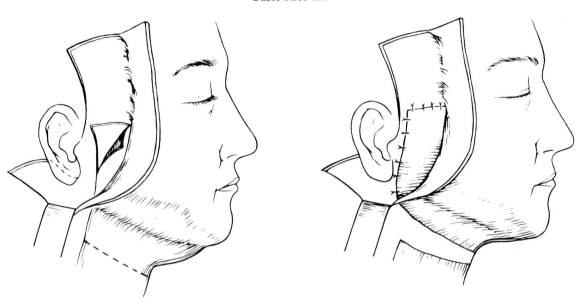

FIG 12–1.
Incision design for SMAS dissection and elevation: a two-directional face-lift.

to other fascial layers. Both methods have many and experienced followers. The classic experiment of performing one method on one side and the other method on the opposite side has not been done with *long-term* follow-up. The results of each technique have been compared to not performing the technique, but there has been no comparison of the two different techniques.[5, 6]

Owsley has published twice on the subject: first in 1977, just a few years after Mitz and Peyronie's original description of the SMAS, and again in 1983 with an update and modifications.[7, 8] He wisely states that one operation will not serve all patients. The amount of submental laxity and fat, the depth of the nasolabial fold, and the loose skin on the neck are factors that dictate which operation is necessary. When the submental area is free of fat (either naturally or after liposuction) but still sags, or if the skin is heavy and sags with loss of the cervicomental angle, a suspension of the floor of the mouth is helpful. Pulling the skin flaps posteriorly corrects the loose skin on the neck and the jowl and sometimes the nasolabial area, but does nothing for the submental area. Pulling the skin flaps upward and posteriorly may help the submental area redundancy temporarily, but does little for the neck, jowl, and nasolabial areas.

Therefore, a bidirectional lift is recommended.

In the bidirectional lift, the SMAS-platysma is incised in a vertical line just in front of the ear (Fig 12–1). The incision starts just inferior to the zygoma and extends inferiorily to about the angle of the jaw. The SMAS-platysma flap is undermined for 4 or 5 cm, or to just behind the anterior margin of the parotid, where the facial nerve is still protected by the gland. After the flap has been elevated, the lift on the flap is directed primarily upward. This creates maximum tension in the submental region, extending from the chin posteriorly to the cervicomental angle, producing a bilateral sling. This sling also tightens the anterior jowl region. After appropriate resection of the SMAS-platysma flap, which is usually a triangular excision at the lateral extension of the incision, the flap is sutured closed along the L-shaped incision, with the horizontal limb just under the zygoma and the vertical limb in the pretragal line. The skin flap is undermined as needed to free up attachments on the cheek, the jowl, and the nasolabial fold. Then the skin flap is pulled mostly posteriorly in the direction that best corrects the slack skin of the jowl and neck.

If there are prominent platysmal bands in the submental region, these can be treated while the SMAS-platysmal flap is open. With the aid of good lighting and long scissors, approach the flap posteriorly and transect the platysma, starting 2 cm below the superior cervical crease. Leave it attached to the SMAS and the fat above it. The muscle will gape open but will still be attached to the overlying fat. Make the cut low enough in the neck so that when the flap is pulled up, the now superior leaf of the muscle does not end up overlying the angle of the jaw and the transection does not overlie the submandibular triangle.

The most serious complication of opening and dissecting under the SMAS-platysma is nerve damage. The facial nerve is protected by the parotid gland and careful dissection with a good headlight avoids it. Other complications such as hematomas have not developed more frequently with this type of surgery than with others. A pseudoparalysis of the mandibular branch of the facial nerve has been reported.[9] This weakness of the depressor muscle activity of the lower lip is self-limiting and disappears completely in 8 to 10 weeks. It may be secondary to platysmal muscle manipulation rather than a result of nerve injury.

Each surgeon develops individual variations of this technique. One of these is the more extensive posterior movement of the platysma in what is called the "two-layer, four-flap rhytidectomy."[10] The SMAS is incised and undermined and pulled up as described above. The vertical limb of the incision is extended more inferiorly over the sternocleidomastoid and the platysma is fully undermined from the neck. Thus, the four flaps: two of SMAS-platysma and two of platysma. The lower flap of muscle is pulled posteriorly and sutured to the fascia overlying the sternocleidomastoid. This technique is helpful for patients with heavy, redundant neck skin.

The other wing of this controversy is the strong evidence by Webster that undermining the SMAS does not enhance the positive effect on the nasolabial fold, the jowls, and the submental area.[5] He suggests that for immediate postoperative results, undermining the skin to the level of the anterior edge of the parotid and plicating the SMAS achieve the same degree of improvement. The Webster technique is far eas-

ier and carries less potential complications. The skin flap is developed and the exposed SMAS is picked up and plicated to the preparotid fascia, the sternocleidomastoid fascia, and the mastoid fascia. The superior edge of the SMAS flap is pulled superiorly to support the submental area and to sharpen the cervicomental angle, while the mastoid edge of the flap is pulled straight posteriorly to reduce the slack skin of the jowl and the nasolabial fold.

Webster showed that the nasolabial groove is actually deepened if the overlying skin is not first undermined before the SMAS is pulled, and that SMAS plication plus pulling the undermined skin no more anteriorly than the anterior edge of the parotid produce the same diminution of the nasolabial groove depth as do the procedures that undermine the SMAS-platysmal flap. He emphasizes that this comparison is immediate postoperative and not long-term. Nevertheless, it is an important study because Webster's technique is so much more simple and less prone to complications.

Long Flap and Short Flap

These variations are considerations in this discussion. How much of the skin should be undermined? Before liposuction, rhytidectomy had to deal with the submental fat and the jowl fat one way or another. The most common way was to undermine completely, down to and through the submental region. An incision had to be made to remove some or all of the fat. This direct approach produced problems: postoperative bleeding, hollowness or a long, unsightly scar running across the cervicomental angle. Also, if there was excess fat on the skin of the flaps from the jowl down onto the neck, it had to be trimmed under direct vision, which was hard to do and get even, and made bleeding a greater problem. It also necessitated a long flap — undermining the skin all the way to the oral commissure in some cases, and certainly down onto the neck. Leaving the fat meant trying to suspend a heavy flap, and a less sharp jawline was the result.

The short flap was developed before the introduction of liposuction and was applicable only to those patients with thin, fat-free skin that was loose and moved easily over the underlying structures. After liposuction was introduced, the short flap became practical for many more patients. In this method, undermining starts at the preauricular incision and extends anteriorly to the anterior border of the parotid and masseter muscle — nearly the same anatomic line. (The masseter is easier to palpate in most patients.) Undermining is carried inferiorly about 2 cm anterior to the angle of the jaw and back to the anterior border of the sternocleidomastoid. From this dissection, the skin (and SMAS if desired) is simply pulled posteriorly and superiorly. The attachments of the skin to the underlying structures must be loose, or long, or both, because the redundant skin pulls out nicely. Some believe the skin not undermined pulls the subcutaneous fat back more smoothly than the undermined skin. There is a contention that the fat just posterior to the nasolabial fold pulls out with less rolling when it is not undermined.

The short and long flap design variations do not include the malar prominence and the nasolabial fold. Undermining the skin over the malar prominence allows the skin there to move more easily. However, there are some vessels that perforate the muscle and if transected are a cause of difficult-to-control bleeding. This area is where the temporal branch of the facial nerve comes into the superficial fascial plane. Transsection of that nerve often produces brow paralysis. Other cutaneous nerves there, if cut, produce numbness that can last for many months. Also, if the malar skin is undermined and moved with the rest of the flap, it often crowds the lateral eyelid skin and distorts the area of the crow's feet.

The nasolabial fold continues to be one of the most difficult facial lines to correct. A face-lift usually removes that position of the line that extends below the oral commissure. It may sometimes soften but it rarely removes that portion from the commissure up to the halfway mark on the line between the ala and the commissure. But properly done lifts almost never correct the upper one-half of the line. Also, the mound of fat that builds up posterior to the line is not affected by undermining alone and is very difficult to dissect out with scissors or with the

liposuction cannula. We have all seen the wind-blown-looking faces that were pulled too tight directly posteriorly in order to flatten out the nasolabial fold. Mallard has recommended dissection of this fat with a technique that carefully marks the fat with sutures.[11] It is a difficult, time-consuming technique that carries a greater potential of nerve damage.

Liposuction With Rhytidectomy

The value of fat suctioning to a face-lift was appreciated almost immediately. The submental incision and resulting scar was always an inherent problem, and many different designs attempted to reduce the scar's visibility. The early liposuctions were most successful under the chin because the fat pocket comes out so easily. Therefore, submental liposuction became the first step in rhytidectomy for many surgeons.

A few years later, more extensive neck and face liposuction became commonplace. To our knowledge there was never any problem with more extensive neck and jowl suction because physicians were advancing the new technique conservatively. As the safety and ease of neck and jowl fat suction came to be appreciated, more and more of the fat was suctioned through the submental opening instead of by time-consuming cutting and picking when the flaps were opened.[12, 13] When more powerful machines were developed, the fat could be suctioned from the back of the flaps as they lay back. In other words, the suction was so powerful that a closed system was not necessary. The value of removing excess fat from the flap, from the jowl, and from the submentum and neck can be best appreciated in the finer contouring of the neck and jawline.

The area that suction did not improve was the nasolabial fold. As discussed in Chapter 13 on liposuction, suction removal of the nasolabial fat has led to an unacceptable number of poor results.[14] It remains the most troublesome feature of the aging face.

The cheeks flaps developed in rhytidectomy have long been undermined with blunt-tipped scissors. Several designs of these scissors are popular: The Webster is narrow, with a 4:1 leverage ratio at the fulcrum; Castañares scissors are blunt, with a short cutting surface exposed to the tip; and Metzenbaum scissors come in several sizes. But basically the technique is to push rather than cut, first to create tunnels under the skin and then to join the tunnels until the flap is free and elevated. Luikart designed a special instrument for undermining face-lift flaps which he called the "Iconoclast."[15] It has two long, narrow, blunt-tipped blades which are separated once they are pushed under the skin. The hand-grips are designed to be heavy and have a good mechanical advantage, so separating the blade tips requires little work. This instrument helped to demonstrate that face-lift flaps were best developed by blunt undermining.

Because the liposuction cannulas were sitting on the table and had just been used on the chin and jowl, it seemed logical to use them for undermining the cheek flaps. They have been tried and they work well — very well. The blunt-tipped, narrow, long, strong tube with a good hand-grip became a perfect instrument for developing tunnels just below the skin. In time, a technique was developed in which the cannula is inserted through small openings made first in the same line that the proposed incision is to be made. Cannula undermining is easier if the skin is still attached. Once the entire area is tunneled, the full incision is completed and the flap lifts up easily by simply cutting the strands between the tunnels. The only place where cannula undermining is not a help is at the base of the mastoid bone where the skin is stuck down. This is a difficult area no matter what instrument is used.

Basic Technique

Rhytidectomy is such a long procedure that having two surgeons, one working on each side, is advantageous. For years, this operation has been done well with one surgeon and assistants, but it also adapts well to two surgeons.

All of the preoperative procedures have been covered in other sections of this book: the necessity for patient consultation, photographs, physician visit and history review and postoperative plans. These procedures are the same or very similar for rhytidectomy, except for management of the hair and placement of the head. Once the incision line has been marked, the hair must be secured. The hair anterior and inferior to the incision line is separated and twisted into little pigtails, each fastened by a small rubber band. The hair posterior and superior to the incision is drawn back, covered, and well secured out of the way. Tightly wrapped towels are then clipped into place. One suggestion is to use sterilizing tape around the head with the towels sutured to the tape.[16] The head should be positioned so the patient's neck is comfortable, but also so the surgeon and staff can work closely and easily on both sides. This operation should not be attempted on just any surgical table. The table needs to have special support and access for the patient's head and neck. If two surgeons are working, the head should be supported by a special head holder such as a Berman-Monell. Pitanguy folds a surgical towel and places it against the patient's head once he has turned the head to where he wants it.[17]

Anesthesia

The best anesthesia for face-lifting is local with epinephrine. With local, the facial muscles retain some tone, and the whole face is not so slack. This helps the surgeon carefully drape the cheek flaps up and back. Also, the patient can help a little by turning and lifting the chin. The epinephrine obviously is absolutely necessary. Once the patient has been given the premedications of choice, the surgeon may prefer that the patient be asleep or fully awake; it is entirely the patient's and surgeon's decision. The local anesthesia is administered through a long, 22-gauge, disposable spinal needle. A little blast of lidocaine through a Dermajet or Madajet to the needle entry site further reduces the patient's discomfort. The anesthetic cocktail is lidocaine 0.5% to 1%, epinephrine 1:100,000 to 1:200,000, and Wydase if desired.

Incision Line

The recommended placement of the incision line changes frequently. All recommendations are well-meaning. Each adjustment is an attempt to overcome some of the inherent problems associated with such a long incision on the face. The incision begins with the anterior-superior pole, and the physician's first decision is whether to start in the hair or just below it (Fig 12–2). For women, permanent alopecia just anterior to the incision is not an uncommon side effect in the temple region. The hair follicles must be sensitive there, because there really is not much if any pull on the flap. Therefore, the incision design has been modified to place it further posteriorly, almost vertically above the ear; others place it horizontally forward at the line of the top of the pinna. Others stop at the top of the pinna if they determine that there is not any reason to pull loose skin from the temple. Of course, whether or not a coronal brow-lift is part of the planning will make a difference in the incision's location.

For men, the amount of hair dictates somewhat where the incision can be located. It can go up into the hair posterior to the temple, or it can turn and become horizontal at the sideburn. The latter design preserves the sideburns but means that most of the skin movement will be in a posterior direction, which is a problem if the whiskers on the lateral cheeks are thick. The skin just anterior to the ear is glabrous, or non-hair-bearing; if the whiskers are moved back to just in front of the ear, it looks artificial. Whatever the location of the incision in the hair, it must be beveled in order to transect as few follicles as possible.

When the incision reaches the top of the ear, it is placed into the preauricular fold and carried down around the anterior crus of the helix to the tragus. Whether the incision goes behind, over the top, or anterior to the tragus depends on the size and shape of the tragus. If there is a pretragal fold, place the incision there. If the tragus is prominent, the incision should go behind it.

The next decision is how to deal with the earlobe. If the lobe is ptotic and floppy, it should be reshaped as part of the operation (Fig 12–3). The lobe is picked up between the thumb and index finger and trimmed as needed. Sometimes it is just the length that needs cutting: other times, the attachment to the face is opened and the lobe is reshaped.

The incision continues around the earlobe and up onto the posterior concha — not in the postauricular sulcus. By placing the incision over the midposterior concha, it will eventually be pulled into the sulcus. Also, when the line crosses the sulcus, putting in a dart or notch helps avoid scar contracture at that point.[23] The incision travels superiorly until it is at the level of the external auditory canal, and then turns 90 degrees posteriorly and spans the mastoid and travels into the hair. If it is anticipated that there will be a lot of loose neck skin to be pulled back, extend the incision 5 to 6 cm into the hair behind the ear. If there is little neck portion to the operation, the incision can follow the hairline inferiorly — just inside the fringe hairs. This latter design makes it easier to suture and avoids a notch at that point.

Liposuction

If the patient needs it, submental, neck, and jowl liposuction can be performed at this time. The technique is the same as if a lift were not also going to be undertaken, and is fully described in Chapter 13.

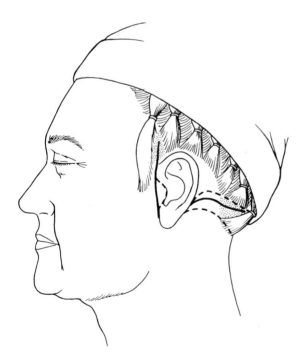

FIG 12–2.
Incision line variations; in the temple and mastoid regions, the incision may follow the hairline or go through it.

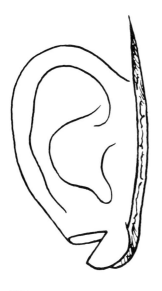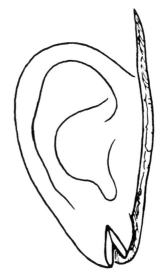

FIG 12–3.
For many patients the ear lobe also needs "lifting." It can be trimmed around its lower edge, or a wedge can be cut out of it.

Undermining

We start the full incision by making three small incisions, each about 1 cm long, in the line for the long incision. The first small incision is pretragal; the second is at the earlobe; the third is at the mastoid hairline. The skin is carefully incised and a hemostat or scissors is used to find the correct subcutaneous plane (Fig 12–4). It is possible to go right through the parotid fascia and under the SMAS unless great care is taken. The SMAS and parotid fascia are usually tough, thick, and glistening in the preauricular area. Once the plane is established, a 3- or 4-mm blunt-tipped liposuction cannula is inserted and pushed forward to the level of the anterior edge of the masseter at the midcheek and to a line at the anterior one-third and middle one-third junction along the jawline. The machine is turned on and the cheek area is suctioned if needed.

The cannula is withdrawn and inserted through the earlobe opening. From this vantage point, the cannula is pushed over the angle of the jaw and makes tunnels through the submandibular triangle to the anterior edge of the sternocleidomastoid. The cannula is then withdrawn and inserted in the third or mastoid hole.

Here, the dissection is difficult and the cannula may need to be smaller — possibly 3 mm. As much as possible, free up the skin over the mastoid and sternocleidomastoid muscle and join the tunnels made from the earlobe opening. This area is often so stuck down that sharp dissection with a scalpel may be necessary. Some surgeons always use a scalpel on this area.

The whole length of the incision is now made, joining the small incisions (Fig 12–5), and the flap is elevated with large rakes (Joseph or Senn types) or clips (Fig 12–6). The tunnels are joined by cutting the remaining strands with scissors (Metzenbaum, Webster, Castañeres) and the entire flap is freed up. It is not uncommon to have to do direct-vision, blunt-scissors dissection of the anterior edge of the mastoid bone and careful blunt dissection over the sternocleidomastoid. Hemostasis is obtained with the instrument of choice. Good lighting — using head lamps, fiberoptics, or hand-held automobile headlamps — is important for fully inspecting under the flaps for bleeders, and for completeness of dissection. Also at this point, additional fat may need to be trimmed from the back of the flap or from the surface of the SMAS.

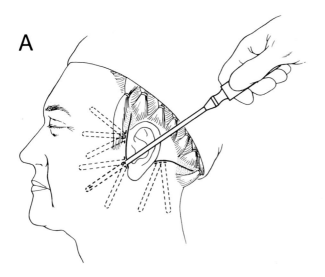

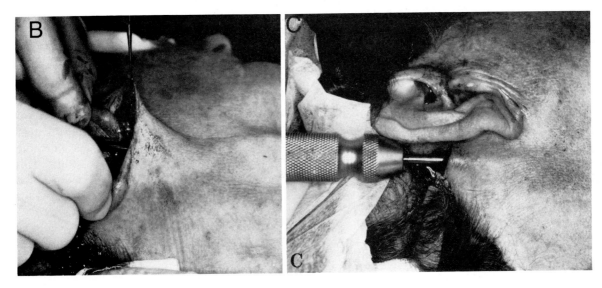

FIG 12–4.
A, three entry openings are made for undermining with the liposuction cannula. **B**, scissors such as Metzenbaum or Webster scissors work well for undermining. **C**, the cannulas also undermine well.

SMAS Plication or Imbrication

The SMAS is incised and undermined as described above, if such is the plan of the surgery. Or, the SMAS is plicated. It is identified by picking up various sites with forceps (Fig 12–7). When the SMAS is picked up, the pull is transferred through the system and movement is seen on the neck and lower cheek. When the location of the SMAS and where it seems the strongest are found, it is pulled up and sutured (it is not an entirely consistent structure and in some people is quite thin and weak in certain areas) (Fig 12–8). We plicate it in four or five different locations using a permanent suture such as Supramid or clear nylon. The most superior leaf is pulled upward to the level of the upper pinna and fastened to the lower edge of the temporalis fascia. The second suture is at the level of the lower tragus and earlobe; the third and fourth pull more posteriorly and fasten to the sternocleidomastoid fascia. These sutures can be pulled

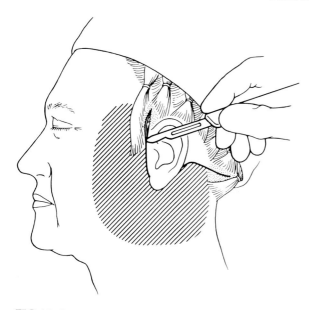

FIG 12–5.
After the flaps are undermined, the three short openings are connected along the proposed incision line.

tightly and, at least at the time of the surgery, tighten the SMAS and platysma enough to sharpen the cervicomental angle, pull out the inferior portion of the nasolabial furrow and fold, and smooth out the cheek sags. These sutures are placed with the knots down. Any fat that rides with the SMAS and that bunches up is

trimmed. The technique is less complicated than SMAS imbrication or a two-directional lift. Also, a short cheek flap is all that is needed to accompany it.

Skin Draping and Closure

The skin is draped back over the cheek and perhaps pulled a little, although much pulling is not helpful or necessary. The most important decision is about the angle of the redraping. Should the skin be laid straight back, or will it be laid with an upward rotation (Fig 12–9)? The answer depends on where the patient has the greatest need and in which direction the most improvement can be accomplished. Before SMAS-platysma fixations were practiced, the direction of pull on the skin was much more important than it is now. Drape the skin back and pull it up, or back, or both, and decide which gives the best improvement (Fig 12–10). Most of the time the direction of pull will be a combination of backward and upward pulls.

Place a stay suture or staple to hold the flap at the upper pole near the temple hairline and another suture or staple over the mastoid at the other end of the incision to hold up the neck portion of the flap. Cut through the flap perpendicular to the edge at the level of the earlobe, with the cut aimed toward where the earlobe

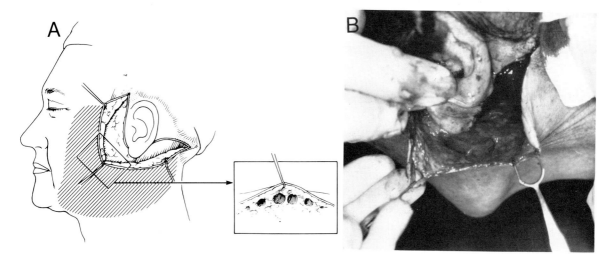

FIG 12–6.
A, when the flap is opened, the tunnels created by the cannula or scissors are visible. **B,** the flap is completely undermined under direct visualization.

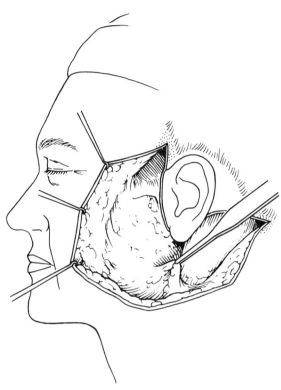

FIG 12–7.
The SMAS is identified by picking up the fascia in the pre-parotid area with forceps and pulling up. When the SMAS is picked up, large sections of the lower cheek and submental region will move with the pull.

will join the cheek (Fig 12–11). Be conservative with this cut. Test its position frequently by pulling the lobe up and over the flap to be sure that the junction is correct. It should be a little tight and have no pull on the lobe. With gravity and scar contracture, that corner may move inferiorly and anteriorly and cause the lobe to be pulled and elongated. When that corner is sutured, work on either end of the closure (Fig 12–12). Next, we like to trim and close the upper or temple part of the flap. It is pulled up with minimal tension and trimmed in whatever way will preserve the most hair and cause the least amount of notching. The portion of the incision line within the hair is stapled (Fig 12–13).

Next, we close the preauricular portion by making cuts into the flap every 2 to 3 cm to check for the correct amount of flap to be sacrificed. If the incision has been made behind the tragus, the skin which will be moved to lie over the

tragus should be defatted so it will not be bulky. This portion is closed with 6/0 nylon or Prolene, using running and interrupted sutures. Finally, we close the posterior limb of the flap. Again, take out a dog-ear wherever that is most advantageous: within the hair-bearing scalp, just anterior to the hairline, or even in the postauricular sulcus. This area is stapled closed except on the ear, where a 6/0 suture is adequate.

Dressings and Postoperative Care

While cleaning up the patient, inspect for bleeding several times before covering the wounds with dressings. The operation is so long that the epinephrine effect will wear off the first side at about the time the second side is done. One of the advantages of having two surgeons is that the operation will be completed and the patient dressed and quiet before the effect wears off. Another phenomenon of local anesthesia also occurs about this time; the local will have infiltrated into the facial nerve and the patient will have developed a slack face and or Bell's paralysis. This can be upsetting to patient and doctor, but is self-limiting within a few hours.

The most common place for bleeders is around the ears, and the blood drains down and pools on the neck or over the mastoid. Sometimes this area must be opened and a bleeder coagulated. Rarely a drain is necessary, but when it is, it is worth the trouble. A closed-system, self-containing suction system can be constructed with scalp vein transfusion tubing and a Vacutaner. Or, several commercial systems are available.

A multilayered, complete head wrap is indicated (Fig 12–14). Telfa or other nonstick dressing is placed over the suture lines and openings. The mastoid and periauricular areas are padded with gauze squares. The hair is combed out and cleaned and arranged so it will be comfortable under the dressing. The turns of the dressing go over the head and under the chin and behind the ears so that pressure is applied in those two areas.

Recovery, ambulation, and postoperative medications depend on the level of anesthesia used. We always personally inspect the patient the next day and are available for any calls that come in before then (Figs 12–15 and 12–16).

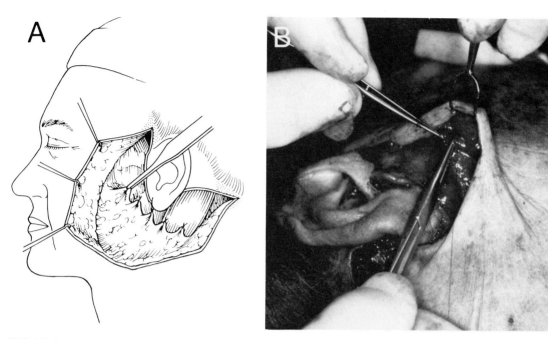

FIG 12–8.
A and **B**, plication of the SMAS; it is pulled up, folded on itself, and sutured in several places.

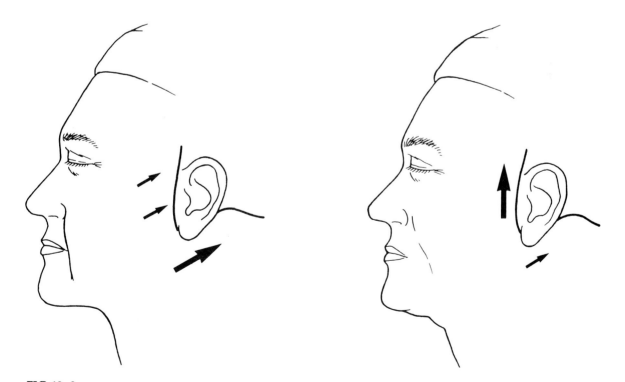

FIG 12–9.
The direction in which the flap is pulled is determined by the location of most of the sagging skin. If the flap is pulled upward, the loose skin of the neck and submental regions are tightened. If the flap is pulled posteriorly, the cheek and nasolabial fold are tightened.

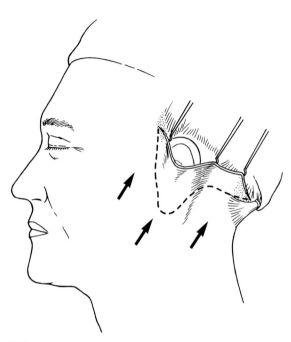

FIG 12–10.
The flap is pulled up and back over the ear.

Two-Staged Face-lift (Tuck-up)

Even before SMAS-platysma fixations were a regular part of face-lifting, surgeons recognized that a second lift or a re-do often produced a tighter, smoother face than the first procedure. The face could be pulled much tighter on the second operation by locating the layer of scar tissue that developed where the flap was undermined, and by suturing that scar to the pre-parotid fascia or the sternocleidomastoid fascia.

The second-stage operation must follow a primary operation that was widely undermined so that a sheet of scar tissue will have developed under a broad cheek flap. The incisions for the tuck-up are relatively short, starting in front of the ear and curving around the lobe and onto the posterior concha. Only the skin should be dissected up for about 3 to 4 cm, and just enough to locate the scar sheet and to free it from the skin and underlying tissues. With forceps, pull on the scar sheet to determine what tissues will move with it. This exercise is similar to pulling

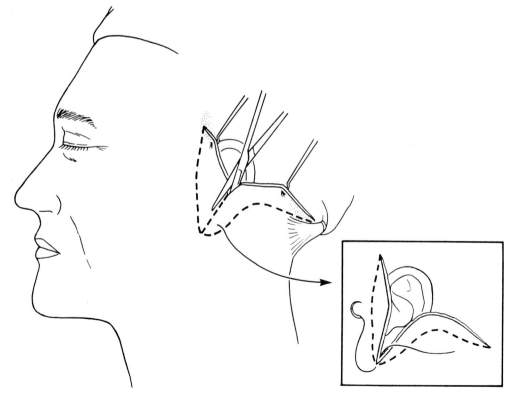

FIG 12–11.
A cut is made in the flap toward the junction of the lower pole of the ear and the cheek and a suture is placed at that location.

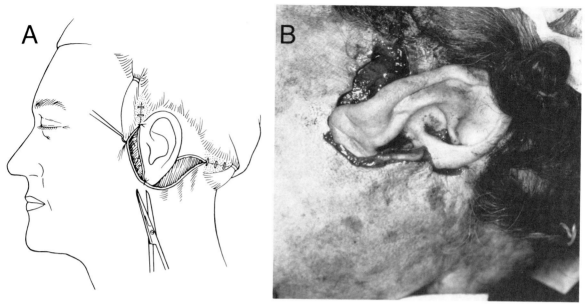

FIG 12–12.
A and **B**, suturing of the flap; staples are used in the hair-bearing areas.

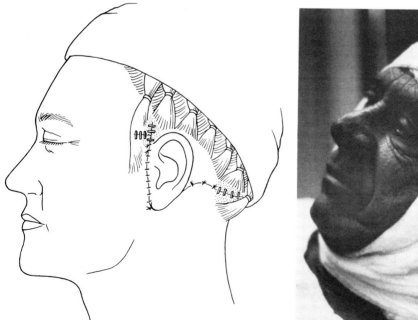

FIG 12–13.
After the flap is completely sutured and stapled down.

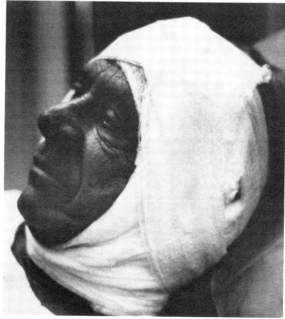

FIG 12–14.
A full, firm, bulky dressing is constructed to provide pressure and to protect the suture lines and the flap.

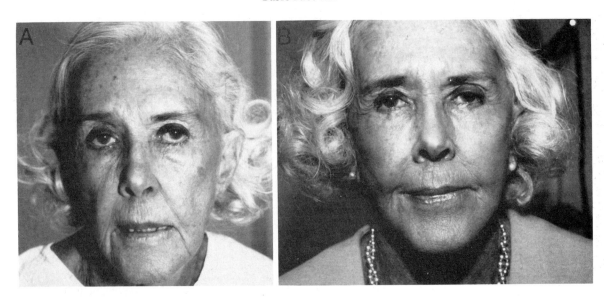

FIG 12–15.
A, woman, 63 years old, before surgery. **B**, 2 months after a face- and neck-lift.

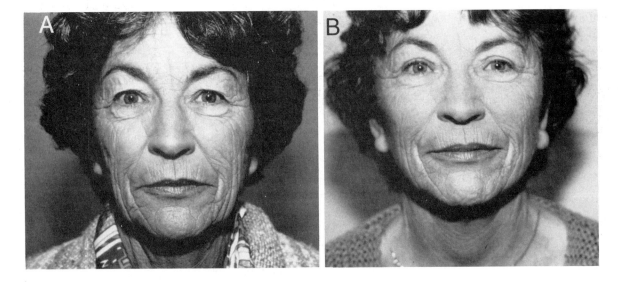

FIG 12–16.
A, woman, 57 years old, before surgery. **B**, 3 months after a face-lift and conservative upper lid blepharoplasty. These pictures show the correction of the gravity changes, but also show that this woman needs a chemical peel to correct the sun-damaged skin.

on the SMAS in the primary lift. A little more undermining and dissection of the scar sheet may be necessary to take advantage of it in several directions — at the cheek, jawline, and neck. Estimate how much of the sheet can be excised so that it can be pulled tightly but still closed.

Excise that strip of scar and close side to side with permanent sutures. Drape the skin over the incision, trim as needed, and close the skin.

In their consultations with patients, any number of surgeons discuss face-lifting as a two-staged operation. Certainly all face-lift surgeons know that a re-do some months or years later will have the advantage of utilizing the scar tissue as a second SMAS for strong subcutaneous fixation.[18, 19]

Combined Procedures

It is regular practice to combine a face-lift with a blepharoplasty, a brow-lift, facial implants, and a rhinoplasty. Whether or not to combine procedures depends on the patient's wishes and the doctor's stamina. However, there is one combination of procedures of which we strongly disapprove. That is a lift and a perioral dermabrasion or peel. We can understand how physicians get talked into that combination. The patient hates the perioral radial lines (and does not see in the mirror other sun-induced wrinkles or lines) and wants them corrected at the same time the lift is done. The physician knows it is not wise to perform peels and dermabrasions on skin that may be undermined during the lift. However, the doctor tries to appease the patient by offering to treat the cutaneous upper lip with a peel or dermabrasion during the lift.

The result is that same horrible result that any spot dermabrasion or peel on sun-damaged skin can produce. The demarcation line between the treated and untreated skin is striking, even if a color differentation does not develop — and it usually does. If patients need treatment for sun-damaged skin, they most likely need it on more than just the upper lip, which is the only area that can be treated simultaneously with a lift. Tell patients they will need a second procedure which can be performed three to six months later, and stick to your advice.

Complications

Some papers indicate that the complications of rhytidectomy are as high as 20%, while others report 4%. Regardless, either number is significant (Table 12–1). Although we doctors may look at complications as an expected risk a certain percentage of the time, and manage them much the same as we manage problems after nonelective or noncosmetic surgery, the patient's original reason for coming to us was to look

TABLE 12–1.
Complications of Rhytidectomy

Bleeding
Skin slough
Nerve damage
Hair loss
Asymmetry
Infection

better. If a complication interferes, it is a serious delay or obstruction to a goal for which the patient has sacrificed time and money. The first rule for treating complications from cosmetic surgery is availability and the second is deep concern. If your are so concerned that the patient feels the need to tell you, "It's not that bad, doctor," then you have properly communicated your feelings.

Bleeding

An expanding or large hematoma should be opened and drained as soon as it is discovered. The areas must be irrigated, the bleeder identified, and the wound closed. It is best to see patients whenever they call to report what sounds like bleeding. If it turns out to be just an edge, so much the better. If it is a large hematoma and you did not see it at the first call, any further damage from the pressure such as flap necrosis, nerve damage, or toxic substance release as it organizes becomes your direct responsibility. For a procedure as complex as a face-lift, failure to discover aspirin ingestion, a tendency to bleed, or use of anticoagulants prior to surgery are serious physician errors.

Skin Slough

Both large and small sloughs may develop in the first 7 to 10 days postrhytidectomy.[20] Small sloughs about 1 to 2 cm may develop around a suture line when the skin has been under tension or rotated at that point. Small areas may show up when the skin is thin and at the tip of a large flap, such as over the mastoid or postauricular area. These areas usually heal without much trouble or sequalae.

Large areas — 4 to 8 cm — develop most commonly over the angle of the jaw or behind the ear over the mastoid. There are many theoretical causes and most are probably true in one patient or another: skin flaps dissected too thin, acute angles in the postauricular incision design that leave narrow pedicles, pressure from instruments or fingers during the surgery and hematomas afterwards, excessive tension on flaps and at suture sites, improperly placed dressings, pressure from head position on pillows, and smoking.

The evidence that smoking causes slough is fairly well documented. Rees et al. proved the higher incidence of sloughs in smokers,[21] and Webster et al. traced out the scientific papers that identify the mechanism.[22] The evidence is adequate to ask patients to stop smoking before and for several weeks after a lift or, if there are other possible complications, not to lift a patient who smokes.

Nerve Damage

Fortunately, most nerve injuries are temporary, self-limiting, partial paralyses. Weakness of the lower lip is more common when the platysma is transected or when liposuction has been performed along the jaw. Permanent nerve injury is more common (although most uncommon) when the dissection is under the SMAS or anterior to the anterior edge of the parotid gland. Undermining in the temple region sometimes transects the temporal branch of cranial VII.

Because the skin is so adherent at the anterior inferior edge of the mastoid, it is not uncommon to transect some of the cutaneous sensory branches of the greater auricular nerve. This leaves a nearly permanent numbness over an area inferior to the lobe. This problem is a small bother, but better tolerated by a patient who has been forewarned. This paresthesia may resolve with the passing of many months or years.

Hair Loss

Permanent or temporary hair loss in the temple region anterior to the incision line is found in as many as 15% of face-lift patients. If the incision stops at the top of the ear or turns posteriorly or anteriorly on a horizontal plane, the incidence is nearly zero. It is doubtful that there is direct trauma to the follicles from undermining. Instead, it is a traction alopecia that shows up some months after the procedure. The hairs thin or fall out completely.

Hair loss seems to bother patients inordinately. We have seen more than a few women distraught about the loss of hair, yet they have to pull their hair back to show us the problem. It is difficult to repair this hair loss. Transplants help a few, but it is hard to recreate the density and the natural curved and tapering hairline. Nondelayed hair-bearing scalp flaps turned down from above the ear or from the temple build a better hairline and are well-tolerated by women. Such flaps are possible only on men who have appropriate hair density and pattern. We have not tried minoxidil for this problem.

Asymmetry

There are several steps in the operation where obvious asymmetry can result: any work with the SMAS or platysma can fall or not be even. If the skin flaps are pulled and rotated differently, redundancies and sags become different on the two sides. Trimming and reshaping the earlobes must be carefully done so they hang the same.

If there is gross asymmetry, a second procedure should be done to correct it. If it is only a matter of skin laxity, time may even things out. If it is obvious that the plication or imbrication sutures did not hold on one side, open the flap and try again.

Infection

This rare event after face-lift usually responds to the appropriate antibiotics. Do not forget the old aid of applying heat to the infected area. It speeds resolution and gives patients something to do to contribute to their recovery.

References

1. Guerrero-Santos J, et al: Muscular lift in cervical rhytidoplasty. *Plast Reconstr Surg* 1974; 54:127–131.
2. Skoog T: *Plastic Surgery: New Methods and Refinements*. Philadelphia, WB Saunders, 1974.
3. Mitz V, Peyronie M: The superficial musculoaponeurotic system (SMAS) in the parotid and cheek area. *Plast Reconstr Surg* 1976; 58:80–88.
4. McCollough EG, Perkins SW, Langsdon PR: SMAS suspension rhytidectomy: Rationale and long term experience. Presented at American Academy of Facial and Reconstructive Surgeons spring meeting, May 10, 1986, Palm Beach.
5. Webster RC, Smith RC, Papsidero MJ, et al: Comparison of SMAS plication with SMAS imbrication in face lifting. *Laryngoscope* 1982; 92:901–912.
6. deCastro CC: The role of the superficial musculoaponeurotic system in face lift. *Ann Plast Surg* 1986; 16:279–286.
7. Owsley JQ: Platysma-facial rhytidectomy: A preliminary report. *Plast Reconstr Surg* 1977; 59:843–850.
8. Owsley JQ: SMAS-platysma face lift. *Plast Reconstr Surg* 1983; 71:573–576.
9. Ellenbrogen R: Pseudoparalysis of the mandibular branch of the facial nerve after platysmal face lift operation. *Plast Reconstr Surg* 1979; 63:364.
10. Kamer FM, Hunter D: The two layer, four flap rhytidecomy technique. *Laryngoscope* 1981; 16:829–832.
11. Mallard DR: A challenge to the undefeated nasolabial fold. *Plast Reconstr Surg* 1987; 80:37–46.
12. Newman J, Fallick H: Lipo-suction tunneling in conjunction with rhytidectomy. *Am J Cosmetic Surg* 1984; 1:28–32.
13. Teimourian B: Face and neck suction-assisted lipectomy associated with rhytidectomy. *Plast Reconstr Surg* 1983; 72:627–633.
14. Aronsohn RB: Lipo-suction of the naso-labial fold: A preliminary report. *Am J Cosmetic Surg* 1984; 1:22–27.
15. Luikart R: The "Iconoclast" a superb instrument for undermining. *J Dermatol Surg Oncol* 1978; 6:274–277.
16. Kamer FM, Garcia MA: A head drape for rhytidectomy. *Laryngoscope* 1978; 88:2036–2038.
17. Pitanguy I: Face lift. AAFPRS meeting. Indianapolis, Indiana, March 1988.
18. Kamer FM: Sequential rhytidectomy and two stage concept. *Otolaryngol Clin North Am* 1980; 13:305–319.
19. Anderson JR: The tuck-up operation, a new technique of secondary rhytidectomy. *Arch Otolaryngol* 1975; 101:739–743.
20. Fredricks S, Faires R: Postauricular skin slough in cervical facial rhytidectomy. *Ann Plast Surg* 1988; 16:195–200.
21. Rees TD, Liverett DM, Guy CL: The effect of cigarette smoking on skin flap survival in the face lift patient. *Plast Reconstr Surg* 1985; 73:911–914.
22. Webster RC, Kazada G, Hamdan US, et al: Cigarette smoking and face lift: Conservative versus wide undermining. *Plast Reconstr Surg* 1986; 77:596–602.
23. Tardy ME, Klingensmith M: Face-lift surgery: Principles and variations, in *Dermatologic Surgery* Roenigk RK, Roenigk HH (eds) New York; Marcel Dekker, Inc., 1988.

Thirteen

Liposuction

This relatively new surgical procedure has from its inception caught the interest of dermatologic surgeons. Some of the first physicians to visit the French and Italian originators of the technique were U.S. dermatologists. Initially, fear of fluid-balance problems forced surgeons to undertake the procedure only in a hospital operating suite until Illouz' "wet technique" and refinements in local anesthesia infusion became a reality. After only a few years' experience with extensive infiltration of a local anesthesia cocktail, liposuction surgery has become a safe and effective *outpatient* procedure. Because it involves only skin and subcutaneous fat, because it is a local-anesthesia procedure, and because additional surgical procedures are not necessary in conjunction with it, liposuction is a natural addition to a cosmetic dermatologic surgery practice.

History

Dr. Josef Schrudde, professor of plastic surgery in Cologne, West Germany, curetted fat from hips, thighs, knees, and ankles through a small incision. He presented his work in 1972 at the meeting of the International Society of Aesthetic Plastic Surgery in Rio de Janeiro. The description of his early work states that after the incision, a tunnel was formed by scissors 1 cm below the skin surface. Fatty tissue was removed from both sides of the tunnel, first by small and then by larger curettes. Remaining particles of fat were removed by irrigation and suction. He called this procedure "lipexeresis," from the Latin for "removal of fat."[1]

It was Giorgio Fischer in Rome who developed special instruments for fat removal. First, he developed a planotome, which created an intra-adipose plane about 9 to 13 mm below the skin surface. Second, he made the cellusactiotome, which removed fat with a grinding motion that chipped fat in a way similar to quarry mining. This instrument had a blunt tip, a blunt opening, and suction (all of which proved to be correct) although the cutting apparatus made this a sharp instrument. Cutting fat creates a pocket within the transected tissues which leads to excessive seroma and hematoma formation. The story is told that when Fischer visited Illouz and Fournier in Paris and realized that tunnel formation was all that was necessary, he went back to Rome and discarded the cutting part of his instrument.[2] He later described these changes in his equipment.[3]

In the mid-1970s, Kesselring of Lausanne, Switzerland, also published his work, which added suction to a 40-cm-long cannula that had a tapered tip and a cutting surface on the opening.[4] The sharp cutting of fat has since been found to be too traumatic and thus is not part of present-day liposuction. However, Dr. Kesselring used the instrument differently. He would treat trochanteric fat by putting the cannula right on top of the tensor fasciae latae with the opening upward. He would carefully shave and aspirate fat at the same time. He then put on a tight dressing which stayed in place for two weeks.[5] His patient selection, technique, and follow-up probably eliminated the problems others have had with a sharp instrument.

Yves-Gerard Illouz in Paris knew of Fischer's technique and also of his instruments, but was not able to obtain them easily in France. He therefore used what was available to him — the high-powered Berkely suction machine used for obstetrical work, and a Karman cannula, which was blunt-tipped and had a blunt opening. He also used that instrument in the only way he could, creating tunnels through the fat.[6] Thus, all the elements were in place for the birth of modern liposuction surgery.

Once the news of fat suctioning spread beyond France and Italy, cosmetic surgeons the world around became interested, as did instrument manufacturers. First came the pilgrimages to France, where physicians of all specialties and all nations were welcomed, and then invitations were issued to the originators to present and teach in the U.S. Liposuction surgery went into a logarithmic growth phase, and is one of the most frequently performed cosmetic surgeries today.

With this procedure, the genesis of which can be closely documented, the silliness of the so-called turf battles among various specialities performing cosmetic surgery is completely exposed. Whether or not one group had the better invited speaker two weeks or two months before the other hardly gives that group the right to proclaim primacy and thus ownership of a technique. Practioners who have had the most deaths and the most grievous complications from liposuction have most frequently been the very specialists who insist that a doctor from any other discipline is unqualified to perform liposuction. Dermatologists have had an excellent record in the progress of liposuction: we have a sterling safety record, we have significantly contributed to the refinement of the technique, and we have encouraged the outpatient performance of the operation.

Equipment

The critical features are blunt-tipped can-

nulas, no cutting surfaces, and suction. Among instruments, however, there are many variations. The central direction of the changes has been toward smaller-diameter cannulas and less-traumatic cannula tips. At first, stronger suction machines were recommended, but now that feature seems less important as operating room wall suction and even syringes have been shown to be effective (although some physicians still prefer strong suction). Once liposuction, like so many operations, was understood, it was realized that good results could be obtained in various ways.

The cannula tips were originally quite blunt; cannulas were 6 to 8 mm diameter measured on the outside walls. These instruments were so hard to push through the fat that surgeons went to the gymnasium to strengthen their muscles for the procedure. Liposuction was the only surgical procedure that required more physician exertion than cardiopulmonary resuscitation. Rapidly, improved cannulas came on the market. It was not unusual during the first five years that liposuction was performed in this country to have cannulas become completely out-of-date within one year. The tips became less blunt, though never sharp, and some were tapered in one axis (spatula type) or two (tapered type). The number and shape of the openings ranged from one ventral port to three, from partial to nearly open front ends, and with the growth of the "wet technique," the diameters routinely used were smaller — 4 to 6 mm. These changes greatly reduced the work (and the trauma) and increased the efficiency of liposuction. The number of ports and their location must influence the efficiency of fat removal, but with individual stroke variations in speed and repetitions the number probably makes no practical difference. For large-volume removal of fat, such as from a big abdomen or thigh, a cannula of 6 mm diameter, with the front end partially open and with two or three ventral ports, will pull a lot of fat out quickly. For more subtle work such as on the ankles or knees and for feathering the edges of an area, smaller and less efficient instruments are indicated.

The handle end of the cannula also has many variations. There are detachable handles so the suction end of the cannula can be changed with-

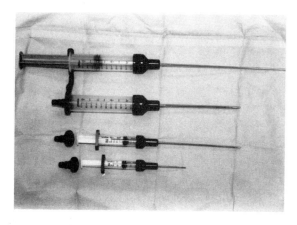

FIG 13–1.
The Tulip design by Pierre Fournier for syringe liposuction.

out changing the connection of the suction hose. These cannula tips snap on and off or screw in, and give the surgeon the ability to quickly change cannula diameter and length as needed. Some of the detachable handles are designed for disposable shafts which may be of more value than they first appear because the cannulas are not easy to clean well. Many of the cannulas are not polished on the inside walls, which means that the metal is porous. It is further gouged by passing brushes through the tube. The design of cannulas in the future will include better inside polishing and finishing and better ways to get them completely clean. The handles vary in grip size and design, but all have a thumb indicator to signal the position of the opening(s), which should be down. A variation is a Swan-necked handle which is designed to help the physician keep the length of the cannula parallel to the skin surface yet provide plenty of hand room so the knuckles clear the skin surface easily.

The syringe method will be discussed below. There are specially designed systems for this technique (Fig 13–1). The disposable syringes are locked into holders that attach to cannulas or fit into cannulas designed with a proximal end to fit onto the syringe. There is a range of cannula lengths, widths, and tip designs comparable to machine systems. There are also adapters that allow aerobic and sterile transfer of fat from the collection syringe to other syringes for use in fat grafting.

The first requirement for the suction ma-

chines was bigger, stronger, faster suction. The dead space and airflow needed to draw a vacuum when a 40-cm-long, 8-mm wide cannula was used demanded a powerful machine. As physicians developed techniques which called for pulling the cannula out and repositioning it, the machine also had to develop a vacuum quickly. Industry responded, and several companies built reliable and powerful suction machines. We have tried and used several different brands of machines and all seem adequate. It becomes a matter of personal choice, and of how it sounds, and of how many whistles, buttons, and lights it has to make the physician happy. The question most recently asked is how much of a vacuum is really needed — .75 or .5 of .25 of an atmosphere? Smaller-diameter cannulas and closed systems need less suction power. This part of the procedure is very much in flux as this text is being written.

Equipment for local anesthesia will be discussed below. Dressings have changed and improved in the past five to seven years. There has been no question from the beginning — even though the theories of what is actually happening to the fat have changed — that the treated areas need even and firm support that lasts from the time of surgery to several weeks afterward. At first the suctioned areas were taped, but it was soon realized that form-fitting garments were both easier to remove and more comfortable than tape. We settled on the French elastoplaste (distributed as Elastoplast in the U.S. by Smith and Nephew) as our favorite brand.

An area of improvement is the availability and design of tight-fitting garments. Depending on the volume of liposuction done, it is wise to have several sizes and shapes of garments available to put on the patient immediately after the procedure. The cost of the garment is built into the fee and the doctor has the luxury of knowing the garment fits properly and supports the treated area well. Many companies show their garments at meetings and they are no longer any problem to buy.

We now tape abdomens, thighs, and love handles and put the patient immediately into a tight garment. The tapes come off in a week and the garments stay on for a month. For knees, ankles, and submental fat, we use the tape.

The specific instruments and equipment for liposuction surgery mentioned above are available and highly advertised in medical journals, and because of the competition, priced fairly. The rest of the equipment needed depends on the type of anesthesia used and the volume of fat to be removed. The room where liposuction surgery is done should be a designated surgery large enough to accommodate the level of sterility necessary. Assistants need to be trained in sterile preparation of themselves, the room, and the patient, including cleansing, draping, and gowning. The table must be movable, comfortable, and able to position the patient in a reverse Trendelenburg position if necessary. Lighting must be adequate.

IV capabilities and monitoring equipment commensurate with the level of anesthesia to be used are required. Fluid replacement and colloid supplement depend on the volume of fat removal anticipated and whether the wet or dry technique will be used. We may not start an IV at all, or will start one if the case is going to involve more than 1,500 ml of fat removal. We replace fluids parenterally if the amount is larger than 1,500 ml, if any dissociative drugs are given, if any IV anesthesia is used or if we anticipate the need for IV analgesia. A blood-pressure monitor is used if there is a special reason to expect a problem. A cardiac monitor and finger-pulse oximeter are used on cases involving more than 2,000 ml fat removal of if any IV medications are used.

Heavy twilight anesthesia should be administered by a second physician or a nurse anesthetist; general anesthesia should be administered by an anesthesiologist. Cases of more than 1,500 ml fat removal and with IV medications should be followed appropriately in a designated recovery room (it may be the surgery room) until these patients have recovered and been transported on a gurney or in a wheelchair to the car that waits to take them home. If general anesthesia is used, the facility should meet appropriate standards for general anesthesia.

A large percentage of our cases and indeed a large percentage of all liposuction cases fall into the category of local anesthesia only and involve less than 1,500 ml of fat removed.

Anesthesia

When Illouz first developed the wet technique formula, he included epinephrine for control of hemorrhage. When some surgeons in the United States first tried liposuction, they put the patient under general anesthesia and used the "dry technique."[6] However, problems of fluid and blood loss with the dry technique mandated the use of local anesthesia with epinephrine used more for vasoconstriction than for anesthesia. It was quickly recognized that fat was easily anesthetized, and that a local was fully adequate for small cases such as removal of submental fat or fat from knees. Pierre Fournier and other French liposuctionists realized that local injections were adequate total anesthesia for the procedure.[7, 8] General anesthesia then became a matter of choice for the patient and/or physician as it is today, except in the largest cases or in combined procedures.

Because it is both anesthesia and an important adjunct to fat removal, the wet technique will be discussed here. Illouz probably started this procedure by injecting hypotonic saline into the area to be treated; he called this "lypolysis."[8, 9] His solution was saline, distilled water, and hyaluronidase. The variations of the solutions used for the wet technique were so numerous and so quick to appear that an exact history of their introduction into liposuction surgery is impossible and not really important (unless it is possible that someone has made an important individual contribution, and to that person we apologize). Soon the cocktail contained lidocaine and epinephrine, just like Illouz's original. The formula we settled on and still use today is shown in Table 13–1.

TABLE 13–1.
Wet Technique Anesthetic Solution

Ingredients	for 100 ml	for 1,000 ml
0.9% NaCl	80 ml	800 ml
1.0% lidocaine	6 ml	48 ml
Sterile water	20 ml	160 ml
Epi 1:1000	0.1 ml	0.8 mg
Wydase	100 I.U.	800 I.U.

This formula has one gram of lidocaine in the full liter bag and the epinephrine concentration is 1:1 million. There are variations. Some physicians do not add the hyaluronidase, but we and others who have used it on one side and not on the other are certain it greatly helps the lidocaine and epinephrine disperse evenly through all of the tissues. Some add distilled water for injection or use one-half the normal saline to make it more hypotonic, believing this reduces blood loss. Sodium bicarbonate reduces some of the sting from the lidocaine. Some physicians add less epinephrine. We do not add the Wydase when we use this formula for removing fat we plan to harvest for microlipoinjection (see Chapter 7).

As best we know, early on we and all others injected the fat to be suctioned with this solution through a regular needle, for example a 19- to 21-gauge disposable. We added a three-way stopcock on the syringe and connected one opening to the bag of solution, the other to the syringe, and the third to the needle. We would draw up a syringeful, twist the valve, and inject the solution into the patient. Then we changed to a 50-ml syringe. Next, we added a short IV tube between the syringe and the needle; the assistant would hold the 50-ml syringe and draw up the solution, the doctor would insert the needle when required, and the assistant would depress the plunger. It would take 15 minutes to inject an abdomen.

The next improvement was substituting a McGahn tissue expander filler (McGahn Medical Corporation, Santa Barbara, California) for the syringe and three-way valve (Fig 13–2). This apparatus is a disposable 10-ml spring-loaded, pump-action syringe with a comfortable hand grip, which makes it possible to quickly draw from the bag and inject about 8 ml with each pump stroke. It is rapid and easy and not tiring to anesthetize a large area. A 19-gauge needle or a 3- to 4-inch spinal needle can be attached to this pump.

Klein developed a special instrument for fluid injection and used it for what he called the "tumescent technique" for liposuction surgery.[10] The instrument is made by welding a blunt-tipped 30-cm-long stainless steel needle with an outside diameter of 4-mm and an inside diameter of 1

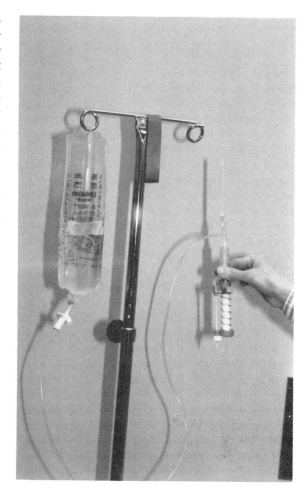

FIG 13–2.
The injection system we use with a McGahn disposable spring-loaded syringe originally designed for filling tissue expanders. The spring-loaded syringe is attached to an IV fluid bag.

mm to 10-cm-long hollow handle which accommodates a 60-ml disposable Luer-Lok syringe. Between the needle and the handle is a fluid-intake port which connects to the bag that contains the local anesthetic solution. A flow-regulator clamp and a check valve are put on the line from the bag, which limits the rate of flow and prevents retrograde flow.

The needle is inserted through the same incisions and infiltration travels along the same pathways intended for the suction cannula. The blunt tip reduces trauma and nearly eliminates the possibility of intravascular injection. The method of passing the needle along the same plane that the cannulas will later pass assures uniform infiltration of anesthetic.

Since Illouz first introduced the wet technique, the trend has been to use more and more solution to fill the fat space. This fluid loading not only provides anesthesia, but it also vasoconstricts and softens the fat, which allows the cannula to penetrate much easier and for the fat to be suctioned out more easily and quickly. The more the fat is fluid-loaded, the more it comes out in a homogeneous, small-particle form. The properly loaded fat flows into the suction tube like a slurry, not in large, dry, fat globules that come out in fits and spurts as with the dry technique.

Having the fluid chilled at refrigerator temperature may help reduce blood loss and actually provide cryoanesthesia. This is the method of Pierre Fournier but our patients complain of the cold and a few actually chill. We have done it with fluid at room temperature or chilled. Both methods seem to work well.

The amounts of fluid cocktail used for various anatomic fat compartments are listed below.

Abdomen	600 to 1,200 ml
Two lateral thighs	600 to 1,000 ml
Two medial thighs	400 to 800 ml
Two love handles	400 to 800 ml
Two knees	300 to 500 ml
Submental area	50 to 150 ml

After an area is loaded, we massage or knead it to spread the fluid evenly throughout. The saddlebag area is deeply massaged and rolled. The abdomenal skin is picked up and rolled between the fingers. This step and a 15- to 20-minute wait ensure good anesthesia and hemostasis. Our patients are so comfortable that we have been using less and less intramuscular analgesia and sometimes none at all. The first few needle sticks hurt, but after that we are injecting through skin that is already partially numbed. If we encounter a bit of fibrosis, we inject a bolus just before it, wait a minute or two, and push on. If the patient has discomfort while we are suctioning, we reinject that area,

move the suction to another spot, and come back later (Fig 13–3).

There are several valuable advantages with the local method. The first, mentioned above, is the even consistency of the removed fat. Next, patients are mobile; they can turn, bend, or roll as the surgeon requests. This is a *great* advantage. When patients are asleep, moving them is difficult and dangerous because of the problems with ventilation, the physical task of moving all the tubes with them, and making sure that in the new position all pressure points are padded. Another advantage is the ability to get the patient up to see what has been taken out. We will discuss below how to test the adequacy of removal, but nothing fully replaces having the patient stand at the side of the table. (Fig 13–4). Symmetry or the lack of it becomes immediately obvious. Also, missed areas are outlined when gravity pulls on the skin. Fluid problems seem to go away when the wet technique is used more vigorously. It has not yet been proven exactly what features of the wet technique lead to the surprisingly little total fluid loss experienced. Surely there is less blood loss as a result of vasoconstriction; the fluid-filled fat area may not be as traumatized as the dry and therefore there is subsequently less serum leakage. Some fluids may be absorbed in a mechanism like clysis.

Blood loss was a much more serious problem

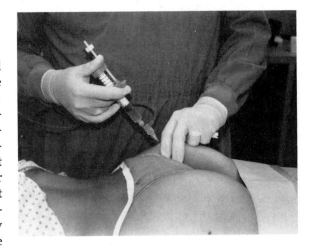

FIG 13–3.
The wet technique anesthetic solution being injected, using the McGahn system.

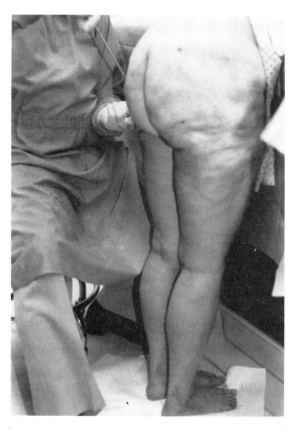

FIG 13–4.
The patient may be asked to stand up during the operation so the effects of gravity can be assessed and symmetry can be achieved by suction.

when the dry technique was first used. Hematocrit reductions of five to seven points after surgery were not uncommon.[19, 20] Careful protocols have been published about fluid and colloid replacement; although these have disappeared recently because of the efficiency of the wet technique. Recent studies have verified that blood loss is only 30 to 50 ml and that patients show little hematocrit loss when it is measured one week later after the fluid system has stabilized.[10, 12] Patients who have had nothing to eat or drink for 12 hours before surgery are already dehydrated. Replacement of fluids and electrolytes may be indicated in cases where more than 1,500 ml has been removed. But with the wet technique cocktail, including epinephrine, blood loss and fluid balance problems seem to be minimized.

One troublesome question about the wet technique — the possible danger of lidocaine toxicity — has nearly been answered. Although no physicians have reported real or apparent lidocaine toxicity when the wet technique was performed, a study appeared in 1987 by Piveral in which he injected 800 mg of 1% lidocaine with epinephrine 1:100,000 subcutaneously and 15 minutes later obtained a central blood level of 4.2 μg/ml. A second patient developed a central blood level of 6.3 μg/ml 15 minutes after 1,350 mg of 0.5% lidocaine was injected. These levels are just below the dysrhythmic level of 5.0 μg/ml blood level. However, the levels fell very rapidly after the first 15 minutes. It was assumed and hoped that the more dilute solutions would not be absorbed as rapidly.[11]

Klein reported that in 26 patients a mean total dose of 1,250 mg of lidocaine (range 825 to 3,100 mg) was infiltrated into the subcutaneous space over a one- to five-hour interval.[10] The mean serum lidocaine level one hour after the completion of infiltration was 0.336 μg/ml and the highest serum level was 0.614 μg/ml. Lillis expanded Klein's study by administering larger volumes of lidocaine and removing more tissue.[12] In his study, 20 patients were given an average of 3,550 mg of lidocaine in the subcutaneous spaces (range 2,000- to 5,600 mg). Blood was drawn 15, 30, and 60 minutes after the completion of infiltration. The highest blood level obtained was 1.7 μg/ml (safe levels are considered to be below 5.0 μg/ml).

These two studies proved well that lidocaine levels do not raise dangerously within the first few hours after injection. But where does the lidocaine go? Skouge partially answered the question by measuring the amount of lidocaine in the aspirant.[13] He found only trace amounts, so it was not simply suctioned back out with the fat. Currently, both Klein and Lillis are checking lidocaine blood levels 6 to 12 hours after the procedure. Early indications show that it peaks at 10 to 12 hours. These levels are still well below the toxic range, but it does answer the question of what happens to the lidocaine. It is very slowly absorbed and excreted in the usual manner. The addition of epinephrine affects the lidocaine levels by causing slower absorption, which peaks at a lower blood level only at 12 to 14 hours. The total amount absorbed is the same with or without epinephrine.

General Technique

Liposuction surgery is a tactile process. A patient may have bulges and pouches that look like they should come off, but until the physician has felt them — has pinched up and actually handled those pouches — it is impossible to predict whether or not they will respond to liposuction. The fat pockets that are best treated are just that — pockets. It is nearly always possible to feel the margins of the pocket that will suction out easily. Ask the patient to do the same. As you pinch up and determine which fat will come out, also have patients do this so they can appreciate what is to be expected. The same technique is used just before surgery to mark the areas. We usually mark with the patient standing, which accentuates all the fat pouches. Be sure the patient sees and agrees with the markings. As discussion progresses through the various anatomic areas, the unique features of each area should be mentioned.

Liposuction is a two-handed operation (Fig 13–5). The right hand (dominant hand) pushes the cannula or syringe. It is the power. It also detects resistance or irregular pressure. The left hand (nondominant hand) is the "smart" hand or the "eyes" for the procedure. The left hand is always just above the tip of the cannula. It feels where the tip is, and determines the distance between it and the tip (which tells how deep or shallow the dissection is progressing).

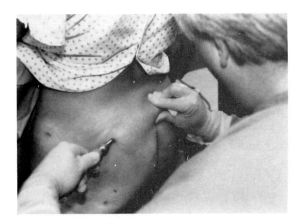

FIG 13–5.
The right hand pushes the cannula and the left hand is the "smart hand" that constantly controls the location of the cannula tip under the skin.

It picks up a fistful of fat and the cannula gradually suctions it away. When it presses its palm flat, it can feel the cannula tip moving below. It also is a stabilizer to hold skin steady. It pinches around on an area already suctioned to test for evenness or missed pockets.

Liposuction requires close attention to the sterility of the procedure. More than for any other operation discussed in this book, full-body draping, full gowning, and proper skin preparation at the entry sites are indicated. Some of the few disastrous complications have been from infections. The patient is asked to shower as usual on the morning of surgery. When the patient comes to the operatory the doctor discusses the procedure (again), checks for changes in the patient's health, makes sure that postoperative care is available, and marks the areas to be suctioned. We generally start the patient on antibiotics orally — cephalosporin, erythromycin, or semisynthetic penicillin. If not done previously, photos are taken — which we recommend. Preoperative medications are given, monitors applied, and the field is cleansed with chlorhexidine (e.g., Hibiclens) which has a long-lasting antibacterial effect. Other antiseptics of choice are certainly acceptable. The patient is draped and the administration of the local anesthesia — the wet technique — is started (see Fig 13–3). It is wise to have several sets of small drapes available, because they will need to be reinforced after the local is given because of leakage. Also, as the patient is turned from side to side, it is good to have fresh drapes to put down.

A tiny incision is made in the skin with a #11 blade. The entry site is determined during the marking and is indicated by a circle rather than a line or dot. That eliminates any chance of tattooing the skin by sticking the scalpel point through the marking ink. Entries are planned so most areas are accessible from two directions. That way, the direction of the cannula strokes will be at nearly 90-degree angles to each other. Once under way, if more openings are necessary, make them. We make the incision with the #11 blade and follow with a hemostat to stretch the opening. This is followed by probing the fat space with scissors or a longer hemostat to be sure we are in the correct pocket. Fournier recommends using an awl to make the opening and then using several dilators to bring it up to size.[14]

The skin is picked up with the left hand, near the opening, and the cannula is inserted. The opening may require a bit more dilation, which can be done by the cannula tip itself. The tip should not be aimed downward toward a viscous or deep structure, but rather toward the palm of the left hand which holds the skin up and away from the body. This provides protection from perforating a deeper structure and gives the freedom to push the cannula in with one smooth movement. The first few strokes are made to establish the proper location of the tip and to check the anesthesia. Some recommend that one to ten strokes be made at each new area before the suction pump is turned on.

At this point we will mention some of the theories about what really happens with liposuction and how those theories relate to proposed techniques. Possibly when looking at tissues that had been suctioned (after an abdomen was first treated with suction, followed by a lipectomy) it was noticed that there were tunnels through the fat. These tunnels were visible only when the skin was picked up above the fat. Thus, the theory that liposuction cannulas only create tunnels by separating fat cells, and when many tunnels are made, the remaining fat collapses around the tunnels and produces the effect. It is our contention that the holes in the fat are just what can be expected from running a cylindrical stick through fat and really are "tunnels." When the treated skin is palpated, the fat is gone — not perforated. When the fatty skin is picked up and the suction cannula is worked through the fat between the fingers (one of the standard techniques), that fat goes. It goes until the fingers almost touch. When an area that has been treated is palpated, if any lumps or thick parts remain, they are resuctioned until smooth. The fat is not tunneled; it is removed. Additionally, damaged fat is also absorbed over several days, postoperatively.

Empirically, experienced liposuction surgeons have reported better results when an area is cannulated from two directions. Because each area for treatment has several entry sites, the cannula tracts overlap at nearly a 90-degree angle. It is understandable that a thin tube wound create and recreate pathways that make it dif-

ficult to suction out the walls of fat between strokes. Coming in another direction certainly increases the amount of fat recoverable from a given area, although not all liposuctionists recommend this. The two-directional method also further disproves the "tunnel" theory.

Giorgio Fischer recently stressed that whenever possible, try to align the direction of the cannula strokes in the vertical axis of the body.[15] He believes this is most important on the saddlebag area. He does not know the reason why it happens, but has the experience to justify his contention that vertical strokes give better results.

For most large pockets, anesthetize a wider area than you estimate will be needed, so the edges can be tapered or feathered. When the edge of a pocket has been adequately suctioned, extend every second or third stroke further into the normal subcutaneous fat. These extensions should be made with cannulas of slightly smaller diameter. This technique reduces a step-off between the treated and untreated areas. The lateral thighs and the gluteal furrow are where this problem arises most.

Antibiotic prophylaxis is the physician's choice. If antibiotics are to be used for prophylaxis, the drug should be in the patient's body before the surgeon is. Broad-spectrum antibiotics of choice are acceptable. Because there have been a few infections and because infection can become overwhelming before the first symptoms appear, it is not unwise to have the patient start the antibiotics on the day of surgery or to give IM cephalosporins before the surgery begins.

Preoperative laboratory work may include a CBC, SMA 18 or 24, UA, and evaluation of the clotting system with platelets, prothrombin time, fibrinogen levels, and clotting time, depending on the patient's history. If the patient is younger than 45 years old, only a hemoglobin assay is necessary.

Suction Machine vs. Syringe Suction

Following the suggestion of Fournier, the use of a syringe to provide suction to harvest or collect the fat has become popular.[14, 16, 17] The proponents of syringe liposuction tell us that all of the same areas and the same-sized cases are treated just as well without the machine pump. Anesthesia is by infiltration. Cannulas recommended are from the smaller end of the scale: 3.0 and 4.0 mm in external diameter for the trunk, and even smaller ones for the face and neck. The cannulas have the same design requirements: blunt tip, ventral ports, and no sharp edges. The length is the same—15 to 24 cm.

After the site is numbed, a small incision or opening is made. A few ml of saline are drawn into the syringe to eliminate the dead space so that when the plunger is pulled, the suction is full and instantaneous. The saline also cushions the first fat harvested in the event that it is to be used for fat grafting. The cannula is inserted and the plunger pulled. The plunger can be held by hand, which is not too difficult, or held out with a locking mechanism. Some of the holders have a specially designed lock or a metal ratchet that flips onto the plunger stem to hold it out; a hole is easily drilled so that a metal rod can be pushed through; or, a needle can be pushed through the soft plastic. The vacuum created by the syringe is just as effective as the vacuum created by a powerful pump. The pump must work against a huge dead space in the cannula, the tubing, and the bottle, whereas the syringe has no dead space as soon as a little saline is drawn up. Stroking begins at once, and the fat flows easily into the syringe. When the syringe is full, it is replaced or emptied.

An advantage of the syringe is that less equipment is necessary: no pump or tubing are required. The cannulas may be easier to clean completely on the inside. Also, the fat harvested is less traumatized and better for fat grafting. It is practical for two physicians to work, because two pumps are not necessary, and achieving symmetry is easy because the volumes extracted are more readily measured. Proponents like the control they have with the light weight and the lack of long hoses. They believe they can sculpt and not so much suction fat as extract it.

Specific Areas for Liposuction

Specific areas for liposuction are listed in Table 13–2.

TABLE 13–2.
Areas for Liposuction

Abdomen
Thighs
Buttocks
"Love handles"
Knees
Ankles
Breasts
Face and neck

The Abdomen

Many patients develop abdominal fat that is external to the abdominal muscles and highly resistant to diet and exercise. To assess this pocket, pinch from one side across the abdomen to the other side. The pocket will be definable and the skin on both sides will have less pinchable subcutaneous fat. The thickness of the skin on the sides will be the endpoint of liposuction. If this skin is also thick, realize — and share this with the patient — that this patient has both a fat pocket over the abdomen and generalized fatty skin. Also test to determine how much fat is superficial to the abdominal musculature and how much is behind it. At the same time, examine muscle tone and shape. Obviously, the fat in the omentum behind the atonic muscles or a naturally protuberant abdominal muscle wall will not be helped by liposuction of subcutaneous fat.

Skin tone affects the outcome of all liposuction, but makes more of a difference in some areas. The abdomen is one of these. If patients want a better profile *in clothing*, abdominal suctioning usually works. If they hope to look better in a bathing suit, however, the skin must tone up. Age is not the absolute prognosticator, but generally as patients get older, the skin becomes more slack. For most areas treated by liposuction, the skin will tighten up adequately or so little actual change in skin size will occur that there will be no problem. The abdomen, however, may need a combined or — even better — two procedures: liposuction and abdominal lipectomy. In the latter operation, excess skin and fat are excised and the whole abdominal apron is reduced. It is a major operation with attendant complications and scarring. It also carries the highest incidence of embolic phenomenon when the liposuction and the abdominoplasty are done concurrently.[18]

The fat superior to the umbilicus is often more difficult to extract than the fat that is inferior to it. It is technically more difficult to remove this fat because on some patients the skin above the navel in the V of the rib cage is not easy to pick up. Also, the inferior border of the diaphragm may be low and have little overlying muscle protection. Before liposuction was fully understood, diaphragmatic perforations occasionally occurred with abdominal liposuction.

One or several entry sites through the umbilicus used to be the favorite approach for abdominal liposuction, and there is nothing wrong with that portal today. Now, two lateral suprapubic entries are more often used (Fig 13–6). Suprapubic entries make it easier to suction the fat around the navel itself. This was hard to do through a navel entry site because the portals on the cannula can slip out of the skin as it is stroked and suction can be lost. The bilateral portals also provide easy access for criss-crossing the field.

The abdomen is one area where it is especially important to keep the cannula on a horizontal plane. Most physicians pick up the skin away from the abdominal wall and suction between their fingers. If the skin is not loose enough to do that, upward pressure should be kept on the tip so that it follows a course under the skin and does not dive to or through the peritoneum. Holding the tip upward is tiring on the surgeon's wrist, but necessary. Fischer designed the swan-neck cannula for just this problem. It is easier to keep the swan-neck cannula tip parallel with the skin surface without as much wrist pressure. Doing the abdomen with the patient under only local anesthesia provides added protection: if the cannula tip goes below the numbed fat, the patient will feel it and complain. It can be much easier to perforate the peritoneum or diaphragm with the patient asleep.

The results of abdominal liposuction have been gratifying (Fig 13–7, A and B). If the patient has one of those little weight-reduction-resistant pockets, it can be removed and the patient is back in a bikini. If there is a thick layer of fat across the abdomen, the patient has a better profile in clothes and more choice of clothing.

Thighs, Lateral and Medial, and the Bermuda Triangle

The lateral thigh area is one of the best for happy results from liposuction. The congenital/familial fat pocket over the trochanteric head of the femur, extending down the lateral thigh and/or around into the gluteal furrow, seems to be almost a separate anatomic structure. It appears on some young women during the teens even before they put down other secondary sex-related fat deposits. It makes it necessary for some women to have different clothing sizes for their upper and lower bodies, and it makes the silhouette from behind look lumpy, too broad, and unattractive. Although patients may be slightly dissatisfied with the symmetry or amount of fat taken out, their exuberance after saddle-bag removal is high (Fig 13–8). From the surgeon's point of view, it is pure cosmetic artistry because

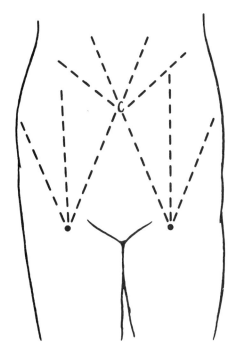

FIG 13–6.
Entry sites and direction of cannula strokes on the abdomen.

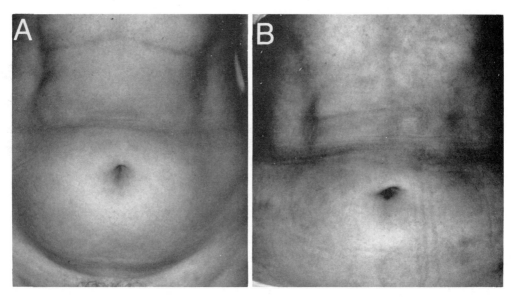

FIG 13–7.
A, woman, 44 years old, before liposuction surgery on the abdomen. **B**, 4 months after surgery.

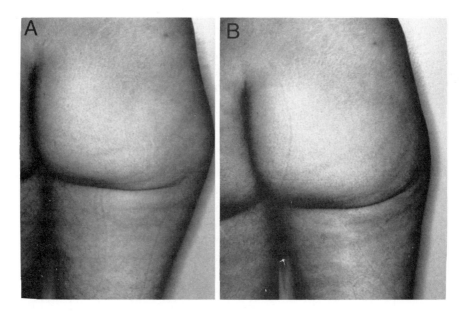

FIG 13–8.
A, woman, 29 years old, before liposuction of the hips. **B**, 10 weeks after surgery.

the lateral thigh fat overlies the tensor fascia lata — there is a strong, almost impenetrable, protective (in this case) sheet, there is almost no other anatomy of any consequence, and the fat pocket is fairly well-defined.

When examining a patient for liposuction on the lateral thighs, the pinch technique works for much of the examination. There is usually a sharp step-off at the edge of the fat pocket and the commonly ample subcutaneous fat over the rest of the thigh. Be sure the wideness of the hips indicates fat and not a widely splayed ilium. The patient must palpate the iliac crest with you so that no change in the bony pelvis will be expected. The only complicated area is an extension of the fat pocket onto the posterior thigh just inferior to the gluteal furrow. There may be a mount of fat running from the inferior gluteal furrow superiorly and laterally to join the trochanteric fat pad. Particularly when it is palpated and outlined with the fingers, this area feels like, is shaped like, and is appropriately called "the banana." When the patient stands, it does not always show. Therefore, the patient is asked to bend at the waist, and this stretches the skin of the back and buttocks enough to outline the banana. Another maneuver (both should be done) is to have the patient pinch the gluteal muscles together. This action will define the gluteal crease more sharply, which then accentuates the infragluteal fold of fat. If this feature is not discovered and treated, it will be very obvious after the lateral thigh fat is removed.

Some patients have huge thighs that have no real definition among the anterior, lateral, and posterior fat pockets. Actually, no pockets are discernible, but instead, there is a seemingly continuous layer of fat that encircles the entire thigh. These people can be helped, but success is relative. The thigh can be reduced but it will still be large, and there is no natural stopping place as there is when the lateral thigh fat is in a well-defined pocket. Also, skin so stretched does not tighten adequately. Removing fat on the anterior and posterior surfaces of the thigh seldom produces great-looking legs. Liposuction can be done to reduce some bulk and to prevent the thighs from rubbing together, but those are the only realistic goals.

For the extremely large patient, liposuction is even less helpful. A few protuberant lumps can be removed, but these patients will remain very large. Experience has helped all surgeons realize that liposuction is not a procedure for reducing the patient's weight or size, but for refining the patient's shape. Experience has also shown that removing great amounts of fat (4,000 to 6,000 ml) is accompanied by difficult-to-manage fluid imbalances and also by massive skin redundancy.

The fat of the medial thigh is soft, but so is the overlying skin. Thus, it is more difficult to obtain a smooth-appearing medial thigh after suction unless the skin is almost as thick as it is over the lateral thigh. Patients like to grab a fistful of skin and fat on the upper medial thighs and say "This is what I want removed." That is a fair request but not so easy to respond to. When that fat is suctioned, the skin becomes slack and tones up slowly or never. We are not saying this area should not be suctioned, but be sure you and the patient consider the problems that will occur when this thin skin remains loose.

The "Bermuda triangle" is an isosceles triangle with its base on a verticle line of the lateral thigh; the superior arm crosses the edge of the buttock and the inferior arm crosses the infragluteal furrow to meet at the apex on the gluteal furrow at about the midbuttocks line. (This triangle crosses the banana but is a different problem.) Liposuction surgeons appreciate — and are appreciated for — the salutary changes they make on patients' shapes. One figure fault deformity we have tried to correct is the "saggy butt," (what else to call it?). It seems as though it should be easy to run the cannula in the gluteal crease and make it deeper, thereby creating a nice smile and deeper furrow.

It turns out, however, that this may be exactly the wrong thing to do. The furrow is most likely created by fibrous bands that hold the skin in that area, and suctioning creates the very real risk of breaking the very bands that are accomplishing what you are trying to achieve. This theory is supported by the fact that several surgeons have been unhappily surprised to find that their gluteal fold suctioning has produced more sagginess than was present before. Thus, the danger zone — the Bermuda triangle. This area has so traumatized Giorgio Fischer that he now recommends that no suction be performed in the triangle.

Analysis of saggy buttocks reveals several causes. A shallow or lacking gluteal furrow is one. If suctioning produces no response, garments designed to crease this area are probably the best answer. Another cause is gluteal muscles that may be undertoned and hanging. A trip to the gym may help some patients, although we have seen ballet dancers with saggy butts. Excess fat that overlies the gluteals may weigh it down, and this problem can be helped

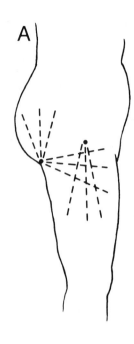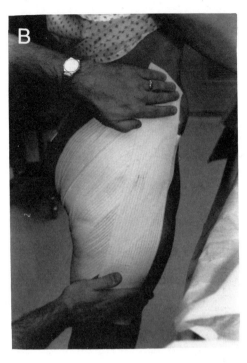

FIG 13–9.
A, entry sites and direction of cannula strokes on the thigh. **B**, the thighs after taping.

with liposuction.

The liposuction surgeon is bombarded by questions from the public and the lay press about "cellulite." This puckered and wavy skin is found on the thighs, almost exclusively in women, and more frequently on heavier thighs. As best we can tell, cellulite is an individual variation on the fat septae attachments to the undersurface of the skin. Weight gain and fat deposition probably aggravate and emphasize it. On many patients, it may be caused only by the septae and not aggravated by any external events. The fakers have tried to make something out of this condition and promise cures through the use of creams, exercises, or special diets. If the puckers and waves are accentuated by fat, removal of the fat may reduce or relieve the appearance. If septae are the cause, the liposuction cannula may transect some of them and help. However, the very success of liposuction is the removal of fat without trauma to the other structures such as nerves, vessels, and septae.

The patient should be marked while standing and the markings should include a gradual feathering. The entry sites are high on the tro-

chanteric area under the bikini line, and for the banana and for criss-crossing the thigh, somewhere in the gluteal furrow (Fig 13–9, A and B). The operation is fortunately straightforward: the anesthesia is not too painful, the access is good through those two portals, the patient moves easily from side to side, and by lying on the side completed provides good hemostasis for it while the other side is treated. When liposuction is done in these areas, we can happily stand the patient up to compare the two sides and also to check the fat pocket, which moves with different leg positions. Once the patient is cleaned up, a firm-fitting garment — panty-girdle-shaped — is pulled on, or the area taped, or both, and the patient walks out. The patient is also advised to cut the crotch out of the garment so it does not need to be removed except for showering. During the first few days when the skin is sore, patients appreciate not having to remove the garment frequently.

Buttocks

First determine if there is excess fat over the

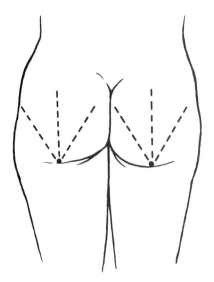

FIG 13–10.
Entry sites and direction of cannula strokes on the buttocks.

gluteals by pinching them and by having the patients tighten the muscles. The fat is not as compartmentalized over the buttocks as it is in other areas, and is more or less very thickened, subcutaneous fat. The fat needs to be thick enough so that the cannula will fit between the muscles and the necessary layer of fat that will be left.

The entry sites are in the gluteal crease at the midline of both buttocks (Fig 13–10). The

cannula strokes are directed superiorly and fan across the entire buttock. Even though the buttock may be large and fatty, the skin is often thin. Be careful to leave an adequate fatty cushion for function and cosmesis. Work hard to leave an even layer of subcutaneous fat (Fig 13–11). This area remains sore for a long time after suction, and patients may want to wear the support garments for several months.

Love Handles

We really do not know a better name for these rolls of fat at the waist, and this term is so well-known that we expect everyone knows what we are talking about. Patients frequently request liposuction in this area, and it is a common request from men. Many men have love handles even though they are otherwise in perfect trim and have flat abdomens. It is difficult to impossible to dermine clinically how much of the roll is fat and how much is skin. Even if a lot of fat is palpable, the skin is so heavy that the results may take months to realize, and of course the operation does nothing for redundant skin.

The entry site is at the mid-lower back bilaterally. The cannulas are worked around the sides in the love-handle roll. The fat is fibrous and does not come out easily. Here more than in any other area, repeated stroking is necessary.

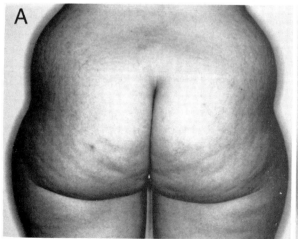
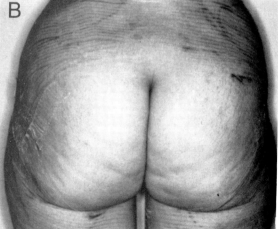

FIG 13–11.
A, woman, 34 years old, before liposuction surgery on the buttocks. **B,** 14 days after surgery.

Also, the operation may best be performed with the patient seated and the physician working from the back and side. If the operation is done with the patient lying on the side, be sure to ask the patient to sit up to check for symmetry and completeness. If the rolls extend anteriorly, second entry sites from the front may be helpful. There is no single best type of instrument to use, only whatever works: large-diameter, small-diameter, open-tipped, or closed-tipped.

After surgery, the area can be taped, or a back-brace-type of garment will be satisfactory. Most patients will want to wear the garment for several weeks to reduce the soreness. When the area is healed, it may be as long as 6 to 12 months before the final result is seen. Suctioning love handles is a good and safe operation, but the work is hard and the results are slow to appear.

Knees

The fat pockets on the medial knees are a good place for a beginning liposuctionist. The pockets are well-defined and the fat comes out easily. The fat is whiter and less dense than abdominal or thigh fat, for example. Some patients have a fat medial thigh that extends to and becomes part of the medial knee fat, but these are exceptions. Usually, the bulge on the medial knees is discrete. In women patients, even if the upper thigh is large, improving the shape of the knee is helpful because it allows these patients to wear knee length skirts instead of only long skirts.

Liposuction is not limited to the medial pad. The suprapatellar fat pad is often excessive. This area also suctions well but because it is not as sharply demarcated, more judgment is called for when deciding just how much fat to take out. To help you sculpture the suprapatellar area, talk with patients about what bothers them specifically.

The anesthesia and wet techniques are the same as described elsewhere (Figs 13–12 and 13–13). A small incision is made on the medial calf just inferior to the lower edge of the pad. A small cannula is inserted and the fat flows out quickly and easily. We often use a 3-mm short cannula or even a microcannula for the suprapatellar area. The knee is an area we still tape, and close-fitting

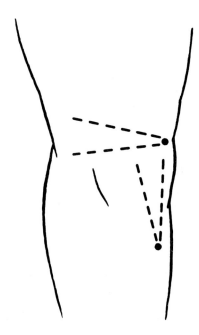

FIG 13–12.
Entry sites and direction of cannula strokes on the knees.

garments work well. We use Elastoplast tape, starting on the medial thigh, and pull it across the medial knee where we work and down onto the midanterior leg. A few strips are adequate and the tape stays on for only three to five days.

Ankles

The fat pads that lie on the posterior calf just superior to the perioneal muscles add unsightly bulkiness to some people's ankles. The pad may extend down to the pseudofossa posterior to the malleloli, making the lower ankles look heavy. The improvement that results from removing this fat is subtle but effective (Fig 13–14). The skin on the lower posterior calf is often thick, and therefore the fat is more difficult to appreciate. It may be difficult to determine if it is fat or muscle. If it turns out to be muscle, the operation does not disfigure or lead to any complications but it does not help the patient. Conversely, the skin over the malleloli is often thin, and suction should be performed carefully with a small cannula.

Entry sites are on both sides of the ankle just posterior and superior to the malleloli (Fig 13–15). This gives access to the peroneal fat and the

the ankles. A few veins may be superficial but the nerves and arteries are deep. Stay in the subcutaneous plane. The actual volume of fat recovered is small. It is not unusual to see only a few globules of fat in the suction tubing or the syringe, but not to worry — there is not much. We also tape this area after suction. Both the suprapatellar knees and the ankles may develop some interstitial edema which takes a long time — months — to resolve. In some patients, the final result will not be seen for three to six months.

Arms

If arms look like legs, they respond well to

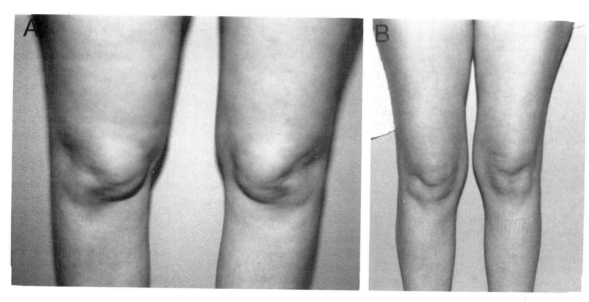

FIG 13–13.
A, woman, 26 years old, before liposuction surgery on the knees. **B**, 4 months after surgery. The knees showing less puffiness and a more gentle curve on the medial thigh/knee junction.

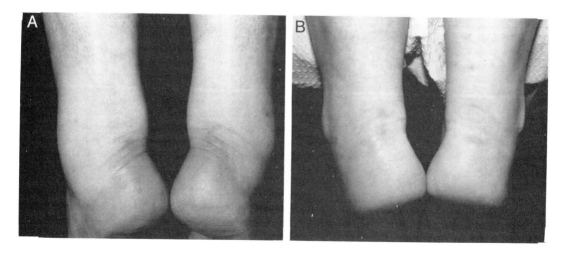

FIG 13–14.
A, woman, 29 years old, before liposuction surgery on the ankles. **B**, 3 months after surgery.

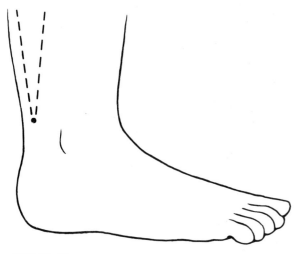

FIG 13–15.
Entry sites and direction of cannula strokes on the ankles.

liposuction. This means that if there is a discrete fat pocket, usually on the lateral triceps or deltoid areas, suction is safe and effective. However, many patients come in with sagging skin (and fat) on the medial arms near the axilla. This is 90% skin and some fat. Regardless of the proportion, this operation will not remove the main problem, which is excess skin. If the surgeon wants to undertake a combined operation of liposuction and skin removal, treatment of the medial redundancies is possible.

When the arm does have designated fat pockets, the procedure is the same as it is else-where. The fat comes out easily, and the ample muscles below the fat make the limits of the operation obvious. Also, there is little anatomy that can be injured by the cannulas.

Breasts

For women who want and need breast reduction, liposuction is sometimes combined with one of the many standard mammary reduction techniques that are beyond the scope of this book. For males with gynecomastia, liposuction is a valuable tool (Fig 13–16). For males of all ages plagued by prominent breasts, this operation removes the fat without telltale and unsightly curved scars below both breasts or on the peri-areolar area. Do an endocrine workup to make sure the enlarged breasts are an isolated problem. The wet technique is the best approach because the fat under the breasts is fairly fibrotic. The entry site is the anterior axillary line far enough posteriorly so that fat can be suctioned from the tail of Spence. In this location, the spatula-shaped cannulas seem to have some advantage.[21]

The fat in this area is difficult to suction and becomes bloody, and the fat comes out in globules rather than like the smooth, small-curd cottage cheese of the thigh or abdomen fat. It is sometimes difficult to determine where the back of the breast tissue ends and the fat underlying it begins. Ideally, the best plane for the cannula

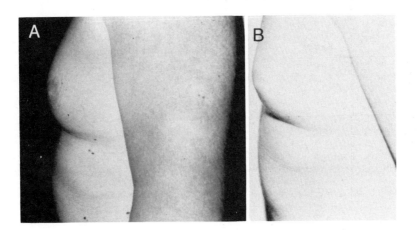

FIG 13–16.
A, man, 27 years old, before liposuction for gynecomastia. **B**, 3 months after surgery.

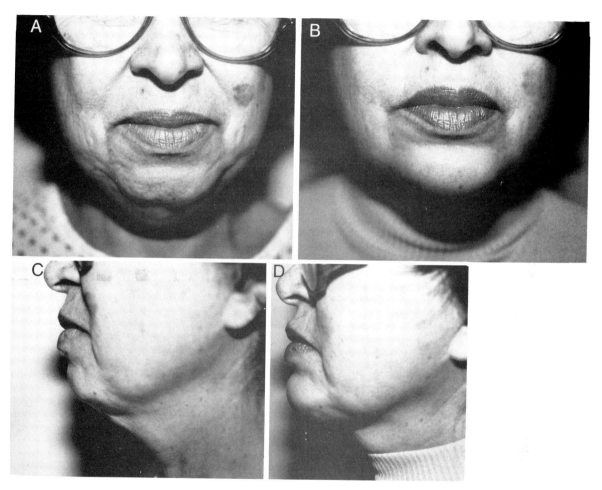

FIG 13–17.
A, woman, 53 years old, before liposuction surgery of the submental region and neck, frontal view. **B**, 2 months after liposuction and chin implants, frontal view. **C** and **D**, lateral views of same patient.

is just superior to the pectoralis muscles. Patients are sore for a while after this procedure, but it is far, far better than the direct approach under open-skin incisions.

Face and Neck

The submental region was one of the first to be appreciated as ideal for facial liposuction. The fat that accumulates in the midline submental region is acquired by many patients, but is congenital in some. This simple operation has made drastic changes in the appearance of those patients with congenital pads that become apparent in the late teens (Fig 13–17).

There are many different patterns of neck fat. The submental regions may be limited to the

midline and several centimeters on each side. This fat is palpable between the finger and the thumb. Another pattern is a wide band of fat that lies under the skin and above the platysma muscle. This band may extend as far laterally as the angle of the jaw and the anterior edge of the sternocleidomastoid muscle, and as far inferiorly as the supraclavicular fossa. In some patients, there is a second layer of fat that lies between the medial margins of the platysma and is deep to the muscle. All of these pockets are treatable with liposuction. We usually use a modified wet technique for the neck. Lidocaine 0.5% with epinephrine is infiltrated into the areas to be treated. If, however, the neck is full and large, we may use the full wet technique cocktail or formula.

For midline superficial fat, the best approach

is through a small incision just behind the mental crease (Fig 13–18). A 3-mm spatula cannula slips in and the fat comes out quickly with only a few strokes. There is not a large volume of fat. As with the ankles, only a few globules of fat appear in the tubing, but that is adequate. Palpation of the skin will prove that the fat is gone. The rest of the neck is accessible through the same entry. Carefully tread the cannula subcutaneously, and the fat as far posterior as the sternocleidomastoid muscle and to the supraclavicular fossa will come out easily. Obviously, the cannula ports should all be ventral and should be kept pointed away from the back of the skin because the skin is so thin.

Recently, it has been recommended that the neck be treated with criss-cross strokes as well. The second entry site is just posterior and inferior to the angle of the jaw. Some even recommend that the whole neck can be done from that one opening.

A high percentage of people who need neck liposuction also need a rhytidectomy or platysmal work.[22] In addition, *all* neck patients must be prepared for the possibility that the skin will not tighten up adequately, and they will need more surgery.[23] Neck suction has become a part of the vast majority of face-lift procedures, with the suction preceding the lift or performed through the open face-lift incisions (see Chapter 12).

The marginal mandibular nerve courses just inferior to and deep to the inferior margin of the mandible. There are some variations to the branches of this nerve, and therefore a rare patient might have nerve that lies more exposed and lower. The wise technique is to keep the cannula tip elevated and away from the underlying structures. The skin is thin and plastic, so the tip is always visible through it.

If the patient has a ptotic chin pad, it will suction. A small, 3-mm cannula pushed anteriorly through a submental opening into that chin pad will disrupt it some and will suction some fat away. This area sculptures well.

Ptotic jowl fat also suctions out. It is only a little awkward to thread the cannula over the jaw from the submental portal. Pick up the jowl fat — it is a discrete structure — between your index finger and thumb and run the cannula between your fingers. Gradually the fat will disappear. Keep the whole process out and away from the nerve and bone. Small cannulas — 3 mm — are better for this type of facial sculpturing. We once used a 4 mm-cannula and the entire jowl pad popped out in one piece; it was nearly impossible to get the other one out, and the patient was unhappy with the asymmetry.

Facial liposuction created interest at first, but some scarring and flat facies caused most of us to hesitate using it. Recently, with the development of small cannulas, syringe suction, and lipoinjection, it is generating more interest. The entry through the pyriform aperture just inside the nostril provides good access to the nasolabial fold. However, suction there does nothing for

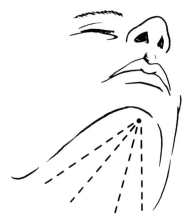
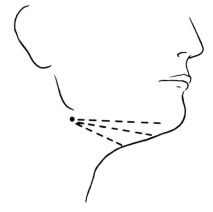

FIG 13–18.
Entry sites and cannula strokes for submental region and neck.

the redundant skin, which is probably more of a problem than the fat. Nevertheless, 2- and 3-mm short cannulas on a syringe, with entry through the skin just lateral to the oral commissure, allows suction of the various small fat pockets around the mouth and cheeks.

We are just on the threshold of realizing the possibilities of facial sculpturing. As soon as fat grafting is better understood, replacing facial fat, along with the removal of sagging fat and skin, will make true rejuvenation possible. Until now, many operations have had the serious limitation of creating false or unnatural-looking faces.

Other Applications

The most common noncosmetic application of liposuction is for removing lipomas. It is useful for the giant variety and for multiple lesions.[24-26] The traditional removal of large lipomas is by excision, which is straightforward but leaves a long scar; also, because of the dead space, seroma and hematoma are sometimes problems. Multiple lesions pop out through a small opening but also leave multiple scars. When the lesions are angiolipomatous, they are more fibrotic and have a greater vascular supply, which makes them much more difficult to remove. The necessary hemostasis precludes getting them out through a very small opening.

For giant lipomas, the wet technique will soften them enough so that with multiple strokes, usually in two directions, the tumor is delivered. The cannula acts as a dissector, a suction apparatus, and a stick to beat the tumor into pulp (literally). The physical work is worth the result of avoiding a long, wide scar. We always advise patients that if there is significant bleeding or if we are not satisfied with how the lipoma is coming out, we may have to revert to the standard, open-excision technique. A pressure dressing is wise afterward.

Several multiple lesions are removed by suction through one entry.[27] Short cannulas are used for close lesions, and long cannulas for distant ones. Again, the technique is trauma and suction together. Some fibrotic lipomas can be squeezed with the fingers into the cannula and delivered.

Liposuction cannulas, either with or without

suction, are handy dissectors. Blunt dissection has long been part of surgery, and each surgeon has a favorite instrument. With its blunt tip and long length, the cannula introduced an instrument more practicable than long scissors or hemostats. In the face-lift, the cannula can undermine the whole cheek and submental flap before any flaps are lifted. It speeds the operation and definitely reduces the chance of undermining in the wrong plane. Flaps for reconstruction on the face are often bulky, and therefore undermining the flap and suctioning some of the fat from it is a time-saving and useful step.

Recently, the cannula has been used in axillary hyperhidrosis.[28] It is inserted under the axilla and the suction port is turned toward the skin. It is also used in a windshield-wiper fashion. The purpose is to cut off or remove the many eccrine sweat glands located in that skin. The procedure literally converts the axillary skin to an attached "graft." The skin becomes dusky for several days, and it is almost impossible to cut the glands from the back without some perforations healing in. We have not tried this technique, and it is hard to imagine that it is better than a vault resection, which is effective and has few side effects.

Complications

The risk-benefit ratio for liposuction has been acceptable since the beginning. Serious complications — and there have been some — are terribly unsettling, but the procedure has been of such value to so many thousands of patients that we accept the risks. Both the rate and severity of complications are diminishing to a point where almost all problems are now minor and reversible to some degree.

Dermatologists have had a remarkable history of safety with liposuction. Bernstein and Hanke published a study of complications encountered by dermatologists and found that of the 9,478 cases reviewed, approximately 3% had local complications such as irregularity, hematoma, seroma, or edema.[30] All other types of complications such as blood loss, infection, emboli, perforated viscus, or paresthesias had an

Liposuction

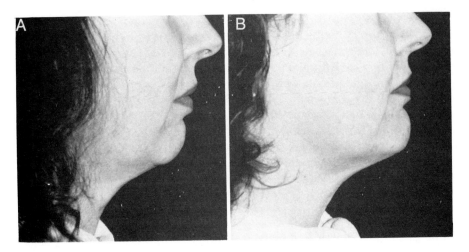

FIG 13–19.
A, woman, 48 years old, before liposuction surgery of the submental region. **B,** 3 months after liposuction and chin implant.

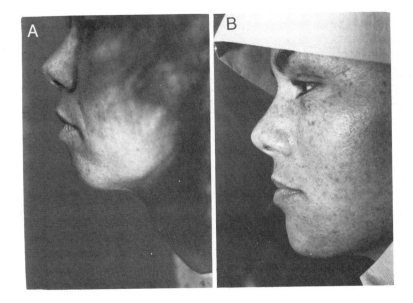

FIG 13–20.
A, woman, 24 years old, immediately before chin implant only. **B,** immediately after chin implant only.

incidence of less than 0.5% and in many categories the rate was zero.

The many changes and improvements in the technique, particularly the wet technique described above, have contributed to the gratifying reduction of problems. A report in September 1987 by the Ad Hoc Committee on New Procedures of the American Society of Plastic and Reconstructive Surgeons reviewed the complications of liposuction surgery. This group reported more serous complications than the dermatologists, but found that the rate had significantly decreased since their report five years earlier.[31]

The most serious complication, death, has resulted from perforation of a viscus, infection, fluid loss or shifts, or an embolic phenomenon. As we become more skilled and experienced and as more cases are performed under only local anesthesia, or local and light anesthesia, the incidence of perforation, although now very low, will become even lower. Infections will always occur, but quicker recognition and the use of prophylactic antibiotics will surely keep that problem minimized. Embolic problems have already been solved to some degree. Review of the cases suggests that almost all of the emboli occurred when liposuction was combined with some sort of abdominoplasty.[18, 31, 32] More careful or more conservative skin removal, or even separation of the operations, may eliminate this complication. When the procedures are combined, close observation and preventative measures are possible.

Infections have been either of no consequence like a small entry-site erythema, or have been disastrous. Fasciitis, abscesses, diffuse intravascular clotting, and massive, overwhelming sepsis have been the course.[33] These cases have been reported by the lay and medical press and have certainly encouraged the practice of sterile techniques. Some of the cases were most likely caused by poor physician management of sterility, and some by undiagnosed patient medical conditions. Regardless, the incidence of infection has always been very low. There will always be an infection rate, but with good technique and a lack of other complications, infection can be prevented or managed well.

Intraoperative problems with fluid balance and blood loss are rare nowadays. Use of the wet technique, pre- and intraoperative fluid replacement, colloid replacement when more than 1,500 ml of fat is removed, and better patient selection (patients with discrete fat pockets and not the obese patients who were treated when the procedure was first introduced) all have helped reduce fluid problems. In those rare instances where blood replacement might be needed, banking the patients own blood is recommended, although we certainly believe that the nation's blood supply is safe.

Hematomas and seromas will always occur, but the epinephrine in the wet-technique cocktail and use of better-fitting pressure garments have lowered and will continue to lower the incidence of these problems. Both should be managed in the usual ways. Large or expanding hematomas and seromas should be drained. Small ones usually should be allowed to absorb.

The most common complication is contour irregularity. Some irregularities are only asymmetries resulting from unequal volumes of fat removed. Most result when fat is removed too close to the skin or from ridges of fat left below thin skin. Irregularities can be a mild nuisance for both patient and doctor, and time softens some of them. Massage probably helps a little, and fat-grafting works most of the time. Resuctioning will even out those areas where fat was left or where there is asymmetry *and* fat remaining. If the back of the skin has been excessively thinned, only time will help. This is the most difficult of the contour complications to deal with.

Numbness or hyperesthesia are not uncommon sequelae. It is assumed they occur from transection of cutaneous nerves. They almost always go away five to six months after surgery without any treatment. Forewarning is the best treatment, but patient support is usually satisfactory.

Persistent edema can be a complication if the doctor has not anticipated it. As mentioned above, some areas such as the love handles and ankles may stay swollen for many months. In treatment of male love handles, the value of the surgery may take a year to appreciate. If the patient has not expected this, it becomes a complication. Sometimes a lateral thigh or abdomen will stay swollen, and there is nothing to do but wait it out.

Chin Implants

A discussion of submental liposuction and the problem of the cervicomental angle is not complete without mentioning chin augmentation. At the time of the submental liposuction, through a slightly widened submental incision, using sterile technique, a pocket can be created just anterior to the pogonium of the chin by bluntly dissecting the overlying muscle away from the underlying bone. The pocket is carried laterally just short of the point at which the mental branches of the mandibular branch of the facial appear. A specially designed, hard acrylic implant, or a softer, more malleable silicone implant can then be placed into the pocket to augment the anterior projection of the chin, bringing it more into line with the vertical projection of the lower lip vermilion. Bringing the chin forward helps accentuate the result obtained from the liposuction, restoring a more youthful appearance to the face (Figs 13–19 and 13–20). The technique is underutilized, and careful clinical examination of many patients who present for submental liposuction will in fact benefit greatly from augmentation. Readers are referred to other references for more complete descriptions of this technique.

References

1. Schrudde J: Lipexeresis as a means of eliminating local adiposity, in *International Society of Aesthetic Plastic Surgery*, vol 4. Amsterdam, Springer-Verlag, 1980.
2. Fournier PF, Otteni FM: Traitement chirugical des adiposities localisees par aspiration, la technique seche. *J Chir Esthet L'Hospital de Montreuil*, Nov 9–11, 1981.
3. Fischer A, Fischer GM: Revised technique for cellulitis fat reduction in riding breeches deformity. *Bull Int Acad Cosmetic Surg* 1977; 2:40.
4. Kesselring UK, Meyer R: A suction curette for removal of excessive local deposits of subcutaneous fat. *Plast Reconstr Surg* 1978; 62:305.
5. Grazer FM: Discussion: Suction-assisted lipectomy, suction lipectomy, lipolysis, and lipexeresis. *Plast Reconstr Surg* 1983; 72:620–623.
6. Fournier PF, Otteni FM: Lipodissection in body sculpturing: The dry procedure. *Plast Reconstr Surg* 1983; 72:598–609.
7. Otteni FM, Fournier PF: Les procedes mixtes (dans la Chirgure esthetic de l'abdomen: Techniques and indications. *Rev Chir Esthet Fr* 1983; 7:19–26, 32.
8. Illouz YG: Reflexions apres 4 ans d'experience at 800 cas de ma technique de lipolyse. *Rev Chir Esthet Fr* 1982; 6:27.
9. Mladick RA, Morris RL: Sixteen months' experience with the Illouz technique of lipolysis. *Ann Plast Surg* 1986; 16:220–234.
10. Klein JA: The tumescent technique for lipo-suction surgery. *Am J Cosmetic Surg* 1987; 4:263–267.
11. Piveral K: Systemic lidocaine absorption during liposuction (letter). *Plast Reconst Surg* 1987; 80:643.
12. Lillis PJ: Liposuction surgery under local anesthesia. Limited blood loss and minimal lidocaine absorption. *J Dermatol Surg Oncol* 1988; 14:1145–1148.
13. Skouge J: Lidocaine in the liposuction aspirant. Presented at International Society Dermatologic Surgery Meeting, Edinburgh, United Kingdom, 1988.
14. Fournier PF: Why the syringe and not the suction machine. *J Dermatol Surg Oncol* 1988; 14:1062–1069.
15. Fischer GM: Liposuction. American Society for Dermatologic Surgery, Ft. Lauderdale, 1989.
16. Bisaccia E, Scarborough DA, Swensen RD: Syringe-assisted liposuction: A cosmetic surgeon's office technique. *J Dermatol Surg Oncol* 1988; 14:982–989.
17. Fournier PF, Otteni FM: Liposuction in body sculpturing: The dry procedure, in Hetter G (ed): *Lipoplasty — The Theory and Practice of Blunt Suction Lipectomy*. Boston, Little, Brown & Co, 1984.
18. ASPRS Ad-Hoc Committee on New Procedures: Five-year updated evaluation of suction-assisted lipectomy. Sept 30, 1987.
19. Dolsky RL, Fetzek JR, Anderson R: Evaluation of blood loss during lipo-suction surgery. *Am J Cosmetic Surg* 1987; 4:257–261.
20. Goodpasture JC, Bunkin J: Quantitative analysis of blood and fat in suction lipectomy aspirates. *Plast Reconstr Surg* 1986; 78:763–769.
21. Dolsky RL, Fetzek JR: Gynecomastia: Treatment by lipo-suction. *Am J Cosmetic Surg* 1987; 4:27–34.
22. Dido DD: Liposuction and the platysma muscle. *Arch Otolaryngol Head Neck Surg* 1986; 112:306–308.
23. Lewis CM: Lipoplasty of the neck. *Plast Reconstr Surg* 1985; 76:248–257.

24. Kanter WR, Wolfort FG: Multiple familial angio-lipomatosis. Treatment of liposuction. *Ann Plast Surg* 1988; 20:277–279.

25. Carlin MC, Ratz JL: Multiple symmetric lipomatosis: Treatment with liposuction. *J Am Acad Dermatol* 1988; 18:359–362.

26. Coleman WP: Noncosmetic applications of liposuction. *J Dermatol Surg Oncol* 1988; 14:1085–1090.

27. Spinowitz AL: The treatment of multiple lipomas by liposuction surgery. *J Dermatol Surg Oncol* 1989; 15:538–540.

28. Field LM, Skouge JW, Anhalt TS, et al: Blunt liposuction cannula dissection with and without suction-assisted lipectomy in reconstructive surgery. *J Dermatol Surg Oncol* 1988; 14:1116–1122.

29. Shenag SM, Spira M: Treatment of bilateral axillary hyperhidrosis by suction assisted lipolysis technique. *Ann Plast Surg* 1987; 19:548–551.

30. Bernstein G, Hanke CW: Safety of liposuction: A review of 9478 cases performed by dermatologists. *J Dermatol Surg Oncol* 1988; 14:1112–1114.

31. Grazer FM, Mathews WA: Fat embolism (letter). *Plast Reconstr Surg* 1987; 79:671.

32. Christman KD: Death following suction lipectomy and abdominoplast (letter). *Plast Reconstr Surg* 1986; 78:428.

33. Bello EF, Posalski I, Pitchon H, et al: Fasciitis and abscesses complicating liposuction. *West J Med* 1988; 148:703–706.

Fourteen

Sclerotherapy

Sclerotherapy is a new old subject for U.S. dermatologists. It is old in that the French journal *Phlebologie* is in its forty-first year of publication; it is new in that the North American Society of Phlebology was established in 1988 and already half of the organization's members are dermatologists. The current resurgence of interest in sclerotherapy is well under way, but why now, and why interest was lost in the late 1950s, are unknown. Many thousands of women particularly are grateful to find competent physicians who can safely and fairly quickly remove ugly vessels from their legs.

As interest in the subject has grown, so has the scope of the field. Historically, dermatologists have wanted to treat the small (less than 1 mm diameter) sunburst vessels but not the larger veins and true saphenous varicosities. Becoming facile in treating small veins does involve some progression into larger ones: for instance, how many of the small ones are caused by or at least related to subclinical perforator incontinence? Some may be, but not all, and how many? Eventually, better agents will be coming from Europe where the science is far more advanced than it is in the U.S. There is no doubt that the management of veins by dermatologists will grow into treatment of blue veins (1.0 to 2.0 mm) and eventually varicosities. However, this discussion is limited to treatment of the small sunburst telangiectasias.

History

In 1925, Jausion used chromicized glycerin to treat varicosities, but the dosage needed for this mild agent was large — so large that patients sometimes developed hematuria.[1, 2] Therefore, it was eventually used only for small-caliber veins. It was quite viscous, which was the primary drawback, but it could be diluted with lidocaine or water. Extravascular injection did not produce slough.

Biegeleisen developed a technique for treating telangiectasia that was published in 1933.[3] However, problems resulted from agents that were overly strong, and complications of slough, pigmentation, and allergy were too common. It was not until the 1950s that milder agents were discovered for treating small vessels, and with these developments, sclerotherapy for sunburst or telangiectactic vessels became popular.[4]

Polidocanol (Aethoxysklerol) was developed as an anesthetic agent for both topical and injectable routes.[5, 6] It was first used as a sclerosant by Eichenberger in Germany in the 1960s.[7] Several others in Europe soon reported its use in the successful treatment of small vessels. Higher concentrations were used for large varicosities with much less success.[8–11]

Vessel Classification

The names for the vessels treated by sclerotherapy include sunburst vessels, telangiectatic vessels, unwanted leg veins, or spider veins. These small, superficial, and visible veins are the topic of this chapter. We will not discuss the etiology or treatment of varicose veins, which

TABLE 14–1.

Vessel Classification*

Type	Size	Description	Color
1	0.1 to 1.0 mm	Telangiectasis or spider veins	Red to cyanotic
1A	<0.2 mm	Telangiectatic matting	Red
1B	0.1 to 1.0 mm	Telangiectasis in communication with varicose veins	Red to cyanotic
2	1.0 to 6.0 mm	Mixed telangiectatic and varicose not communicating	Cyanotic to blue
3	2 to 8 mm	Superficial, reticular veins	Blue
4	>8 mm	Saphenous varicose veins	Blue to blue-green

*From Duffy DM: Small vessel sclerotherapy: An overview, in Callen JP, et al (eds): *Advances in Dermatology*, vol 3. Chicago, Year Book Medical Publishers, 1988, pp 221–242. Used with permission.

are much larger, symptomatic, probably representative of familial valve weakness, and/or pressure related. We will call these veins sunburst telangiectasia—which seems to be the most common name in use recently.

Duffy proposed a classification that is reproduced here and is the best attempt yet for defining the various vessels commonly visible on the legs[12] (Table 14–1).

Histologically, leg telangiectasias are widened venous vessels with irregularly thickened walls that usually lie 0.2 to 0.4 mm below the stratum granulosum. They are a part of the superficial vessel network, and the vessel walls contain collagenous and muscle fibers. Electron microscopic studies reveal an interfibrillar collagenous dysplasia, lattice collagen, and some matrix vesicles.[13] The meaning of these findings is unknown, although some of the same alterations are found in the walls of true varicosities. The irregular thickness of the vessel wall could be a manifestation of pressure within the vessel or of changes in support of the surrounding tissues.

Etiology of Sunburst Telangiectasias

Currently, there are only theories about the causes of these vessels. They are so common that it is hard to say they are familial. Certainly they are usually more common in females. Saphenous varicosities are fairly well established as secondary to congential or acquired abnormalities in the deep venous system, the venous valves, or the vessel walls.[14] However, pressure does not seem to play a role in the small vessels unless they are directly related to true varicosities, although some investigators believe this must be the case.[15, 16] There have been too many examples of vein incompetence or postthrombotic syndromes that did *not* develop telangiectasia. External pressure does not consistently produce vessels, nor do the greatest majority of vessel patients have any deep vein abnormalities.

Although it has not been statistically verified, many women believe they develop more vessels during pregnancy. The best theory to date is that estrogen plays a role in neoangioneogenesis, although relaxin produced during pregnancy causes some vein dilitation.[17]

A physician extremely experienced in treating telangiectasia and varicosities, Lester Mantse, has come to the conclusion that trauma is at least one etiology for these vessels.[18] He has seen many cases where new vessels arise in trauma sites on the legs, at the sites of stripping of varicosities, and at the sites where his own sclerosing agents were strong enough to cause some sloughing. In the section on complications, below, we discuss the "matte effect," a recognized effect of sclerotherapy, which is the appearance of many tiny new vessels at a treatment site.

Mechanism of Sclerosing Agents

Studies from as early as 1920,[19, 20] including an excellent comparative study by Goldman et al.,[21] all come to similar conclusions. The mechanism of action for all sclerosants injected into veins is basically the result of injury. Endothelial damage occurs almost immediately after injection or after one hour in all cases. This is followed by the rapid onset of vascular thrombosis with subsequent organization. Depending on several factors, one of which is the concentration and irritancy of the agent, some of the vessels will recanalize and others will scar down as fibrous bands or cords — the desired result.

The induced endothelial damage results in the activation or release of thromboplastic activity. Also, the same endothelial damage exposes collagen fibers, which leads to platelet adherence, which in turn initiates the intrinsic pathway. Thus, intravascular clotting begins by one or both of the pathways.

The thrombotic effect starts within a few seconds and is complete after four hours. In most studies the formation of a fibrous cord or the recanalization was complete by 45 days.

Sclerosing Agents

This section will include discussions of hypertonic saline (HS), salt and sugar solutions, polidocanol (aethoxysclerol) (AES), sodium tetradecyl sulfate (Sotradecol) (SOT) and sodium morrhuate (Scleromate). It is no surprise that each of the agents has some strong proponents and some detractors. Because all agents have similar mechanisms of action, choosing one and learning how to use it well and being comfortable with the results and complications is an acceptable goal. The careful, blind, paired comparisons needed to really understand if one agent is better than another are lacking and are not likely to be done. How the physician views the incidence of untoward results, including poor response, determines to a great degree that doctor's satisfaction with the various agents. We do not like complications when we are treating benign, strictly cosmetic problems. There is not much trade-off in the risk-benefit ratio. Therefore, we happily use a less potent agent of salt and sugar and like the low-to-zero complications.

Hypertonic Saline (HS)

This agent is approved by the U.S. Food and Drug Administration (FDA) as an abortifacient but not as a sclerosant. It is used at a 20% to 23.4% solution and is sold as Heparsal. Some experienced doctors like it best.[22, 23] It is very effective and may have one of the highest success rates of all of the agents used for sunburst telangiectases. There is no potential for allergic reaction and it is inexpensive.

The disadvantage is the pain.[24] It stings or burns on injection and the pain lasts from three to five minutes. Also, if much is infiltrated around the vein, the solution should be diluted immediately with 1% lidocaine. Nevertheless, there is still a significant incidence of slough that sometimes leads to small scars. It is obviously important to inject HS only into the vein.

Salt and Sugar Combinations

There are several formulae for salt and sugar solutions, and they are marketed under several different names: Sclerodex, Dextroject, or Vari-

TABLE 14–2.
Agents for Sunburst Telangiectasias

Agent	Active Ingredient	FDA-Approved	Pain
Hypertonic saline	Saline 20% to 23.4%	No	Moderate
Sclerodex/Dextroject	Saline and sugar(s)	No	Mild
Polidocanol (AES)	Hydroxypolyethoxy-dodecane	No	Moderate
Sotradecol	Sodium tetradecyl sulfate	Yes	Mild
Sodium morrhuate	Cod liver oil fatty acids	Yes	Moderate

sol. The Canadian formula for Sclerodex and Dextroject is dextrose 250 mg/ml, sodium chloride 100 mg/ml and phenethyl alcohol 8 mg/ml as a local anesthetic and preservative. This is essentially a hypertonic solution with action similar to HS. Abbott Laboratories used to make and sell Varisol, which to the best of our knowledge was the same as Anodyne. Abbott took the product off the market in the late 1950s, presumably because the FDA said it would require a designation of investigational new drug for the product. The formula for these products is glucose 150 mg/ml, fructose 150 mg/ml, sodium chloride 100 mg/ml, phenethyl alcohol 10 mg/ml, and propylene glycol 0.1 mg/ml of final concentration.

We have always preferred one of these combinations. They cause almost no pain when injected. Occasionally a patient will state that one vessel hurt a little; we assume that occurred when we tapped into a large feeder vein and several proximal veins were infused at the same time. Also, there is a very low incidence of complications with this agent. We are not aware of any allergic reaction, hyperpigmentation nearly always fades, and slough is rare. The results are a little slower to appear than with AES or HS, but they are generally good. In this area, we are willing to trade a slower and slightly less successful treatment for minimal complications and pain.

Our experience is shared by Dr. Mantse. Below are two paragraphs from a letter he wrote to the *Journal of Dermatologic Surgery and Oncology*.[18]

> "Two years ago, I was treating the spider veins exclusively with 1% trombovar (Sotradecol). Due to the high rate of severe complications — including ulcers — I stopped using the 1% trombovar. Using the aethoxysclerol for a short period of time, I was still unable to eliminate the severe complications.
> "Since then, my working agent has become "Sclerodex" which contains 25% dextrose and 10% sodium chloride in 0.8% phenethyl alcohol, as local anesthetic. I was able to almost totally eliminate the severe complications with Sclerodex and drastically reduce the "new" small spider veins, which

I had noticed sometimes after using 1% trombovar for the treatment of spider veins."

Polidocanol (Aethoxysclerol) (AES)

This is a popular agent in the U.S. and one study rates it the best.[24] It is not FDA-approved but is sold by Dexo Laboratories in Nanterre, France. Recently some shipments have been confiscated by the U.S. FDA, but many others pass without difficulty. It is unlikely that a patent could be obtained by a U.S. company and the product now costs so little per patient that there would not be a large enough profit margin. For these reasons, it is doubtful that AES will be submitted to the FDA for licensing by any U.S. company.

This agent is available in several strengths but most frequently used for sunburst telangiectasias in concentrations of 0.25% or 0.5%. Norris et al.[25] performed a human comparison study of efficacy and discomfort with increasing concentrations of AES. This study confirmed the popular notion that concentrations of 0.25% and 0.5% worked well but have far fewer complications, such as slough and hyperpigmentation, than higher concentrations.

AES was introduced in Europe in the 1960s and has been commonly used since, with minimal problems of toxicity, pain, necrosis, or hyperpigmentation.[26] Allergic reactions are extremely rare.[27]

Sodium Tetradecyl Sulfate [(Sotradecol or Trombovar (SOT)]

This agent is a long-chain fatty acid of an alkali metal and therefore has the properties of a soap; it is a surface-active substance. It was first used for sclerosing in 1946[28] and first described in the dermatology literature in 1982 as an agent for sunburst telangiectasia.[29] It is approved by the FDA for treatment of sunburst telangiectasias. It is distributed by Elkins-Sinn, Inc., Cherry Hill, N.J.

This agent was first used in a 1% concentration but there was such a high rate of superficial necrosis that the recommended concentration now is 0.33%. The frequency of hyperpigmentation and necrosis makes it far less

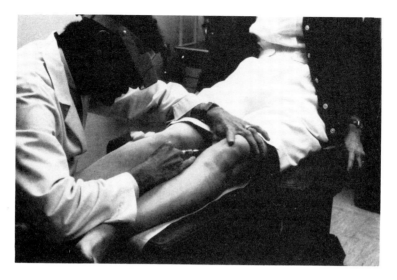

FIG 14–1.
Physician is seated and using magnification and good lighting, and has the ability to move to both sides of the patient when administering sclerotherapy.

popular than NS or AES. There have been reports of anaphylactic shock and generalized urticaria and edema.[30–33]

Sodium Morrhuate

This mixture of sodium salts (manufactured as Scleromate, Palisades Pharmaceuticals, Inc., Tenafly, N.J.) is made of the same saturated and unsaturated fatty acids present in cod liver oil. It was first reported in use as a sclerosant in the 1920s.[34, 35] Because of the many reported cases of anaphylaxis, and the severe necrosis that occurs if any is injected perivascularly, this agent is reserved for treatment of large-vessel varicosity.

Injection Technique

The patient is placed supine on the table but advised that turning frequently will be necessary. A pair of shorts is the best clothing for the patient to wear. Before we start we always remind the patient that the veins will look worse for several weeks but will gradually fade. (Many women come in at the start of the summer, hoping for a "quick fix." It's best to find out their vacation plans before performing a procedure that will create purple veins for 6 weeks.)

The physician should be seated and be able to sit on both sides of the table (Fig 14–1). It is best to have a movable table so the doctor's elbows can rest on the table. Magnification of 2 to 3 diopters with a 14- to 18-inch focal length is necessary for all physicians except those with perfect vision. Ideally, lighting should be from two directions to eliminate shadows. The area to be injected is then liberally doused with alcohol, which makes the skin more transparent and which seems to alter the refraction coefficient of the skin, thus making the vessels more visible.

Different doctors have strong opinions about whether to start at the thigh and work down, or start at the ankle and work up. We doubt if it makes any difference. The best place to start is with the veins that bother the patient most. We ask patients which veins we should treat during a particular session. There are usually some veins that bother patients more than others, and it is frustrating to use up the allotted time only to have patients bemoan the fact that you did not treat the "right" veins. By outlining which groups will be treated during a given session, a natural quitting point is built in and patients feel they are given proper care.

Because we usually use a salt and sugar combination, we like to use a 3-ml disposable syringe with a Luer-Lok and a 30-gauge disposable needle. The 32-gauge needles are not disposable, are too short, and offer little advantage. The 30-gauge needles should be changed frequently during the injections; they rapidly become dull. If a new needle feels dull or is slightly barbed, use another one. The needle is bent about 30 to 45 degrees at the hub, with the bevel up. This bend helps in several ways: it identifies where the bevel is, and it is up; also, a bend makes it hard to drive the needle too deep. As the doctor's hand and arm move forward, most of the pressure is vectored laterally to the surface rather than pushing the needle deeper into the skin. The single most common technique error is going too deep. Sunburst telangiectasias are *superficial.*

The best position for the syringe is lower than the needle tip so that the injections head upward. That way, the solutions do not leak out as easily and obscure the point of entry. Stabilize the skin in whatever way is most comfortable (Fig 14–2). Some physicians have the assistants hold several-point pressure around the vessel to be injected; we use three-point finger fixation with one hand and the hypothenar eminence of the injecting hand as a fourth pressure point as a resting point for the hand.

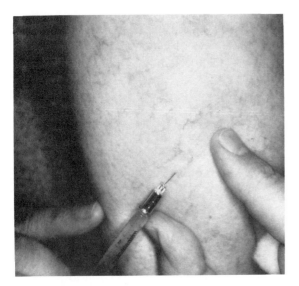

FIG 14–2.
The skin is stabilized with the fingers of the nondominant hand and with the base of the injecting hand.

Another controversy revolves around injecting a small amount of air to clear the vessel prior to injection. This does minimize the risk of inadvertent injection into the surrounding tissues. However, it is a burdensome step before each injection, and when the needle is in the vein, the flow into the vessel is so spontaneous that it is easy to know when you are in the vessel. It might be that this air-block technique was more important when stronger agents were used and any extravascular injection could lead to serious complications.

Regardless of where the treatments are started, all physicians seem to agree that it is best to pick out a large vein in the center of a group or a vein that serves as the feeder for a large group. It is easier to cannulate by visualizing a tree trunk that feeds all of the small branches. The needle is placed just over the vessel and gently nudged in, and slight pressure is kept on the plunger. As soon as the tip enters the vessel, the sclerosant begins to flow in. This can be felt as a loss of pressure on the plunger and seen immediately thereafter as the blood in the vessel is replaced with the clear sclerosant. Inject from 0.1 to 0.5 ml. Although some trunks will feed a large number of vessels, the theory is that vessels more than 1 to 2 cm distant are not injured enough to clot, even though they clear when the agent runs through them.

Keep your eye on the flow of the sclerosant. The needle tip (which sometimes is barely in the small vessel) may wiggle loose. Or, with the increased load, the tiny vessel may burst and the agent may spill into the tissues. Both of these events are common and are the main reason why we use a milder agent. In a given session, we will probably "spill" sclerosant 10 or 12 times. It is good to know that each of these leaks will not produce a scar.

We suspect that more physicians inject toward the heart, with the perceived general flow of the blood. After many patients have been treated, it becomes obvious that in these low-pressure, superficial systems, the blood flows in many directions and the sclerosant will also flow (and seem to work) in many directions. Whatever direction the needle goes in is the best direction to inject. After we have injected an area, we rub it with a gauze to induce some "urtication." We do not know what this really accomplishes, but it does cause the vessel to swell faster. This step seems compatible with the traumatic mechanism of the process.

The safe maximum dose of an agent is not usually discussed. For HS, or salt and sugar, and, we suspect, for the other agents, the maximum dose is far greater than the physician has the patience or dexterity to inject at one sitting. As mentioned above, have a predetermined stopping point, usually a fixed number of minutes per treatment session, or a total amount of agent to be used or areas to be treated. Understandably, patients will want "all of those ugly veins" eliminated at once.

The need for and the effects of pressure have not been verified in the literature. Just after injecting, we or our assistants hold cotton balls over the injection sites. This stops leakage and catches the little bit of blood that does flow back out. These or fresh cotton balls are then taped to each entry site. The value of whole-leg compression is debatable. The patient requires some wrap to hold the cotton balls in place and to prevent staining clothing during the first few hours after surgery. The concept that any dressing can maintain any degree of pressure, much less even pressure, is frequently challenged. Some patients with large legs can receive a tourniquet effect from stockings that apply pressure. If pressure is recommended, be sure to use carefully and professionally measured stockings such as Sigvaris, Jobst, or Medi-Strumpf. The required compression for 24 to 72 hours after treatment is 20 to 40 mm Hg.[26, 36, 37] We wrap the legs with Co-ban self-stick paper roller and tell the patients to leave it on until the next morning, but with the admonition that if there is swelling or discomfort, it is to be removed at once.

In the first few days after treatment, patients are encouraged to engage in whatever activities they like. We believe that light support stockings such as Supphose are adequate. Immediately after surgery, the vessels will look worse: at first they are bright red and urticated. This is replaced with blue clots or red and blue, irritated-looking veins (Fig 14–3). Repeat treatments into the same veins is best after six weeks, after full healing or clot organization has passed. Repeat treatments into other vessels on the same leg

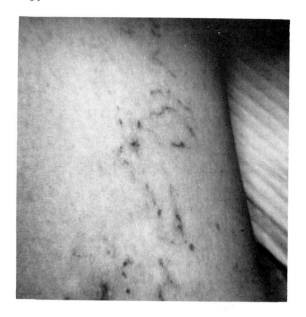

FIG 14–3.
The appearance of sclerosed veins 5 days after treatment. The veins look worse for several weeks, but the clots eventually dissolve out.

can be done as early as two weeks after surgery (Fig 14–4, A and B).

Complications

Hyperpigmentation

It is estimated by some that as many as 30% of the vessels rupture during treatment, which leaves a streak or "flame" of hemosiderin[38] (Fig 14–5). Formerly, this pigmentation was thought to be melanin, but has been proved to be hemosiderin.[39, 40] This hemosiderosis obviously will not respond to bleaching or peeling. Only time, and the body's gradual ingestion of the iron pigment, will erase these small brown spots. They usually show up by the third posttreatment week and persist for six to nine months; some may be permanent.

The depth of the color and the size of the macule are related to the amount of blood that leaked into the tissues and how much tissue damage accompanied it. Tissue damage is related to the strength and dose of the sclerosant. Some patients, however, are easy bruisers, and bruising clears within a week or so.

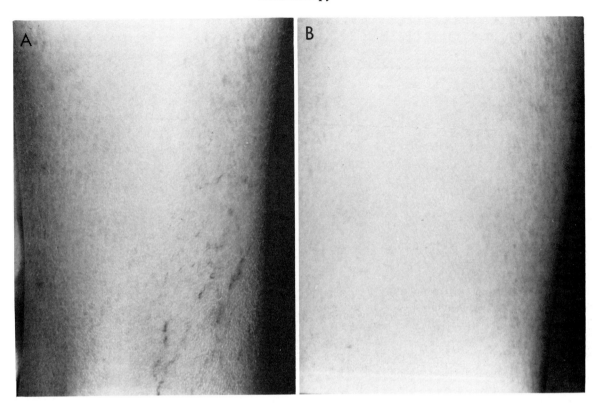

FIG 14–4.
A, before treatment. **B**, 3 months after treatment.

Pain

It is rare for patients to complain of pain much past the office visit. Some of the agents hurt — some more than others, some only when a large vessel is entered, and some only in the popliteal space or medial thigh. However, a few patients report prolonged discomfort. If they do, they should be seen in case there is another complication the physician should observe.

Edema

Pedal edema is common after sclerosing. It is even more common after treatments on or around the ankles, or when large volumes of sclerosant were used. It goes away with supportive care including elevation, Ace wrapping, and time. Alone, it does not indicate any further problem. If edema is accompanied with pain, leg swelling, or fever, however, the patient should be examined for thrombophlebitis.

Thrombophlebitis

This is rare and nearly always a superficial problem. By definition, the treatment causes a thrombophlebitis as it injures, then clots, then organizes the tiny veins. The very small size of the veins, however, makes the reaction minimal. The veins occasionally become red, with a tiny amount of peripheral erythema. Sometimes pressure over a treatment site will cause tenderness. Rarely, a small visible clot is present that may be lanced and drained. We do not recommend incision and drainage because that will surely leave a small scar, whereas spontaneous organization seldom does.

If a true thrombophlebitis with edema, tenderness, erythema, and fever is discovered, immediate and full treatment should be instituted. Consultation with an internist may be necessary. Antibiotics, elevation, anticoagulation, and nonsteroidal anti-inflammatories are indicated.

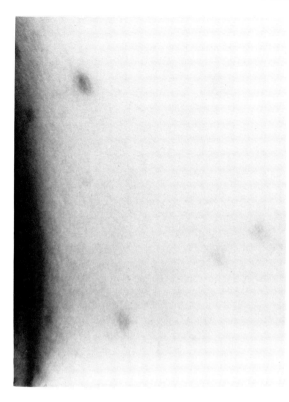

FIG 14–5.
Brown hemosiderin deposits after treatment; they disappear slowly.

of a brisk reaction to treatment of slightly larger veins — those of about 3 to 5 mm diameter. This condition may take more than a year to resolve. Small amounts of triamcinolone acetonide given intralesionally may speed recovery, but this is risky because the lower leg is susceptible to steroid atrophy.

Telangiectatic Mattes

During the course of treatment as many as 5% of patients will develop a network of small veins (0.03 to 0.05 mm) near the treatment site of sunburst vessels (Fig 14–7). These veins can also develop at the treatment sites of larger veins. They are asymptomatic, questionably related to estrogen and angioneogenesis, and about one-half of the time will go away slowly without treatment. Other times they persist, and are frustrating, even though they are much less noticeable than the original veins.

With luck, the tip of the 30-gauge needle will enter one of the veins of the network and a whole matte will blanch as the agent flows through all of the tiny interconnections. Sometimes this will obliterate them. This same technique occasionally works for pre-existing telangiectatic mattes

Slough and Scarring

Uncommonly, the reaction to the agent will be so brisk that the overlying skin breaks down and sloughs. These small, full-thickness injuries heal spontaneously and leave tiny, white, atrophic scars (Fig 14–6). When there is a large slough, the morbidity is greater for the slower-healing, larger scars. This is a predictable but unusual risk that needs to be discussed with the patient before treatment.

To date, there are only theories to account for the more severe reactions. Certainly extravasation of a large amount of the agent, inadvertent treatment of a large but superficial vessel, or predisposition to ulcers around the ankles or skins, are on the list of possible causes.

Nodular Fibrosis

This long-lasting, firm, sometimes tender, sometimes hyperpigmented chord is the result

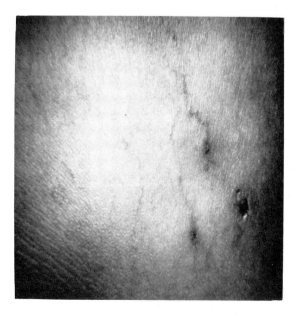

FIG 14–6.
Some areas on the veins have developed small areas of slough. These leave small, white, atrophic scars.

Sclerotherapy

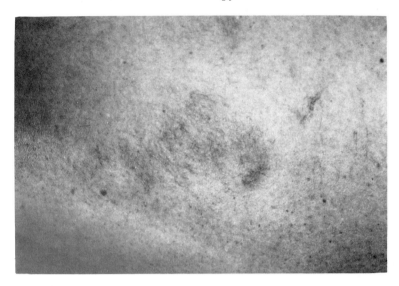

FIG 14–7.
Matte effect that develops after treatment in some patients.

that are the result of other trauma or pressure. Almost blindly push the needle tip very superficially into the center of the matte, and move it gently back and forth while very gently depressing the plunger. Every so often, a vein will be entered and the whole matte will blanch.

Anaphylaxis

This reaction has been reported after the use of Sotradecol[26] and sodium morrhuate.[18] If either of these agents is used, the office should have a protocol for management of allergic reactions.

References

1. Report from the Societé Francaise de Dermatologie, February 1931.
2. Tournay R: De quelques nouveautes — ou soi-distant telles — an phlebologie. *Phlebologie* 1948; 1:12–14.
3. Biegeleisen HI: Telangiectasia associated with varicose veins: Treatment by micro-injection technique. *JAMA* 1934; 102:2092–2094.
4. deGroot WP: Treatment of varicose veins: Modern concepts and methods. *J Dermatol Surg Oncol* 1989; 15:191–198.
5. Schultz KH: Ober die verwendung von alkyl-polyathylenoxyl-derivaten als oberflachenanaesthetica. *Dermatol Wochenschr* 1952; 126:657–662.
6. Soehring K, Scriba K, Frahm M, et al: Beitrage zur pharmkologie der alkylpolyathylenoxyd derivate. *Arch Int Pharmacodyn* 1951; 87:301–320.
7. Eichenherger H: Resultate der varizenverodung mit hydroxypolyzthoxyl-didecan. *Zbl Ogkebik* 1969; 8:181–183.
8. Ouvey P, Chandet A, Guillerot E: First impression of aethoxysklerol. *Phlebologie* 1979; 31:75–77.
9. Cacciatore E: Experience of sclerotherapy with aethoxysklerol. *Minerva Cardioangiol* 1979; 27:255–262.
10. Jacobsen BH: Aethoxysklerol: A new sclerosing agent for varicose veins. *Ugeskr Laeger* 1972; 136:532–534.
11. Hofer AE: Aethoxysklerol (Kreussler) in the sclerosing treatment of varices. *Minerva Cardioangiol* 1972; 20:601–604.
12. Duffy DM: Small vessel sclerotherapy: An overview, in Callen JP et al (eds): Advances in Dermatology, vol 3. Chicago, Year Book Medical Publishers, Inc, 1988, pp 221–242.
13. Wokalek H, Vansheidt W, Martay K, et al: Morphology and localization of sunburst varicosities: An electron microscopic and morphometric study. *J Dermatol Surg Oncol* 1989; 15:149–154.
14. Goldman MP, Fronek A: Anatomy and patho-

physiology of varicose veins. *J Dermatol Surg Oncol* 1989; 15:138–145.

15. Ouvry PA: Telangiectasia and sclerotherapy. *J Dermatol Surg Oncol* 1989; 15:177–181.

16. Davy A, Ouvry PA: Possible explanations for recurrence of varicose veins. Phlebology 1986; 1:15–21.

17. Folkman J, Klagsbun M: Angiogenic factors. *Science* 1987; 235:442–447.

18. Mantse L: More on spider veins (letter). *J Dermatol Surg Oncol* 1986; 12:1022–1023.

19. Burdick KH: *Electrosurgical Apparatus and Their Application in Dermatology.* Springfield, Charles Thomas Publishers, 1966.

20. Kirsch N: Telangiectasia and electrolysis (letter). *J Dermatol Surg Oncol* 1984; 10:9–10.

21. Goldman MP, Kaplan RP, Oki LN, et al: Sclerosing agents in the treatment of telangiectasis. *Arch Dermatol* 1987; 123:1196–1201.

22. Bodian EL: Sclerotherapy: A personal appraisal. *J Dermatol Surg Oncol* 1989; 15:156–161.

23. Duffy DM: Sclerotherapy, Peel and Dermabrasion course presented by American Society for Dermatologic Surgery, San Diego, 1985.

24. Carlin MC, Ratz JL: Treatment of telangiectasias. *J Dermatol Surg Oncol* 1987; 13:1181–1184.

25. Norris MJ, Carlin MC, Ratz JL: Treatment of essential telangectasia: Effects of increasing concentrations of polidocanol. *J Am Acad Dermatol* 1989; 20:643–649.

26. Goldman MP, Bennett RG: Treatment of telangiectasia: A review. *J Am Acad Dermatol* 1987; 17:167–182.

27. Marteau J: Trial of sclerosis treatment on telangiectasis under microcontraction. *Phlebologie* 1974; 27:361–364.

28. Riener L: The activity of anionic surface active compounds in producing vascular obliteration. *Proc Soc Exp Biol Med* 1946; 62:49–54.

29. Shields JL, Jansen GT: Therapy for superficial telangiectasias of the lower extremities. *J Dermatol Surg Oncol* 1982; 8:857–860.

30. Fegan WG: The complications of compression sclerotherapy. *Practitioner* 1971; 207:797–799.

31. Stother IG, Bryson A, Alexander S: The treatment of varicose veins by compression sclerotherapy. *Br J Surg* 1974; 61:387–390.

32. Wallois P: Incidents et accidents au cours du traitement sclerosant des varices et leur prevention. *Phlebologie* 1971; 24:217–220.

33. Reid RG, Rothnie NG: Treatment of varicose veins by compression sclerotherapy. *Br J Surg* 1986; 55:889–895.

34. Ghosh S: Chemical investigation in connection with leprosy inquiry. *Indian J Med Res* 1920; 8:211–215.

35. Cutting RA: The preparation of sodium morrhuate. *J Lab Clin Med* 1926; 11:842–845.

36. Mantse L: A mild sclerosing agent for telangiectasias. *J Dermatol Surg Oncol* 1985; 8:857–860.

37. Crisman BB: Treatment of venous extasias with hypertonic saline. *Hawaii Med J* 1982; 41:406–408.

38. Goldman PM: Polidocanol (aethoxyskerol) for sclerotherapy of superficial venules and telangiectasias. *J Dermatol Surg Oncol* 1989; 15:204–209.

39. Cuttell PJ, Fox JA: The etiology and treatment of varicose pigmentation. *Phlebologie* 1982; 35:387–389.

40. Goldman MP, Kaplan RP, Duffy DM: Post sclerotherapy hyperpigmentation: A histologic evaluation. *J Dermatol Surg Oncol* 1987; 13:547–550.

Fifteen

Cosmetic Camouflage

The proper use of cosmetics elevates the results of cosmetic procedures another increment. It does not matter whether a little bit or a lot of cosmetics are used; what matters is that they should be applied properly and tastefully. In Chapter 3 we mentioned that unsightly benign lesions such as seborrheic keratoses or nevi should be removed so they do not detract from the patient's improved final appearance. The same rationale applies to the use of cosmetics: cover blemishes, hide color irregularities, enhance certain features, diminish other features. The total results are so much better with proper makeup (and the proper coiffure) that after major cosmetic surgery it is well worth the expense for the physician either to provide the patient with cosmetic advice and demonstration or to pay to have a professional aesthetitian do it.

The need of your office for personnel trained in the use of cosmetics depends on how much of your practice is devoted to cosmetic procedures. It might be helpful to have a full-time assistant (or part-time person who comes in on demand) who specializes in cosmetics application, training, and advising. Patient follow-up visits can be coordinated with this staff member. Another possibility is to have one of your regular staff members trained in corrective cosmetic procedures. This person can spend time with the patient before and after cosmetic surgery and help adjust the makeup during all phases of recovery. The same range of possibilities applies to the physical setting. The nearly full-time cos-

metic surgeon will want to set aside a corner or cubicle that is equipped with mirrors, lights, stools, and supplies for makeup application and instruction. The physician who practices cosmetic surgery along with other surgery and general dermatology, however, may only need a makeup case that holds the cosmetics a specially trained assistant will use.

Any discussion of makeup separates into three parts: corrective makeup or camouflage, foundation, and enhancement. Some aspects of all three categories are used for all patients, but different conditions and events require one more than another. For example, after a chemical peel, camouflage makeup is needed for weeks; with the "glow" of the peel showing through, little enhancement is warranted. The difference in makeup requirements between daytime work and nighttime dress-up is the amount of enhancement used on the eyes and cheeks.

Proper Application

The best technique for applying makeup to the glabrous skin has been known for years. Why it is not universally used is perplexing. A makeup sponge is the only correct applicator, and should be a specially designed, tiny-pore, smooth, dense, synthetic sponge. The sponge is held between the thumb and two fingers. The packed powder or creamy cosmetic is picked up onto the sponge, which is then touched to the skin and rolled, or dabbed gently. Applications are repeated until the area is covered. This technique deposits a smooth, thin coat of makeup on the skin. If heavier coverage is needed, several coats can be applied. Smearing with fingers or brushes is not as effective.

The most vociferous complaints about cosmetics, from both wearers and viewers, are about heavy makeup or a theatrical look. This is best prevented by sponge application and by trying to cover only about 80% of any problem. For practical purposes, 80% coverage is the same as 100%. During the course of a day's activities, and during normal movement into and out of various lights and shadows, 80% coverage is all that is necessary. Lighter application avoids the caked-on appearance that results with 100% coverage.

Setting the makeup with powder is another skill all cosmetic wearers should learn. Powder keeps the makeup from running and holds it in place for the whole day. The resistance of younger women to powder is based on the thick, pasty look of powder that is improperly and too heavily applied. Also, older women frequently become presbyopic and apply powder too heavily and unevenly. The appropriate color of translucent powder is selected and it is pressed on with a puff and with an action similar to that used with the sponge. The puff is pressed onto the skin and rocked back and forth to transfer the powder. The powder should not be dusted on with a powder puff. There should be no powder floating around the room.

Corrective or Camouflage Cosmetics

For our purposes, the application of makeup as a camouflage is almost always to hide the early effects of surgery (Fig 15–1, A–C). It is erythema and or bruising that needs hiding. Sometimes there are long-lasting hyperpigmentation problems that also need covering (Fig 15–2, A and B). The general rule for color selection is to choose an opposing color. In the primary color wheel, orange is opposite blue; green is opposite red; and yellow is opposite purple (Table 15–1).

TABLE 15–1.
Color Opposites

Blue	Orange
Green	Red
Yellow	Purple

Thus, a patient with a purple bruise should use a yellow cream over the discolored area. Postpeel patients with red skin should use a lime-green product. Greenish discolorations require a pink cream camouflage. The table of opposite colors works for all except blue, because the orange-colored creams are incompatible with most colors used in the type of foundation makeup that follows camouflage. The best choices for hiding blue are yellow or pink.

Have the patient place the camouflage makeup over the discolored area and blend a small amount of makeup around the area. This will help keep the total amount of makeup as thin as possible and will help to blend the next layer. This is the only additional step required for corrective makeup, and it is tedious and time-consuming.

Foundation

This layer of makeup covers the whole face evenly and includes careful application over the camouflaged areas. The foundation should be a color near the patient's own and is the base for the enhancement makeup to follow. Foundation blends out small blemishes, evens the color, and darkens or lightens the facial color one or two shades depending on the desires of the patient. The foundation can be a liquid, powder, paste, or lotion. The choice is somewhat related to how dry or easily irritated the skin is. Obviously, dry skin calls for lotions or creams and oily skin for packed powders. The same method of pressing and rolling with a sponge insures a thin, even coat of foundation.

Frequently now, and more so in the future, foundations can be expected to contain sunscreens. The titanium dioxide in the foundation itself is somewhat of a block, and the addition of one or several screen agents is a welcome

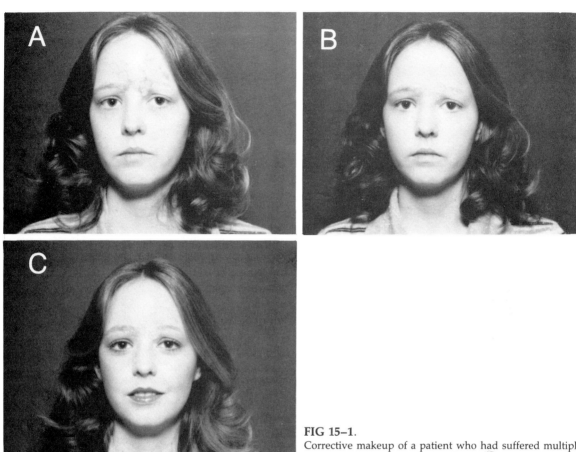

FIG 15–1.
Corrective makeup of a patient who had suffered multiple facial lacerations. **A**, before makeup. **B**, after foundation has been applied with makeup sponge. **C**, color enhancements have been added.

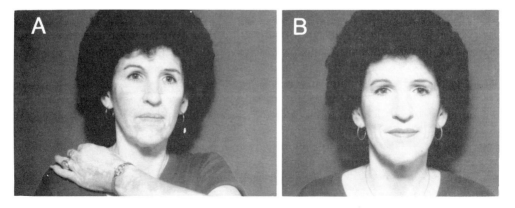

FIG 15–2.
A, woman, 45 years old, with hyperpigmentations. **B**, after application of foundation and color enhancement.

improvement. Cosmetic companies shy away from the p-aminobenzoic acid (PABA) products and keep the suntan photoprotection factor low so stinging is not a problem.

Hair Styles

Hair styling is not a subject we will specifically address in this book, but we encourage all doctors who perform cosmetic procedures to gradually become acquainted with it or make a trained person available to their patients. The hair style the patient chooses makes a huge difference in the overall appearance. The coiffure reflects style and also hides some unsightly features, accentuates other features, and frames the face. Long hair may hide baggy ears and a long thin neck but it may lengthen a long narrow face and accentuate a long nose. Short hair may balance a round face but can highlight a recessed chin.

Hair stylists know how to use the hair style to the patient's advantage. Do not hesitate to encourage patients to have their hair style changed if you think it may help. If they do not like the new style, the hair will grow; if they do, you both win.

Enhancement

This is the fun part of makeup: rosy cheeks, eye blush, highlighting or hiding certain features, and shadowing. This is also the aspect of makeup that changes from day to night and with the style of dress — formal or casual. This is where fads and styles make their appearance. Rouges and eye makeup are enhancement products, and are applied just under the powder or setting layer.

Product Selection

If the physician has a preference for makeup lines or products, it is certainly reasonable to recommend that line. Some lines have more colors to choose from, are generally less oily, or have sunscreens. Although the price range is wide, the true difference in makeups is minimal. Very inexpensive lines are not as elegantly formulated or perfumed or stabilized, and expensive lines "feel" better, are packaged more

attractively, and have a bigger advertising budget. (There may be social value for the patient to be perceived as using "the best" and the "in" products.)

It is good advice to tell patients to use whatever line feels good, covers the way they like, and does not irritate the skin. Getting involved with specific recommendations is something that patients sorely want, but because these recommendations cannot be scientific, making them detracts from your total credibility. Cosmetic manufacturers try to sell a whole line and are able to charge more for "do-something" additives: vitamins, collagen, antiaging chemicals, protein, or wrinkle erasers. These formulations change frequently without any change in the labeling. The physician has no chance to keep up with the changing formulations and should not try to.

Remember that the purpose of cosmetics is to create a guise (or disguise as the case may be). Cosmetics are 100% successful as coverups and color enhancers. They are minimally valid as anything else except as sunblocks. They are fun for patients to use and should not be discouraged.

Postsurgical Cosmetics

Blepharoplasty

The suture lines of blepharoplasty are completely hidden on the upper lids when the eyes are open and somewhat hidden by the lashes on the lowers. Within just a few days after surgery the intense redness (if there is any at all) fades enough so that edema is the only (and often minimal) problem. There is some disagreement about how soon makeup should be applied to a suture line itself, but if there are no unusual circumstances, we believe that it is permissible to apply makeup after the sutures are removed, providing the suture line is not stretched or disturbed.

Use of coverage to hide puffiness or edema follows the general rule for all cosmetics. Darker colors cause features to recede and lighter colors bring them out. Because the eyelids are already swollen, a darker shadow on the upper lids will help diminish their prominence. Another gen-

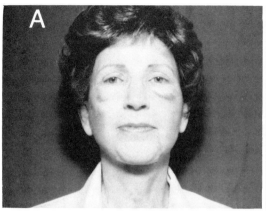 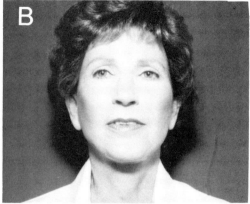

FIG 15–3.
A, woman, 58 years old, seven days after blepharoplasty and face-lift. **B,** after application of a yellow muting cream and enhancement makeup.

eral rule pertains to the finish: a shiny or glowing finish makes a feature appear larger, while a matte finish makes a feature look smaller. Clearly, the upper lids should be made up with a slightly darker matte color when they are swollen.

The lower lids may be bruised for up to ten days (Fig 15–3, A and B). The proper color of camouflage, followed by foundation and enhancement, will hide the bruises well. Sometimes the edema settles along the eyelid/cheek groove and actually accentuates the baggy appearance — the very reason the patient sought blepharoplasty. In this case, a slightly lighter-colored foundation will blend out all the dark shadowed areas and minimize the bags. Heavier adornment to the upper lids and brows may draw attention away from the lower lids.

If there is a slight downward pull of the lower lateral lid — hopefully temporary — the lower lid eyeliner should be very light or avoided entirely, and the lower lid lashes should not be colored. Again, upper lid and brow cosmetics can be emphasized until the sad eye is corrected.

Brow-lift

We pointed out in Chapter 11 how difficult it is to hide the scars from a direct or midforehead brow-lift. If the scar is still red, the color is easy to erase, but if there is a raised or depressed scarline, camouflage is much more difficult. Once the color is blended, the depressed scar does not attract as much attention if there

are other horizontal forehead creases. Failing that, a "wrinkle filler" is available. It is a stiff cream or paste that is spread into the crevice. It hardens and is covered by the foundation. We recommend filling a depressed scar only for special occasions. It is not very satisfactory for daily use, and in a few months the line should settle down.

Women can often select a hair style that covers a good portion of the forehead if necessary. They will sometimes resist, because getting their hair off their foreheads may have been an original motivation for the cosmetic surgery. But encourage them to be patient and to remember that their facial appearance is your advertisement.

Face-lift

By design, the scars from a face-lift are naturally hidden in the hair and behind the ear. All coiffures except a backward sweep will adequately hide the face-lift tracts. The only exposed problem areas are just inferior to the ear, which is often swollen or bruised, and sometimes onto the neck, where some pooled hemorrhage may show bruising. For women, hair styling and scarves and high-collared clothes can hide everything. It is best for men not to use makeup and to have an excuse on the tip of the tongue — hit by a ball; caught head in window trying to escape; in a fight. Makeup on men has too many negative connotations; it also rubs off on shirt collars where it invites the wrong inquiries from the curious.

Chemical Peels

The camouflage requirements after a peel change as healing proceeds from the immediate postoperative period to a normal desired appearance. Just after the crusts come off (after three days with a light peel; after ten days with a deep peel) the skin is pink to bright red (Fig 15–4, A and B). The opposite colors go on first — greens and yellows to neutralize the red — followed by foundations. In the early postoperative days when the skin is very red the patient should not try to hide it all because the colors and foundation will be too heavy and look artificial and removing them will be too abrasive for the tender new skin.

The next period is the hyperpigmentation phase. It is not unusual with a light peel — TCA 20% to 35% — to have a postinflammatory hyperpigmentation period of from 6 weeks to 12 weeks postoperatively. The skin is often blotchy and thus a nuisance to cover first with opaque makeup and then with full-face foundation.

Finally, a significant percentage of patients develop permanent hypopigmentation after deep peels. This presents several considerations for makeup. The demarcation line between the peeled and nonpeeled areas is tough to hide. If the color contrast is great, a lot of coverage is required along the line. The pat-on technique is the best way to deal with this, using makeup a few shades darker than the foundation, which will go on next. Next, if the facial skin has become considerably lighter, the enhancement colors may not need to be too much of a contrast. The reds of rouge and lipstick and the blues of eye shadow could stand out too much on lighter, whiter skin. Because the face will have far fewer wrinkles and a more even coloration after a deep peel, lighter-colored makeup is indicated and the patient's more youthful appearance will carry a light makeup technique better.

The neck and the backs of the hands are often a problem after a peel because they usually have developed sun damage and have not been treated. Makeup on the neck rubs off onto the clothing so it is not the answer to hiding the actinic changes on the neck and the V of the neck. The best solution is to select clothing that will hide and distract.

Dermabrasion

Many postdermabrasion problems are the same as those following a chemical peel. However, dermabrasion is often performed on younger females and men. Both of these groups should be more able to tolerate the recovery period with less camouflage, if only because they may not be inclined to use it in the first place.

As mentioned above, permanent hypopigmentation and demarcation lines are most difficult to camouflage. These are sometimes worse after dermabrasion than after a peel: there may be lines around the lower eyelids and cutaneous upper lip area because these areas are usually peeled rather than abraded.

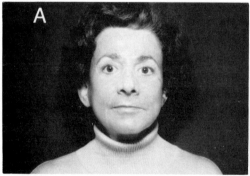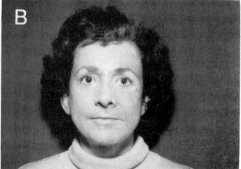

FIG 15–4.
A, patient 14 days after a chemical peel. **B**, after application of a muting cream and foundation.

Milia are another problem more prevalent after abrasion than peel. These are coverable with opaque foundations. It is better, however, to gently open and drain them.

Miscellaneous

Localized bruising after Zyderm collagen, Fibrel, or silicone injections is not uncommon. Sometimes bruises arise immediately, sometimes a few hours later. Bruising also may occur after electrodesiccation of telangiectasias on the face. The opaque cover sticks to hide acne work well to hide small, localized bruises in men, and in women who do not use foundation routinely. Remind your patients: Do not try to completely cover the spot because the coverage will be too heavy. Just hide 80% of it.

Index

Index

Index